CONTRACTING A CURE

Contracting a Cure

Patients, Healers, and the Law in Early Modern Bologna

Gianna Pomata

translated by the author, with the assistance of
Rosemarie Foy and Anna Taraboletti-Segre

The Johns Hopkins University Press
Baltimore & London

This book has been brought to publication with the generous assistance of a grant from the College of Liberal Arts and the Department of History at the University of Minnesota.

Originally published as *La promessa di guarigione: Malati e curatori in antico regime,*
© 1994 Gius. Laterza & Figli
© 1998 The Johns Hopkins University Press

The Johns Hopkins University Press
2715 North Charles Street
Baltimore, Maryland 21218-4363
The Johns Hopkins Press Ltd., London
www.press.jhu.edu

Library of Congress Cataloging-in-Publication Data will be found at the end of this book.
A catalog record for this book is available from the British Library.

ISBN 0-8018-5858-5

For Tom and Catherine,
dearest ones

CONTENTS

ACKNOWLEDGMENTS

This book was started many years ago at the University of Bologna, and it was completed at the University of Minnesota. Meanwhile I piled up a huge debt of gratitude to friends and colleagues on both sides of the ocean. For valuable suggestions, advice, and criticism at various stages of research I would like to offer my thanks to Alberto Caracciolo, Barbara Duden, John Eyler, Lucia Ferrante, Carlo Ginzburg, Ivan Illich, Maura Palazzi, Paolo Prodi, Adriano Prosperi, Nancy Siraisi, and Gianni Sofri.

Part of chapter 4 was first presented as a paper at a seminar of the Istituto per la Storia di Bologna on "Forme e soggetti dell'intervento assistenziale in una città di antico regime" (Bologna, 1985). On that occasion I was lucky enough to receive the perceptive and incisive comments of the late Gina Fasoli. Part of chapter 2 was presented at a seminar organized by John Eyler at the Department of History of the University of Minnesota. The book was completed at the University of Minnesota thanks to the financial support of a McKnight Land Grant Fellowship, which helped immensely with the last two years of research and the final drafting of the manuscript. Kit French was a splendid research assistant, who worked patiently at sorting out mountains of photocopies and microfilms from the Bologna archives and enthusiastically tackled the job of transferring the Italian text from typescript onto disk. I would like to thank her for her precision and assiduity.

Among my colleagues at the University of Minnesota, special thanks go to Bruce Lincoln, the most generous of friends and the most lucid of scholars, who gave me the double gift of his friendly support and his discerning acumen, especially on issues of power and authority, professional or otherwise. And I thank him for speaking impeccable Italian to me when I felt too homesick for (English) words.

Other colleagues helped in encouraging an all too diffident and tardy author to bring the book to completion: in particular I would like to thank Sara Evans and Barbara Hanawalt, who made me feel welcome in my new department, and at home even at temperatures of twenty below.

A very special thanks goes to Natalie Davis — who is, in my opinion, "il miglior fabbro" among present-day historians, and whose work has always been a source of inspiration and keen intellectual pleasure to me. She thoroughly read a semifinal draft of the book and offered numberless critical observations and comments. Her intellectual generosity is unparalleled.

I had the good luck of finding in my Italian editor, Piero Severi, the combined qualities of a skilled editor and a professional historian. I owe him many suggestions for revisions that concerned not only the copyediting of the text but also its scholarly content. I would like to thank Anna Taraboletti Segre and Rosemarie Foy for their assistance with the translation of the book into English. For financial support for the translation, I gratefully acknowledge a grant by the Department of History at the University of Minnesota. Finally, I would like to express my gratitude to my American editors, Jacqueline Wehmueller and Miriam Kleiger, for their careful handling of the manuscript.

But my greatest intellectual and emotional debt is to Tom Dewar. This book was written while we were learning to live together and to be parents together. Each page is charged for me with memories of our daily life — memories of his constant support through the years, of special kindness and reaching out at moments of exhaustion and discouragement. But I owe him gratitude on more counts than that: from his work as a researcher and organizer, and particularly from his critique of present-day professionalism, I learned much that is central to the arguments developed in this book. He gave unconditional support to my calling as a professional historian, and at the same time he urged me to avoid the pitfalls of professional vanity. I thank him from the bottom of my heart.

Introduction

The Voices of the Sick

When I began this research, I was looking for something different from what I ultimately found. I was interested in the practice of popular medicine and its cultural world, as opposed to the learned medicine taught in books and in schools. I was trying to understand how and when the practice of popular healers had been marginalized and outlawed. I expected the relationship between popular and learned medicine to be characterized by a pattern of conflict and repression from above—along the lines suggested by the studies of popular religions in medieval and early modern European history. The records of Bologna's College of Medicine seemed to provide an ideal source for this research project. Here was a city with a strong tradition of medical learning, institutionalized since the Middle Ages by the lectures taught at the university, the Studio. Here was a city with a medical elite organized, as early as the fourteenth century, in a college as exclusive and prestigious as the College of the Jurists. In the second half of the sixteenth century, in Bologna, the medical college acquired exclusive jurisdiction over all matters pertaining to medicine, assuming the authority to define legal and illegal medical practices and to repress the latter through its own tribunal (the Protomedicato). What better observation point could I find from which to retrace the process of control and repression of popular medicine in the ancien régime?

In the records of Bologna's Protomedicato, I encountered several folk healers, both women and men: from itinerant quacks to licensed practitioners such as barber-surgeons and midwives, who were, in some respects, part of the official medical system. The reader also will be able to meet them in the following pages. And yet these healers are not the main characters of this book, just as they were not the real protagonists in the judicial records of the Protomedicato. Another presence dominated these court proceedings—a presence that I did not expect to find, at least not so close by: that of the patients. In trial after trial, the sick speak at length in the records of the Protomedicato. They recount their experiences of illness, their attempts to understand and fight it and, to use their own words, their hopes of being "freed" from it. Clearly and in great detail—with almost legal precision—they describe their involvement with different kinds of practitioners. The figure of the healer is vividly remembered, scrutinized by attentive eyes that carefully noted and weighed every detail of the treatment. Above all, each healer is evaluated not only in terms of the effectiveness of treatment but also in terms of a specific—again, I would say quasi-legal—notion of what constitutes a fair transaction between patient and healer.

At first glance, the patients' presence in these documents seemed of little significance to me, as the patients were obviously summoned as witnesses in the trials against the unlicensed healers. Gradually, however, I noticed that, far from being mere witnesses, the patients were often the plaintiffs who had started the proceedings, setting in motion the Protomedicato's judicial machinery. In this case, also, my initial assumptions were not confirmed. I had expected to find folk healers brought to justice by the licensed professionals, physicians and surgeons, who resented their competition. Partly, this was indeed the case, but only in the late eighteenth century. As we shall see, it was not until then—the last fifty years of the medical college's century-long history—that the trials in the Protomedicato were clearly motivated by the rivalry among different groups of healers, whose ancient hierarchy, balance, and labor division had collapsed. Earlier on, however, things were very different: from the end of the sixteenth century (when the activity of the Protomedicato began to be recorded) throughout the seventeenth century, most trials of healers, both licensed and unlicensed, were filed by patients, or were filed on patients' behalf by relatives and neighbors. The plaintiffs' argument was usually that the healer had violated a commonly recognized principle of fairness between patient and practitioner.

Initially, the fact that patients played such a key role in the process that led to the modern definition of legal and illegal medical practice left me surprised and disconcerted. The patients' abundant presence in these records presented an extraordinary contrast with their nearly total absence in the traditional histories of medicine, which I had absorbed as a student. There is now general agreement that the traditional history of medicine has taught us much about the relationship between doctors and illnesses, but very little about the one between doctors and patients. This deficiency is probably due to the distinctive character that the doctor-patient relationship has assumed in our culture. Namely, this relationship tends to be seen as secondary and as subordinated to the one between the doctor and an abstract entity—illness. Illness, together with its diagnosis, prevention, and treatment, is what attracts the professional attention of the doctor as a therapist and scientist.

The shift from a concept of illness based upon the patient's subjective symptoms to a theoretical framework in which disease acquired individual identity, and the patient became just a carrier or a "case," has been recognized as a crucial moment in the history of European medicine.[1] In his classic synthesis of the history of doctors' attitudes to their patients, Laín Entralgo maintains that the traditional *ego adiuvans,* aimed first and foremost at helping the sick, has been gradually replaced in our culture by the *ego sapiens,* which aims at attaining scientific knowledge and the power to control nature which this knowledge confers.[2] According to Laín Entralgo, this can be seen in the "therapeutical nihilism" (i.e., the lack of interest in therapy) of the great medical scientists of the nineteenth century, who focused on the diagnosis rather than on the treatment of disease and saw the patient primarily as a corpse to anatomize. This attitude led to what has been called "the disappearance of the sick man from medical cosmology"[3]—a disappearance also reflected in the history of medicine, which has characteristically tended to ignore patients. In 1945, for instance, a historian somewhat aware of this problem tried naively to solve it by proposing to set next to each major medical discovery the anecdotal account of its passive object (for example, the first patient to receive the Jennerian vaccination, and so forth).[4] In a history of medicine entirely centered on the advancement of medical sciences, the real protagonists were the medical scientists, and the role of the patients could only be passive and marginal, confined to the triviality of the anecdote.

With the recent development of a social history of medicine, no longer viewed as a branch of the history of science, more attention has been paid to the patients' ordeal. Dorothy and Roy Porter's studies on eighteenth-century England have exemplarily shown that it is possible to reconstruct the experience of patients—their concept of illness and their relationship with their healers—through autobiographies, letters, diaries, and other literary texts.[5] In this field, extraordinarily rich sources are waiting for historians interested in understanding illness as a subjective experience, in spite of the fact that this experience is so difficult to translate from bodily language into words, as Virginia Woolf perceptively noticed.[6] Dorothy and Roy Porter's painstaking reconstruction shows that in the eighteenth century the experience of illness was still substantially defined and controlled by the sick themselves. It was the sick person who first made an attempt at diagnosis and treatment, while the doctor's intervention was often auxiliary and subordinated to the invalid's own initiative in identifying the illness and its appropriate cure. Their studies show the enormous diffusion and importance of self-therapy in the ancien régime—a fact confirmed by the case of Bologna, as the reader will see below. Above all, they show that the relationship between patients and doctors was characterized by a relative balance of power which was very different from the doctor's dominance typical of our culture.

Several years ago, Ivan Waddington suggested that a crucial shift in the power relationship between doctors and patients took place between the eighteenth and nineteenth centuries. According to him, a crucial aspect of medical professionalization in the first half of the nineteenth century was the transition from a situation in which the doctor's behavior depended largely on the conditions dictated by the patient, to one in which the basic rules of medical practice were instead established by a peer group of professional colleagues. In the medical practice of the ancien régime, the patient's dominance had both intellectual and social causes. Medical knowledge was speculative, often ineffective, and, above all, based on a theoretical framework centered on symptoms. Both diagnosis and therapy depended on the patient's subjective perception of the disease. Furthermore, Waddington stressed that practitioners were typically in a position of social subordination to their patients, as most doctors catered to the upper classes and therefore depended on their favors, just as clients depend on their patrons' good will. The patronage relationship between patients and doctors deeply influenced not only the balance of power in therapy but even the internal cohesion of the medical profession. While competing for the favors of rich patrons, ancien régime doctors (being the weak partner in the patronage relationship) were not able to form any professional associations in order to advance their common interests. This changed in the first half of the nineteenth century as a consequence of a larger demand for medical services by the middle classes, and especially the establishment of hospital training as the main path of entry into the profession. In hospitals, doctors found a new patient — no longer a patron who might grant favors, but a "poor," or at least, weak, member of the social order, possibly an object of experimental and clinical manipulation. Most of all, hospital training led to a more thorough standardization of medical practice than the one consequent to a shared academic curriculum. Therapy also was standardized, no longer depending on the patient's whim but now resulting from the uniform application of medical doctrines based on clinical experience and scientific experimentation. By the mid–nineteenth century, the power relationship between doctor and patient, once dominated by the patient (in the role of patron), had been overturned in favor of the doctor. A fragmented clientele of patients belonging to various social classes faced a medical community solidly united by shared professional and scientific interests.[7]

Waddington's thesis deserves credit for relating the inner changes in the doctor-patient relationship to the broader dynamics of power and authority among social groups. It is an interesting and, in some ways, convincing thesis. Yet, as is often the case with historical reconstructions that view the past as an incubator for the present, we should ask whether this view does justice to the complexity of medical practice in the ancien régime. Unfortunately, it is based on the rather unsound assumption that physicians catered only to the higher classes—a widespread assumption that is nevertheless unsupported by the historical evidence on medical practice in the early modern age.[8] Archival research on medical practice in France, Italy, and England from the Renaissance to the end of the ancien régime has shown that physicians, even those belonging to the academic elite, could have a socially broad clientele.[9] In Renaissance Florence, for instance, the renowned doctor Antonio Benivieni counted among his patients not only the members of the Medici family and other patricians but also a butcher's son, a carpenter, and his baker's wife, as shown by the records of his clinical cases.[10] In eighteenth-century Bologna we will see how the distinguished doctor Giovanni Antonio Galli, a member of the College of Medicine and the founder of Bologna's School of Obstetrics, did not mind occasionally dispensing advice about a sore throat to a poor widow, a shopkeeper.[11] It has often been assumed that medical practice in the ancien régime was primarily directed to a private clientele. As a matter of fact, most practitioners seem to have been more or less permanently employed on retainer by the thick web of associations that made up old-regime society: parishes, confraternities, guilds, hospitals, and convents, which often provided medical assistance to their members.

Anachronistically, the role that doctors play in modern society has been projected onto the past, on the assumption that in the ancien régime, as today, doctors related to their community primarily or exclusively in their professional role as therapists. But was this really the case? In 1723 the landlord of an inn named Al Leoncino, near the Hospital of Santa Maria della Morte in Bologna, told how, while suffering from chronic pain *(doglie)*, he had been convinced by a customer to consult a healer, "some barber, named Antonio Arconati." The healer questioned him about his illness and promised to cure him of any ailment, "be it even 'the French disease.'" The treatment was a long one: fifty days of potions made from powders and herbs dissolved in wine, an ointment and a wine bath for his sore arm, "but to no purpose." Despite having been paid in cash and given four gourds of wine, the barber "tried to get more money from me. But I didn't want to give him anything, and told him that I meant to sue him in the Schools, in the Court of the most illustrious Protomedicato, to find out what kind of medication he had given me and to prevent him from killing other people."[12]

The innkeeper told this story to the *protomedici,* the most authoritative members of the Bolognese medical elite. It is, as in many other cases, a detailed account of an unfulfilled promise of a cure. The protomedici heard him in their judicial role, which entailed arbitrating litigation between healers and patients, and protecting the latter group's rights. This judicial role was central among the prerogatives of the Protomedicato, as was typically the case for medical authorities of the ancien régime. In this judicial capacity, as an entity formally holding jurisdictional rather than professional authority, the medical elite was able to have regular contact with some members of the popular classes, either patients or healers. The existence of this institution allows us to look closely into several aspects of medical practice in an ancien régime city—aspects ranging from the personal relationship between healer and patient to the interaction between learned and popular medicine. From this unexpected viewpoint, we can try to examine the microcosm of transactions between patients and healers and to understand the customary rules of fairness and justice governing their relationship.

Most interestingly, the tales that the sick unfolded in front of the protomedici reveal a precise concept of what was commonly considered a fair relationship between patient and healer. The sick appealed to the Protomedicato when they believed their healer had broken a basic rule of fairness. What was this rule? A very simple one (which, however, I had great difficulty in understanding): the healer should be paid for his service only if the treatment had been effective—in other words, patients were to pay only if they had been healed, and not otherwise.

At first, this rule seemed simply unbelievable to me. I became persuaded that I had understood it correctly—that this was really what the patients meant—only when, carrying on my research, I discovered a similar principle in the medieval juridical tradition. In his commentary on the Code of Justinian, the jurist Bartolo da Sassoferrato stated that the doctor should indeed be paid at the end of the treatment, and only if the patient had recovered.[13] I must confess, to my discredit, that I found it easier to believe one jurist than the many people of Bologna, who had told me many times, through the archival records, that this was the rule of fairness with which the healers were supposed to comply and which the protomedici, as magistrates, ought to enforce. (This shows that even those who have an interest in popular culture are not overly ready to trust common people.)

In the early modern age, when European jurists faced the problem of how to regulate the transaction between patients and healers, they rediscussed this ancient principle of fairness. However, as one might expect, they viewed it with growing embarrassment and skepticism. All of this is a little-known aspect of the process we call the professionalization of medicine — an aspect that much pre-dates the nineteenth century, when this process is usually located in time. The professionalization of medicine obviously could not have been accomplished without a widespread social consensus around the principle that medical service should be remunerated irrespective of results. The documents from Bologna's Medical College indicate that, by the end of the sixteenth century, this consensus had not yet been reached. What happened in the courtroom of the Protomedicato in the next two centuries will show us how this principle of fairness was gradually eroded, to be finally completely removed from collective memory. The ancient concept of a fair relationship between patient and healer was replaced by the one we have today, overwhelmingly representing and imposing the perspective of doctors. In the seventeenth and eighteenth centuries, two different concepts of fairness in medical practice met in the courtrooms of the Doctors' tribunal of Bologna. This book will try to reconstruct and understand them both: the viewpoint of the medical elite, their vision of judicial responsibility and a well-regulated medical system; and the viewpoint revealed by the voices of the sick, which was eventually defeated and forgotten.

CONTRACTING A CURE

Chapter 1

A Doctors' Tribunal

Those who feel aggravated in any way by physicians, surgeons, barbers, and others,
because of medications, bleeding, malpractice, or an unreasonable cost
of medicines . . . by appealing to us, will receive swift justice.
—From a public notice issued by the Roman Protomedicato, 1614

I

What were the origins of the Protomedicato, the court used by patients in Bologna, and how did it operate? The Protomedicato was the judicial arm of the College of Medicine of Bologna. For more than two hundred years—from the second half of the sixteenth century to the end of the eighteenth—the doctors serving as protomedici were drawn from among the members of the college by casting lots every three months. In order to understand the Protomedicato it is essential, therefore, to focus first on the College of Medicine.

In the second half of the sixteenth century, when the Protomedicato began to operate, the College of Medicine was one of the two branches of the College of Arts (the other branch was the College of Philosophy).[1] Throughout its long history, from its oldest statutes (1378) to its dissolution following the arrival of the French in Bologna (1796),[2] the College of Medicine was an exclusive body, rigidly limited to fifteen members. Statutory requirements for membership included Bolognese citizenship, a doctoral degree from the Studio of Bologna, and at least a one-year teaching appointment at the Studio.[3] This elite group of lecturers controlled access to doctoral degrees in philosophy and medicine. No one could graduate without the support of two members of the college acting as *promotores,* or without the approval of the college in a formal public examination. In fact, the college (formally joined by the chancellor of the Studio—the *arcidiacono*) was the only institution entitled to confer doctoral degrees.

It is important to emphasize that the college was an academic oligarchy rather than a medical association in the modern sense.[4] All other physicians licensed to practice medicine in the city—including foreigners who had graduated from the College of Medicine of Bologna and doctors holding degrees from other universities—were officially subordinated to the members of the college. The distinction between members of the college *(collegiati)* and nonmembers *(non collegiati)* was clearly indicated in the official listings of all physicians licensed to practice in Bologna in the seventeenth and eighteenth centuries. The lists were posted in the apothecaries' shops as public information. While other groups of practitioners, such as barber-surgeons and apothecaries, had formed their own trade companies within the city's system of guilds since the Middle Ages,[5] the doctors practicing in Bologna did not belong to any association,[6] with the sole exception, of course, of the group formed by the college members.

The medical colleges of the ancien régime seem to have been of two kinds: the professional fraternities developed within the municipal system of the guilds, and the elitist groups created in connection with the universities.[7] For the second kind, the primary goal was not representing the profession but, rather, protecting the academic oligarchy's special interests. This was certainly the case with the College of Medicine of Bologna. Most of the norms contained in its fourteenth-century statutes, as well as in their revised version of 1507, established the college's control over the most prestigious lectures,[8] as well as over the procedure for conferring the doctorate. Much less attention was paid to problems relating to the professional practice of medicine.

The college became even more elitist in the seventeenth and eighteenth centuries. The procedure for admission of new members, as shown by the archival documentation over a period of more than two hundred years, strictly followed the statutory rule limiting the number of members to a maximum of fifteen (twelve numerary and three supernumerary). Occasionally, the number of supernumerary members was raised from three to a maximum of ten.[9] A member belonged to the college for life. Following a member's death, the college, in principle, was to announce a vacancy, to be filled by a supernumerary member on the basis of seniority of doctorate. In practice, the admission procedure most often adopted throughout the seventeenth century was based on so-called multiple admission. The college was periodically expanded with new supernumerary members, who were assigned the thirteenth to the twenty-third positions; with the death of old members, the number of members gradually returned to the statutory limit of fifteen. But, as stated in a document describing admission procedures: "Supernumerary members have only the title of *collegiate* and the hope for succession."[10] The collegiates in the thirteenth, fourteenth, and fifteenth places were the only ones who could share some privileges and tasks with numerary members. For instance, they could become protomedici, although they were not allowed to sponsor students for graduation. A collegiate could very well die while still a supernumerary, well after having paid the considerable admission fee,[11] and without ever having been able to enjoy all the advantages, including financial ones, of membership in the medical elite.

As a result of the practice of multiple admission, the number of members of the college fluctuated from thirteen to twenty-three in the seventeenth and eighteenth centuries (although the number of numeraries was always fixed at twelve). The numerical composition of the college, therefore, remained fundamentally constant throughout these two centuries. But since the overall number of doctors practicing medicine in the territory of Bologna grew constantly during the same period, the college's elitist nature became more marked. While in 1600 the members of the college comprised 30 percent of the total number of licensed doctors practicing in Bologna, in 1772 the collegiates, including supernumeraries, represented only 12 percent of the total number of professional physicians (see table 1).

Another aspect of the college's elitist character is shown by the tendency of a few families to control membership. This tendency can be noted throughout the college's long history; in fact, we may observe it also in other associations: for instance, the same family names appear repeatedly in the membership of the councils of the guilds.[12] In admissions to the college, preferential treatment was given to the sons or grandsons (in the male line) of

Table 1.   COLLEGIATE AND NONCOLLEGIATE DOCTORS IN BOLOGNA, 1600–1772

	Collegiates		Noncollegiates		
	N	%	N	%	Total
1600	13	30	30	70	43
1630	13	31	29	69	42
1659	15	23	49	77	64
1683	13	16	69	84	82
1698	18	17	87	83	105
1727	15	14	93	86	108
1744	19	19	81	81	100
1772	17	12	124	88	141

Sources: Lists of doctors licensed to practice in Bologna, published by the Protomedicato (A.S.B., Coll. Med., bb. 197, 235, 236, 342).

college members. According to the statutes, when the college had no vacancies, room had to be created among the supernumeraries to accommodate the members' relatives. Not all offspring requesting membership were granted admission, but one's chances of entering the college were definitely linked to one's lineage. In 1576, for instance, the supernumerary members complained to the Assunteria di Studio (the senators responsible for overseeing the university lecturers) that the young sons of collegiates were given priority in admission. "[The collegiates] reserved the sixteenth place for their sons, arguing that this was in the statutes; which is not true. Because of this, the young occupy a higher place than the old, and in time the College will be governed solely by the families of the numerary members."[13] To reverse this trend, in 1615 it was established that no more than two members of the same family or agnatic lineage could simultaneously belong to the college.[14]

If we examine the admissions to the college from 1593 to 1793, we find that 23 of the 130 new members were the sons of collegiates. In addition, 9 doctors joined the college following in their grandfathers' footsteps. And this is not all. Three members were admitted because of a paternal uncle, and 2 others thanks to a paternal cousin and a stepfather.[15] Members closely related to other collegiates on their fathers' sides in this period numbered thirty-seven, that is, 28 percent. This figure would be even higher if we also considered the admissions to the College of Philosophy. Although the privileges mentioned in the statutes explicitly referred only to the male, or agnatic, line,[16] in some cases members were admitted thanks to their maternal kin. Ovidio Montalbani, admitted in 1622, probably the most famous protomedico in seventeenth-century Bologna, was the son of Giulia Gibetti, daughter of the college member Ovidio Gibetti.[17] Bartolomeo Ferrari, admitted in 1677, was the maternal nephew of the doctor Alessandro Magni, who sat in the college from 1651 to 1673.[18] As for Antonio Magnani Cartari, admitted in 1691, his double surname reveals the importance of his maternal kin: his mother's brother was the doctor Giovanni Antonio Cucchi Cartari, member of the College of Medicine from 1652 to 1697.[19]

The Cucchi Cartari family is a clear example of the role of dynasties in the history of the college. Between 1576 and 1724, four members of this family sat in the College of Medicine (see table 2); a fifth member, Giacomo, was a member of the College of Philosophy.[20]

The simultaneous presence in the college of several members of the same family was unusual, however. More typical is the successive membership of three generations: father, son, and grandson (or great-grandson). This is seen in the case of the Zoppio family, with Girolamo (who became a

Table 2.   MEMBERS OF THE CUCCHI CARTARI FAMILY IN THE BOLOGNESE COLLEGE OF
MEDICINE AND COLLEGE OF PHILOSOPHY, 1576–1724

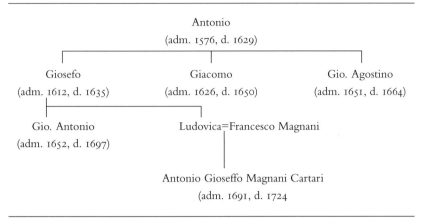

Sources: A.S.B., Coll. Med.—b. 332, "Civilitatis Probationes" of Gioseffo Cucchi; bb. 247, 353, "Civilitatis Probationes" of Giovanni Antonio Cucchi; b. 341, "Civilitatis Probationes" of Antonio Magnani Cartari; b. 250, "Sententiae et decisiones tam in prima, quam in secunda instantia, in causa Excell. D. Io. Augustini Chucchij Philosophi, et Medici Bon. ad favorem ejusdem contra Collegia Bonon. Phil. & Medicinae"; G. B. Guidicini, *Cose notabili della città di Bologna* (Bologna, 1870), 3:178, 4:299.

Abbreviations: adm. = admitted; d. = died.

member of the College of Philosophy in 1591), his son Melchiorre (who became a member of the medical college in 1593), and Cesare, Melchiorre's grandson (who became a member of the College of Medicine in 1651).[21] The pattern was also seen in the Donelli family in the eighteenth century, with Gio. Lodovico (admitted in 1691) succeeded by his son Filippo (1720) and his grandson Benedetto (1751).[22]

The elitist nature of the college was underscored by another, mainly symbolic, privilege. By virtue of the *Privilegium palatinatus,* granted by Charles V to the College of Medicine in 1530, the members of the medical college were officially included in the nobility as knights.[23] As such, the college doctors were entitled to appoint public notaries, legitimize bastards (allowing them to recover their inheritance rights), and finally, in their turn, confer the title of knighthood.[24] The fees for a doctoral degree plus knighthood, which the collegiates had the right to bestow,[25] were slightly higher than the ones for a regular degree—requiring, by the end of the eighteenth century, an extra charge of 86 *lire* and 10 *soldi* in addition to the customary fee of 657 lire and 10 soldi for the simple degree in medicine and philosophy. Like the fees paid by students for their degrees, this money was divided among the college doctors.[26]

Restricted admission seems to have been a common feature of medical colleges in the ancien régime. In the seventeenth century, most colleges in cities other than Bologna were inaccessible to the majority of the medical profession. In a few instances, this oligarchic structure was openly challenged. In London, during the republican interregnum, there was a Puritan-inspired attempt to form a medical association opposed to the Royal College of Physicians, bastion of the traditional medical hierarchy. Founded at the beginning of the sixteenth century on the model of Italian colleges such as Bologna's, the Royal College of Physicians was indeed an elitist institution. With a limited number of members, it epitomized the attempt by the medical schools of Oxford and Cambridge to preserve their hegemony over the medical profession. The Puritan reformers proposed instead the creation of a new college that would be open to any licensed doctor and therefore would represent the interests of the physicians who had been excluded from the traditional college.[27] The plan failed, and one might well say that in the seventeenth century the medical colleges were able to maintain, and even reinforce, their elitist distance from the rest of the medical profession. This is what happened in Bologna. In Bologna (unlike London), the oligarchic nature of the college and its control over other practitioners were never openly challenged, despite some residual discontent.[28]

II

The trend for medical colleges to represent an academic oligarchy to the exclusion of the rest of the medical profession was probably fueled most significantly by the fact that early modern political authorities granted them jurisdiction over medical practice. Thus empowered, the colleges took shape as the representatives of state authority rather than as professional associations. This could only strengthen their oligarchic character. A significant example, in this respect, is Berlin's Obercollegium Medicum. Created by the state in 1685, the college was structured primarily to function as a public authority over medical issues rather than as a professional association, even though doctors had pressed instead for an organization that represented their own interests.[29] As for the College of Medicine of Bologna, its structure reflected the state's granting it a supervisory role over medical practice. Bologna's authorities delegated public jurisdiction to the college: this was the origin of the court of the Protomedicato.

The Protomedicato's institutional profile resulted from a combination of internal developments within the college and this external intervention by the state. Originally, the office of protomedico had been created in 1517 within the college to fulfill what had been until then a role exercised, on occasion, by the dean plus a few members appointed to prosecute empirics and popular healers. Thus, the Protomedicato originated as an extension of the jurisdictional role traditionally held by the dean of the college. In the second half of the sixteenth century, the Senate (the governmental body that, together with the papal legate, ruled Bologna) transformed the Protomedicato into a permanent magistracy with public functions.[30] Together with two other members chosen by lot every three months, the dean formed "the Court called the Protomedicato, which is deputed by the College of Medicine to exercise the powers the College itself obtained *ab antiquo* from the Supreme Pontiff."[31] According to the statutes of the college, the dean held two jurisdictional powers: first, he was entitled to judge, with "summary" (that is, swift and informal) proceedings, any litigation involving the members of the college; second, he could interdict from medical or surgical practice—under penalty of a fine—anyone not licensed by the college.[32] This double jurisdiction, civil (resolution of disputes concerning professional practice) and criminal (control over unlicensed practitioners), traditionally had been performed by the officers of the guilds.[33] The jurisdictional role of the college's dean can thus be seen as equivalent to that of a judge of the guild.

When the Protomedicato was established as a public authority, however, its assigned tasks crossed over into the area of powers traditionally held by the apothecaries' guild and the barbers' guild, as well as by the ordinary courts. This occurred because the political authorities appointed the Protomedicato to rule over the entire field of medical practice "and its appendages," including surgery and pharmacy.[34] In fact, in 1563 the Senate assigned the protomedici an honorarium funded with taxpayers' money, like the salaries of the lecturers of the Studio. This honorarium was meant as remuneration for the public service of controlling the quality and prices of all medicines prepared and sold in the city and its territory. For this purpose, the protomedici were charged with compiling the *Antidotario*—a pharmacopoeia listing the proper composition of medicinal compounds, for the use of the apothecaries. They were also required to visit the apothecaries' shops every three months in the city, and at least once a year in the countryside, in order to verify that drugs were actually prepared according to specifications and with ingredients of good quality. Furthermore, the protomedici were responsible for inspecting drugs and medical substances at the city's customs offices, to ensure that "useless or spoiled medicines" were not brought into Bologna. Finally, they were in charge of establishing the official sale prices that apothecaries were to charge for medicines.[35] As we can see, the Protomedicato performed a public function, which was intended to protect citizens by regulating the quality and price of medicines. Special magistrates carrying out this function can be found in other Italian cities of the ancien régime.[36]

Because of this public appointment that, in a sense, transformed the protomedici into government officers, some historians have defined the Protomedicato as a public health board. This was typically the opinion of nineteenth-century scholars, in keeping with their view that the sanitary policies of the Napoleonic age were simply a continuation of those of the old regime.[37] The importance of the state in the origins of the Protomedicato has been newly underscored more recently. It has been suggested that, by funding the Protomedicato with tax revenue and investing it with public authority, the state was trying to turn this institution into a government-owned agency, removing it from the hands of the college and indeed making the college itself subordinate to it. This attempt, it is argued, was only partly successful, much like other attempts at modern state-building in the Papal States.[38]

I would contend, though, that this attempt by the state failed altogether. In 1563 a conflict erupted between the Senate and the college, when the former claimed the right to appoint one of the three protomedici.[39] But in the end, the Senate's attempt at interference did not succeed, and the appointment of the protomedici remained exclusively in the hands of the college. For centuries, the title of "protomedico" was conferred temporarily on a rotating basis upon the members of the college. The Protomedicato's records from the seventeenth and eighteenth centuries clearly indicate the close link between the Protomedicato and the college and, even more significantly, the constant subordination of the former to the latter.[40] Until 1628, any resolution of the Protomedicato, from the licensing of apothecaries to the granting of permits for the sale of medicines, had to be confirmed by the college. Apothecaries and their apprentices also had to be approved twice, first by the Protomedicato and then by the college. Each decision recorded in the "Acta Prothomedicatus" was properly upheld or overturned by the college in full session.[41] In 1628 the college empowered the protomedici to pass judgment, on behalf of the entire college, in the cases under their jurisdiction, though they were not allowed to pardon or acquit without the college's approval.[42] This was indeed a delegation of power, but, as such, it also signaled that the college remained the true and ultimate source of jurisdictional authority. The following year, the Protomedicato was authorized to license quacks and street vendors wishing to sell medications for external use.[43] This authority was later reclaimed by the college, together with the prerogative of approving "medical secrets."[44]

Significantly, the college reserved for itself the right to examine and license higher-level apothecaries and surgeons, leaving the Protomedicato to deal with lesser practitioners. For instance, in 1671 the college undertook to license master apothecaries, while the Protomedicato was assigned the task of licensing apprentices in that trade.[45] And while barber-surgeon licenses had traditionally been granted by the Protomedicato, after passage of the new laws on surgical practices in 1742 the protomedici became responsible for testing lower-level applicants, while the professional surgeons were to be examined by the entire college.[46] Finally, while the inspection of medicines was a concern of the Protomedicato, it is significant, on a symbolic level, that the college continued to control the preparation of theriac and mithridatium — the two most important medications, the very symbol of the official pharmacopoeia, which were ritually prepared every year in the Studio with a public ceremony.[47]

Clearly, the college viewed the Protomedicato's powers as merely executive, and a delegation of its own authority. It also believed that the public role of the Protomedicato extended and reinforced its own authority and jurisdiction. As a matter of fact, appeals against the Protomedicato's decisions were brought to the college, which acted as "the sole and unappealable judge" on matters pertaining to its jurisdictional domain. The college's decrees and sentences "could not be revoked by any other judge, because he would be incompetent as a result of his not being an expert in the Art and much less knowledgeable in medical matters."[48]

Both in principle and in practice, the Protomedicato was kept well within the college's control. In the case of Bologna, we do not observe the close connection between the state and the Protomedicato which we can see elsewhere — for instance, in the Kingdom of Naples, where the protomedici were directly appointed by the king. In fact, the Neapolitan Protomedicato sometimes clashed with the medical colleges associated with universities, such as the Medical College of Salerno.[49] By contrast, the Protomedicato of Bologna clashed with the city authorities, as it often needed to defend its jurisdiction from their interference.

Some friction between the college and the state authorities (the Senate and the papal legate) was caused by the authorities' meddling with the membership of the college. As already mentioned, in 1563 the college fought successfully against the Senate's attempt to appoint one protomedico out of three. More tension, however, occurred over the issue of the assignment of lecturers in the Studio, which both the Senate and the college wished to control.[50] The college argued that the senators were arbitrarily hiring and assigning stipends or prizes to the lecturers without consulting the college. As the college doctor Camillo Baldi noted in the early seventeenth century, they did so in "their own way, without even taking the trouble to see and listen to what doctors and students were saying and doing."[51] Another source of conflict concerned the administration of the Bolognese Custom House, the so-called Gabella Grossa. This had been assigned in 1509 to the colleges of medicine and law, as a source of revenue to pay the salaries of the university lecturers. The two colleges elected twelve syndics (four doctors of canon law, four of civil law, and four of medicine and philosophy) deputed to administer the revenue from the customs. In 1603, however, Pope Clement VIII decreed that the syndics of the Gabella Grossa should include some senators, thus limiting the autonomy of the colleges in financial matters. Obviously, the colleges did not appreciate this intrusion of the Senate into their money management.[52]

In the history of the College of Medicine of Bologna, there are also some episodes of conflict with the papal legate. In 1630, the college openly opposed a decree by the legate which required the Doctors (i.e., members of the college) to admit Bartolomeo Bonaccorsi, an applicant rejected in 1622. According to the collegiates, Bonaccorsi had not been admitted because "he was, not to mention his other baseborn relations, the son of a man who had been a public constable for ten years in a row, and later became a broker, . . . and he himself has been in youth a low craftsman in the trade of the *Bombasari* . . . and as an adult, the apprentice to an apothecary." In fact, before attaining his doctoral degree in medicine, Bartolomeo Bonaccorsi had apprenticed with an apothecary and had been a member of the council of the guild of the Bombasari, holding the office of *massaro* (steward) in 1611. His father, Pompeo, the son of a weaver, had made a successful career as a "silk broker," eventually counting "even princes" among his customers, as stated by a contemporary witness. Pompeo's influence must have been remarkable if he managed to obtain a decree (issued in 1630 by Cardinal Legate Barberini and confirmed in 1633 in a brief by Pope Urban VIII himself) that forced the college to accept Bartolomeo Bonaccorsi as a member. The college protested against this imposition that, in the Doctors' own words, "stained an honorable and ancient association: no person of such low background has ever been admitted or accepted in these colleges in 1,224 years."[53] (The college dated its mythical origins back to the times of Emperor Theodosius.) In the end, the college had to submit and include Bonaccorsi in the official roll of its members.

Such a direct clash over membership in the college was an exception. But recurrent, chronic disagreements between the college and the legate occurred over another issue, namely, the licensing of popular practitioners. The exclusive right to grant licenses for all kinds of medical practice was formally assigned to the college (and by the college to the Protomedicato) at the end of the sixteenth century. In 1604, the legate further decreed that even licenses previously granted by other legates were to be considered invalid.[54] This is quite significant, if we consider that elsewhere it was not until the beginning of the eighteenth century that the state acknowledged medical colleges' monopoly over licensing. In Piedmont, for example, medical licenses were granted for centuries not only by the colleges but also by the political authorities at the state and local levels.[55]

As a matter of fact, even in Bologna, in spite of the norm that gave the college exclusive rights over licensing, the Senate and the legate continued occasionally to grant licenses for the practice of medicine. These cases, however, involved only folk healers, traveling quacks, and charlatans, and the licenses were usually for a limited period of time. That these cases deviated from the college's rules was often explicitly stated — for example, in the license granted in 1581 to Giovanni Alessi, allowing him "to treat any kind of human illnesses and infirmities with his medical secrets." Significantly, the license included the words "we have notified the Dean of the Doctors of Bologna, and hereby grant it, despite his contrary opinion and opposition."[56] Repeatedly, well into the eighteenth century, the college sent its representatives to the legate to protest this occasional licensing of charlatans.[57]

Aside from this occasional friction, however, it should be pointed out that in Bologna the college's authority over medical matters was generally acknowledged by the state, especially in the jurisdictional sphere. During a case argued in 1670, a lawyer of the college could state as a matter of fact that "the Esteemed Cardinal Legates . . . and other Rulers of the city have always referred to the College's decision the cases of those who had appealed to the Supreme Authorities against the College's own sentences."[58]

All of this shows, in my view, that the Protomedicato was not a public health board or a "sanitary police" (in the peculiar sense that this term had in

the ancien régime)[59] but, rather, a specialized court whose public role depended on the powers given to the college by the state authorities. In fact, in
Bologna the role of public health board was played not by the Protomedicato
but by the Assunteria di Sanità—a governmental body appointed by the
Senate and composed of senators. Although the activities of the Assunteria
di Sanità have not been studied in detail, we know that it dealt primarily with
the prevention and control of epidemics and epizootic diseases (the latter being frequent in the eighteenth century). In times of contagion, the Assunteria inspected letters, merchandise, homes, and barns, enforced quarantine
measures, and routinely monitored air pollution caused by agricultural and
industrial activities (rice fields, paint factories, etc.).[60] In short, it dealt precisely with those public health concerns that were typically placed in the
hands of a sanitary police agency in the ancien régime. While the Assunteria had decision-making and executive powers over these issues, the Protomedicato's role in these areas was merely that of providing advice. Galenism,
the medical doctrine officially upheld by the college until the first half of the
seventeenth century,[61] was extremely sensitive to the role of the environment
in the preservation of health. And the doctors' expertise in this field was recognized by the political authorities. In August 1596, for instance, the Senate
asked the college whether it was safe to proceed as usual with hemp retting,
despite the impending threat of a contagious disease. The college's response
was to recommend against the retting, because it would cause unhealthy
fumes.[62]

Requests for inspections or opinions could be directed to the college as
a whole (as happened in 1680, when another contagious disease was feared)
or to the Protomedicato—as happened in 1729, during a fever epidemic in
the countryside, and in 1748, during an outbreak of disease among cattle,
when the Assunteria di Sanità asked "what to do about hay harvesting in the
affected places, and if it was safe to use [the hay] for beds or fodder."[63] These
were inquiries moved by practical concerns, although obviously involving
medical theories on the modes of transmission of contagious diseases.

There was, therefore, a clear-cut division of labor between the Protomedicato and the Assunteria. The Protomedicato had the practical task of
guaranteeing the supply and quality of medicinal substances available to the
city. In 1743, for instance, the protomedici were requested by the Assunteria
di Sanità to ensure that apothecaries kept in their stores sufficient supplies of
theriac and alexipharmic (antidotes) in the event that the "possible contagion" in Messina spread to Bologna.[64] Above all, the Protomedicato had the
consultative, rather than executive, task of giving medical advice to the city,

as in 1748, during the outbreak of animal disease mentioned above, and in 1720, when the Senate asked the protomedici for "the proper guidelines" to help protect the city from incoming epidemics.[65] But the final decisions regarding, and the implementation of, practical measures designed to safeguard public health belonged solely to the Assunteria. Such a division of tasks — the advising role of the Protomedicato versus the decision-making role of the state-appointed sanitary police — was typical of the Italian political systems of the ancien régime. Even where the Protomedicato was directly appointed by the government, its tasks were quite different from those of the sanitary police, which were usually entrusted to a special governmental board (usually called the Magistrato di Sanità).[66] This was the case outside Italy as well. The Royal College of Physicians of London apparently held a purely advisory role in matters of public health. The Prussian Obercollegium Medicum, from its birth in 1685, was joined by another institution, the Collegium Sanitatis, which acted as sanitary police.[67]

It is misleading, therefore, to define the Protomedicato as a public health board or sanitary police. Rather, it was a court whose specific jurisdiction derived from the college's public responsibility to guarantee the quality of medications (by inspecting apothecaries' shops) and the skill of the healers (by examining practitioners). This task of supervising the entire medical field was warranted by a social need for the protection of the public. This need, in turn, legitimized the college doctors' dominance over all other medical practitioners. By the end of the sixteenth century, the college occupied the highest level in a medical hierarchy formed by several layers of licensed healers — from bottom to top, these were the barber-surgeons, the apothecaries, and the physicians. In this hierarchical system, the collegiates were situated at the top, less as representatives of the physicians as a professional group than as Doctors representing the university's authority, and as public magistrates representing the elite that controlled political office and power in the city.

III

What was the relationship between Bologna's ruling class and the medical elite sitting in the college? From which social classes did the collegiates come? According to the statutes, prospective members of the college had to be born citizens of Bologna and to supply evidence, from four witnesses, of their fathers' (or grandfathers') citizenship.[68] Since witnesses were questioned not only about a candidate's birthplace but also about his social status and his father's (and often his grandfather's) profession, the records of these proceedings to prove citizenship allow us to reconstruct the social background of the college's members.[69] Through this source I was able to determine the paternal status of better than 80 percent of the members of the medical college from 1593 to 1793 (106 of 130 members).

Interestingly, table 3 shows that the social composition of the college was more diverse than one would expect. The sons of collegiates sat next to not only the sons of merchants, notaries, and gentlemen, but also the sons of guildsmen, including members of two trades directly related to the practice of medicine: apothecaries and barber-surgeons. While membership in the medical college, as I have already mentioned, was a way of gaining access to noble rank,[70] the College of Medicine of Bologna was certainly not limited to noblemen. In fact, the collegiates with noble origins were definitely fewer than those belonging to the other two social groups, guildsmen and merchants (who were in many respects interconnected). Among the merchants whose sons gained admittance to the college, the most prominent were those involved in the silk trade—which is not surprising, since Bologna's economy in the early modern period was dominated by the silk industry[71]—and some wealthy grain merchants.[72]

In the college, however, we do find members of Bologna's nobility, such as Giovanni Fantuzzi and Vincenzo Montecalvi, who were admitted in 1612.[73] Sicinio Oretti and his son Francesco, who became members of the college in 1663 and 1698, respectively, came from a "senatorial" family boasting "eighteen generations of citizens," as was claimed in Sicinio's *civilitatis probationes* (although a contemporary genealogist observed that the family was "rather decayed").[74] Other noble families counting a member in the college were the Gandolfi, Belvisi, Odofredi, Bolognetti, and Mattesilani, in addition to the already mentioned Montalbani, Cucchi Cartari, and Magnani.[75]

In addition to these noblemen, however, the college also included several members who came from a humbler background—the trade associations and guilds. Among the collegiates' fathers and grandfathers we find two stewards of the Lana (woolworkers' guild), and one steward each from the guilds of the *pellicani* (furriers), the *bisilieri* (weavers of homespun cloth), the *caligari* (shoemakers), the *salaroli* (grocers), the butchers, and the drapers.[76] Certainly these were families that for generations had held the highest ranks within the guild system, as members of a guild's higher council and often holding the politically prestigious role of *massaro di collegio* (a position that allowed a guild's officer to sit as a magistrate in a court called Magistrato de

Table 3.   SOCIAL BACKGROUND OF THE MEMBERS OF THE COLLEGE OF MEDICINE
OF BOLOGNA, 1593–1793

Father's Status	N	%
Physician		
Collegiate	23	18
Noncollegiate	8	6
Total	31	24
Member of a guild		
Apothecary	8	6
Barber	3	2
Other	11	8
Total	22	16
Merchant	17	13
Gentleman	13	10
Notary	9	7
Rentier	5	4
Treasurer or bookkeeper	3	2
Clerk	2	1
Doctor of law	1	0.8
Choirmaster	1	0.8
Military officer	1	0.8
Architect	1	0.8
Unknown	24	18
Total	130	

Sources: A.S.B., Coll. Med., bb. 196, 208, 234, 238, 247, 250, 259, 332, 338, 340, 341, 342, 348, 353; Bartolomeo Albertini, *Catalogus omnium doctorum collegiatorum in artibus liberalibus et in facultate medica incip. ab A.D. 1156* (Bologna, 1664); G. N. Alidosi, *Li dottori bolognesi di Teologia, Filosofia, Medicina e d'Arte liberali dall'anno 1000 per tutto marzo del 1623* (Bologna, 1623; reprint, Bologna, 1980); P. S. Dolfi, *Cronologia delle famiglie nobili di Bologna* (Bologna, 1670; reprint, Bologna, 1973); G. Fantuzzi, *Notizie degli scrittori bolognesi* (Bologna, 1786–90); B.C.A.B., MS. Montefani, "Bibliografia bolognese," b. 24; and P. Ascanelli, *I fascicoli personali dei Lettori Artisti dell'Assunteria di Studio dell'Archivio di Stato di Bologna* (Forlì, 1968). For details on the types of information contained in these sources, see chap. 1, n. 69.

Note: The honorary members, listed in chap. 1, n. 68, are not included in the table because they did not participate actively in the public functions of the college and the Protomedicato.

Collegi, together with prominent members of the ruling elite, such as senators and jurists). There was nevertheless a great distance in rank between
guildsmen and college doctors, and it often took three generations before a
person whose family included guildsmen could make it all the way into the
college. Take, for example, the case of Gioseffo Maria Garani, who joined
the college in 1691. His grandfather "was an attendant in a grocer's shop and
was several times steward of the grocers' company." His father, Bartolomeo,
"managed a grocer's store" in his youth; he later sold silk and hemp and for
two years directed the post office, eventually achieving the status of one who
"lives on his income" without "having any occupation." Yet the Garanis were
originally a family of artisans in which everyone, men and women alike, used
to work. A witness stated that he had met Bartolomeo when he was six, in
"the year of the plague" (1630), when the witness "used to employ his sisters
and mother in the veil-making business."[77]

In the social background of some of the collegiates, there were also a
few artisans of lower status. The father of Gio. Battista Cortesi, who joined
the college in 1603, was a tailor and "a very poor man." Cortesi had an extraordinary career indeed. As a boy he had worked in a barbershop and as a
public bath attendant. He became a university lecturer in surgery and later a
physician to the army in Bologna. Called to the University of Messina to fill
the prestigious position of lecturer in medicine in 1598, he later returned to
Bologna, joining the medical college in 1603.[78]

Even more remarkable, when considering the doctors' view of the hierarchical ordering of the medical professions, is the presence among the college members of the sons of barbers and apothecaries—practitioners of
trades that were considered inferior and whose guilds were subordinate to the
college's own authority. Indeed, this seems to prove that the college was ac-
cessible (although in a limited way) to people from the lower-status social
world of the guilds. It should be noted, however, that the barbers whose sons
made it into the college had been prominent members of their guild, officers
of the guild's higher council or stewards. Carlo Antonio and Giacinto Maria
Sivieri, who entered the college in 1663 and 1691, respectively, were the sons
of two brothers, both stewards of the barbers' guild (and related in kinship to
wealthy silk merchants). Giacinto Maria's father still ran a barbershop in the
via S. Felice when his son applied to the college for admission. The witnesses
who were called to testify about his citizenship remarked that Giacinto Maria
had gone to live away from his father's dwelling "so that he could attend to
the medical profession in a more genteel way," far from his father's barbershop.[79] The father of Carlo Filippo Brusa, who became a member in 1735,

was also a barber–surgeon. The witnesses pointed out that Brusa's father had not practiced for over ten years but "was living on his income," as a gentleman.[80]

Even more numerous than the sons of barbers who made their way into the college were the sons of apothecaries who did so; this might be expected, since the apothecaries' trade was considered to be of higher standing than the barbers'.[81] In their case, again, we are dealing with very prominent members of the profession, often coming from families that numbered physicians, in addition to apothecaries, among their members. Such, for instance, was the case of the dal Buono family, one of whom, the doctor Gio. Batta, the son and grandson of apothecaries, joined the college in 1593. We even find an apothecary somehow related to a noble family: the father of Alessandro Recordati, who joined the college in 1603, was described in his son's civilitatis probationes as "a merchant" but also as born from a "noble and ancient family."[82] Giuseppe Antonio Monti, father of Gaetano Monti, who joined in 1746, was clearly at the very top of his profession. Although practicing as an apothecary, he obtained a doctoral degree in philosophy, advancing to become a famous botanist and a professor of natural history at the Bologna Institute of Sciences.[83]

Some interesting aspects of the doctors' social background emerge when we analyze separately the data for the seventeenth century and those for the eighteenth (table 4). As we can see, in the eighteenth century the proportion of nobles among the collegiates' fathers decreased dramatically. Guildsmen almost completely disappeared, except for those involved with the practice of medicine, such as apothecaries and barber-surgeons (the proportion of apothecaries among the collegiates' fathers actually increased in this period). In the seventeenth century, many college members came from the families of prominent merchants and guildsmen, who often controlled the prestigious and remunerated public offices in the city government. In the eighteenth century, there were still merchants in the social background of the collegiates, but both nobles and artisans were fast disappearing.

In the eighteenth century we also notice an increase of nepotism within the college: the proportion of sons of collegiates grew from 12 percent to 28 percent of the total membership. We also find a growing proportion of collegiates whose fathers were physicians (although not members of the college); overall, their proportion increased from 17 percent in the seventeenth century to 37 percent in the eighteenth. In the eighteenth century, the college members were more likely to come from families that had practiced medicine or the apothecary trade for generations. We can definitely say that

Table 4.   SOCIAL BACKGROUND OF THE MEMBERS OF THE COLLEGE OF MEDICINE
OF BOLOGNA, 1593–1692 AND 1693–1793

Father's Status	1593–1692		1693–1793	
	N	%	N	%
Physician				
Collegiate	10	12	13	28
Noncollegiate	4	5	4	9
Total	14	17	17	37
Member of a guild				
Apothecary	3	4	5	11
Barber	2	2	1	2
Other	11	13	—	—
Total	16	19	6	13
Merchant	12	14	5	11
Gentleman	12	14	1	2
Notary	7	8	2	4
Rentier	2	2	3	7
Treasurer or bookkeeper	1	1	2	4
Clerk	—	—	2	4
Doctor of law	—	—	1	2
Choirmaster	1	1	—	—
Military officer	1	1	—	—
Architect	—	—	1	2
Unknown	18	21	6	13
Total	84		46	

Sources: See source note to table 3.

Note: The honorary members, listed in chap. 1, n. 68, are not included in the table because they did not participate actively in the public functions of the college and the Protomedicato.

in this period the college members were increasingly recruited from the top levels of the medical professions. In this additional sense, we can justifiably define the members of the college in the eighteenth century as a medical elite.

In the early years of the seventeenth century, the physician and philosopher Camillo Baldi, a member of the medical college, described the social stratification in Bologna as comprising—from top to bottom—first the senatorial nobility, followed by the "gentlemen" (*gentiluomini,* those who "live on their income without having an occupation") and the merchants, then the artisans (*artefici,* "those who work with their hands practicing trades that require manual as well as mental labor"), and finally, lowest of all, the "plebs." If we return to Baldi's classification, we can say that the college doctors came almost exclusively from the middle classes: neither from the highest class nor from the lowest, but from the gentry and the merchants. Some members of the college came from those lower-status groups that Baldi defined as "artisans." Overall, however, in the seventeenth century the college was dominated by representatives of the two classes, gentry and merchants, who enjoyed the political advantages of citizenship — that is, to use Baldi's words, who "could hold public offices in the city, such as those of the Anzianato, Confalonieri del Popolo, Uffici del Contado."[84]

Owing to their family background, most members of the college belonged to the middle class of the city's ruling elite: that patrician-mercantile class that had privileged access to the remunerated and prestigious public offices reserved for the citizens, as well as to some honorific judicial positions, such as the Anzianato (Court of the Elders) and the Tribuni della Plebe (Tribunes of the Plebs). Within the complex web of the city's jurisdictions, a comparison between the Tribunes of the Plebs and the Protomedicato reveals some interesting parallels. The Court of the Tribunes of the Plebs was composed of some stewards of the guilds (drawn, by casting lots, from lists submitted by the guilds themselves) plus sixteen *confalonieri del popolo* directly appointed by the Senate. The tribunes, who held civil as well as criminal hearings, were in charge "of visiting city and countryside in order to prevent fraud by merchants and others to the detriment of the people."[85] Their main responsibility was to control the price and quality of bread and other staple foods. The Protomedicato and the tribunes, therefore, had similar functions. Both institutions were in charge of protecting the public from fraud — controlling food, in the case of the tribunes; and controlling medicines, in the case of the Protomedicato. The two institutions were also similar in their social composition, since in the court of the tribunes guildsmen sat next to senators, jurists, and other "gentlemen and noble merchants" appointed by the Senate.[86] Also among the tribunes, therefore, we find a mingling of the highest officers of the guilds with the patrician-mercantile elite, which, as we know, characterized the social composition of the medical college in the seventeenth century. There were also other links between the two institutions. The offices of protomedico and *tribuno della plebe* often ran in the same families; the records often say that the guildsmen listed as fathers of collegiates served as tribunes — a conclusive proof of citizenship and high social status. Even more significant is the fact that the same person could hold both offices: the doctors of the medical college were often appointed by the Senate to sit among the tribunes (although less frequently than were members of the College of the Jurists). In a list of tribunes from 1593 to 1769, nearly every year we find one or more members of the medical college.[87]

The names of college doctors can also be found among the Anziani, another public role whose functions were mostly ceremonial in this period.[88] For some doctors, therefore, sitting in the college often implied serving in a judicial role as magistrates (even when they were not protomedici). For instance, Ovidio Montalbani not only was a diligent protomedico but also served as a magistrate among the Anziani and, more than once, as a Tribune of the Plebs. We also find him as a judge in the Merchants' Court. Not surprisingly, he held a doctorate not only in medicine and philosophy but also in canon law and civil law.[89] In the seventeenth century, in fact, juridical culture and medical culture presented deep affinities and associations.[90] Another collegiate, Cesare Zoppio, also held doctoral degrees in both medicine and the law and served among the Anziani and the Tribunes of the Plebs. His case shows that one could hold the role of protomedico without having actively practiced medicine. A member of the medical college since 1651, Zoppio stated in 1676 that he had never practiced as a physician but had only "applied himself in examining students, granting degrees . . . and, as a protomedico, inspecting and sentencing barbers, apothecaries, and charlatans."[91] In the eighteenth century, public service as a tribune could still add luster to a physician's professional curriculum. When Domenico Sgargi, a public lecturer and member of the college, asked the Assunteria di Studio to raise his salary in 1778, he mentioned among his credentials having "borne the heavy responsibility of a Tribune of the Plebs" in 1763, 1769, and 1771.[92]

For members of the college, therefore, the professional role of the physician was closely associated with the judicial role of the magistrate. This medical elite formed a group of doctors with a specialized juridical knowledge, who strongly identified with the public role of the city's magistrates, owing also to family traditions and associations. As we shall see, the activity of the Protomedicato cannot be understood merely as a narrow-minded defense of the interests of physicians. On the contrary, the protomedici were inspired by a broader concept of equity related to their role as public magistrates. Certainly, belonging to the college was not only a responsibility but also a financial asset. Being a collegiate and a protomedico was a source of income, authority, and prestige. For every doctoral degree granted in medicine and for every license granted to apothecaries or surgeons, the college received a fee that was routinely shared among its members.[93] As I have already mentioned, the protomedici were also paid for inspecting the apothecaries' shops in the city and countryside.[94] Still, to the doctors of the college, their duty as magistrates was something more than a mere source of power and income: it was the core of their identity, the linchpin of a complex vision of their professional and social roles.

IV

From the viewpoint of the college doctors, the main source of legitimization of the Protomedicato's authority was certainly its public responsibility, its role as a magistracy protecting the community and the sick from the danger of illicit medical practice—a practice based on mere empirical expertise, devoid of true knowledge. In this city that prided itself on having Europe's oldest university, the protomedici, owing to their superior knowledge, guaranteed the protection of patients from the dangerous activities of those who, according to a public notification *(bando)* issued by the college in 1664, "poorly practice the art of medicine, without any knowledge of illnesses and their causes, of the complexions of human beings, and of the virtues of medicines."[95] The college's monopoly over licensing in any branch of medicine—the exclusive authority to pass judgment on every healer's skills—was justified by the its members' academic knowledge, placed at the service of the community.

The public service that the college provided by protecting the sick also warranted the jurisdictional prerogatives of the college and of the Protomedicato in criminal matters. These prerogatives included not only "sending to trial, acquitting, condemning, enforcing sentences and, to this end, issuing executive writs, orders, edicts, and fining" but also "capturing and holding in custody individuals, who will not be able to challenge the college's competence as a judge."[96] This direct jurisdiction over criminal matters was an important extension of the traditional powers of the college, resulting from the creation of the Protomedicato. According to the statutes of 1507, the dean had the authority only to fine those practicing without a license; these fines were to be collected not by the college but by the ordinary court.[97] By the end of the sixteenth century, however, the Protomedicato was able to enforce its own sentences directly. It employed constables to arrest unlicensed healers and seize illicit drugs, and it was entitled to use the prisons of the Torrone (Bologna's criminal court) and of the ecclesiastical court.[98]

Some of the Protomedicato's rules that regulated the activities of the lower-status medical trades were clearly aimed at protecting public safety, in addition to asserting the division of labor among practitioners and the supervisory role of doctors over all medical practice. Hence the prohibition against apothecaries selling "purgative, abortive, and sleeping medicines" without a doctor's prescription, a prohibition that was gradually extended to all kinds of medicines. Another safety rule, often repeated in the Protomedicato's public proclamations addressed to the barbers, forbade the drawing of blood from a woman's foot. This treatment was considered potentially abortifacient, on the basis of medical lore dating back to a Hippocratic aphorism and well known in popular medicine.[99]

The goal of protecting the sick was explicit in the Protomedicato's laws. In the trials for illegal practice, the patient's testimony was considered critical: "We shall hear the report by the patient, and a sworn witness in addition to the plaintiff, whose name will be kept secret."[100] Thus, the patients appeared before the Protomedicato as plaintiffs, and in this role we indeed find them. For instance, in 1593, Bastiano and Camillo Pellicani—"good citizens of Bologna," as they defined themselves—wished "to notify their tribunal—the Most Excellent College—of the danger they incurred when they were treated by a certain Antonio Cardoni, who, not being authorized to keep or administer any kind of medicines, and having nevertheless done it, might very well have given them one medication instead of another." Patients asked the college doctors to establish whether they had been treated according to the rules of medical practice. This indicates public awareness of the protomedici's inspections of the apothecaries' shops and, especially, of the fact that adulterated or poor-quality medicines found in the stores were publicly thrown away. The patients requested justice and, at the same time, protection from endangerment, as the Pellicani brothers conclude in their plea: "We ask that you shall do what, in your opinion, is according to justice, and this we hope because of your integrity, since you are so careful and diligent wherever the poor invalids are in danger."[101]

The Protomedicato was responsible for protecting the sick as consumers, in cases involving not just the quality but also the prices of medicines. It was established that "the *bills* for medicines to be paid by buyers, after being reviewed and checked by the officers of the apothecaries' company, shall be once again reviewed by the Protomedicato, to check that they are in agreement with the *tassa* [the table of prices]."[102] The people of Bologna were aware of their right to buy medicines at a fair price. Thus, in 1588, Donino Zocchini, an *operarius* (handicraftsman), explained in a formal grievance to the protomedici how, "his little girl being sick," he had gone to the apothecary with the "prescription for a syrup." He was given "a small bottle containing some syrup, but if it was the one I had asked for, I don't know." At another apothecary's shop he was told that, in fact, the contents of the bottle had not been made "according to the recipe" and, even more aggravating, that he had been "overcharged."[103]

The patients who filed suits in the Protomedicato viewed it as the magistracy in charge of settling disputes between patients and healers. "It is granted to the College Doctors, the College Dean, and the protomedici to settle and arbitrate any lawsuits and litigations that may arise between doctors and patients." This civil jurisdiction — typical of the medical courts of the ancien régime[104] — was a further development of the dean's statutory power to arbitrate disputes involving college members in their medical practice. As the jurisdiction of the college broadened to include lower-level practitioners, the authority of the protomedici extended to disputes involving apothecaries and barber-surgeons. This jurisdictional power was rooted in the ancient mercantile law of the guild courts, according to which all the people entering into a commercial transaction with a guild member — by buying his goods or hiring his services — could appeal to the guild court for redress. The civil lawsuits heard in the Protomedicato were indeed held "in the manner of merchants": the procedure was swift and informal, or, as they said, without the clamor and ceremony of a formal court.[105] In their lawsuits, healers turned to the Protomedicato to demand fees that their patients had left unpaid. In turn, the patients could ask the Protomedicato to ensure that treatment or medicines were conforming, in quality and cost, to the standards publicly guaranteed by the college, just as the ancient guild courts had upheld standards of quality and fair price for the goods and services offered by their members.

In a letter addressed in 1736 to the Assunteria per il Sollievo delle Arti, the Protomedicato reaffirmed its "ancient and well-founded right . . . to make sure that there are no abuses, frauds, or illegal practices to the detriment of the common wealth." It also defined itself as "a special Magistrate empowered to hear suits and give verdicts and sentences."[106] The vast and complex array of law courts typical of ancien régime society did thus include a special court for patients and healers. Compared to other courts, the Protomedicato was certainly a small tribunal, dealing with a very limited number of cases.[107] It is for this very reason, and owing to the summary procedure followed in the trials, that today we can retrace and reconstruct its activity throughout two centuries — a task that would be impossible with other tribunals.

The records of the Protomedicato during this period enable us to focus on the existence, in the old regime, of a judicial arena corresponding to the field of medical practice, viewed by the college as a hierarchy of three complementary tasks (physic, pharmacy, and surgery). In this judicial arena, the patient's rights were certainly rooted in the mercantile laws of the guilds, that is to say, patients had first of all a right to a standard quality and fair price of the goods or services they purchased. Yet there was something else beside this customary notion, which considered the patient simply as a party to a commercial transaction. There was also a perception by the medical elite that "being sick" implied a condition of weakness and vulnerability. In the old regime, the sick, like the elderly, the poor, women who were virgins or widows, and children in general, were given special legal rights or "privileges."[108] This is signaled by the fact that the lawsuits filed by patients in the Protomedicato were expedited with summary procedure—a benefit also granted to other classes of people regarded as weak: the poor, foreigners, widows, orphans and other children, prisoners, and Jews.[109] The notion of a right as a "privilege," that is, as a corrective to a state of weakness, implies that the bearer of that right has, first of all, a right to be protected. This notion was consistent with the duty to protect society from medical abuses—a duty that the medical elite felt as its own, and on which it based its public authority. This self-imposed obligation to protect the patients was subtly interwoven with the protomedici's interest in protecting their own role as sole medical authority. Yet it was also undoubtedly felt as part of the social responsibility of the powerful toward the weak, the learned toward "the poor, who don't know." It resonated with that culture of paternalism that was, in the ancien régime, a deeply rooted feature of the urban ruling classes' attitude toward the weakest members of the social order.[110]

As magistrates, the protomedici saw themselves as the learned protectors of the patients, who were the weaker partner (weaker also because of ignorance) in the healer-patient relationship. We can now ask: how did the patients act on this judicial stage? How did they view their relationship with their healers? What were their expectations—what did they think of their rights and duties—when they pleaded for justice in the Protomedicato?

Chapter 2

PROMISING A CURE

Agreements between Patients and Healers in the Early Modern Period

To the sick, who hang on your every word, thou shalt promise health.
—*De instructione medici secundum Archimathaeum,* twelfth century

I am not healed, and if you will prove to me that, in fact, I am,
I offer to pay immediately what is fair.
—Paolo Vitali, plaintiff, to the Bolognese protomedici,
in a lawsuit against surgeon Ulisse Parmi, 1574

I

The charges that occasioned the Protomedicato's proceedings from the sixteenth to the eighteenth century were often filed anonymously. Of the signed petitions, however, nearly two-thirds came from patients or their relatives and friends.[1] Thus, sick persons did actually turn to the Protomedicato for justice, leaving records that enable us to understand their viewpoint and to observe the medical system from the perspective of its users. What we notice at first, when we examine the complaints filed in the doctors' court, is that these complaints are framed in the stereotypical parlance of the plea to higher authorities. The plaintiffs are asking for protection, but they also ask for something more. Many appeals involve a specific request, such as, for instance, that of the "humble Laura Diola," who asked the Protomedicato in 1595 for "the refund of three ducats from a Neapolitan man practicing medicine; he having taken to treat said Laura and having crippled her, she wished that her money be returned to her, especially since she heard of the bad practice of said Neapolitan."[2]

The declared aim of these appeals for justice was not only to punish a bad practitioner but also, as in Laura Diola's case, to recover the money spent on ineffective treatment. Patients considered their claims for restitution to be within their legal rights, on the ground that their healers had broken an agreement. They presented themselves to the court as victims of a breach of contract. In 1595, for instance, several claims were filed against a barber, Ludovico Bazano. In one of them, Geronimo dal Usello explained how his wife had been suffering for two years from a "pain in the neck, around the ears":

> About three and a half months ago, I met by mischance this Ludovico who . . . claimed to be a barber. He came to visit my wife Domenica and began treating her, saying that she had scrofula and promising to cure her within two months; and in the presence of witnesses, we agreed on fourteen lire although he ended up taking sixteen. He continued to treat her until he collected all this money and then abandoned her, and for this reason she is crippled and cannot move her neck.[3]

Some features of the transaction between this woman and her healer reappear over and over again in other patients' complaints or depositions. First of all, the promise of a cure, a full recovery within a fixed period of time. On one side, the healer, whether a traveling quack, such as Laura Diola's Neapolitan, or a licensed practitioner, such as the barber Bazano, promises to effect a cure. On the other side, the patient or his or her guardian promises to pay, often in installments, with the balance due at the end of treatment. Most important, the object of the transaction is not just the provision of the healer's services but the positive outcome of the therapy.

Such agreements, or contracts, for a cure have a long history, as testified by many written records. Whereas Laura Diola and Geronimo dal Usello had simply a verbal compact (in Geronimo's case supported by witnesses) with their healers, the stipulation was often written down formally as a contract. Such contracts can be found among medieval notarial records as early as the thirteenth century, and the custom may well be even more ancient, as we shall see. Hitherto these medieval documents have not been studied in depth; they have been viewed mostly as an oddity of past medical practice — worthy, at most, of cursory anecdotal mention.[4] Formally drawn up by a notary, these agreements usually set the terms of payment, the duration of treatment, and the criteria for recovery (often allowing the patient some say over these). Occasionally, they also specified the patient's role in the treatment — for instance, the duty to follow a special diet. Here is one such contract, signed in 1316 in the presence of a notary and witnesses and transcribed in the "Libro dei memoriali" of the Commune of Bologna under the marginal heading "promissio et depositus":

To all readers of these public records: we declare that the learned master Giovanni de Anglio, physician *[medicus]*, has undertaken the treatment and medication of Bertholucio, nobleman, son of the late Guidone dei Samaritani, a citizen of Bologna. Master Giovanni shall pursue such treatment in exchange for fifty good and sound golden florins, weighed Bologna style, at the terms and conditions set herein: that said Master Giovanni has promised to treat and heal Bertholucio from his illness, with the help of medications, waters, and concoctions that Master Giovanni will buy at his own expense; so that in the next forty days Bertholucio will be convalescing and improving, to the point of being again able to partially move his hand, foot, thigh, and leg, to use said hand to dress himself and put on shoes, and to wash his healthy hand with the one which is now ill. These terms being met before the end of the forty days, Bertholucio has promised and agreed to promptly compensate said master with twenty-five golden florins out of the total amount of fifty, in payment for the medications already administered and those still needed in order to complete his recovery. Said master has also promised and agreed to treat, medicate, and completely cure Bertholucio in such a way that he will clearly feel well in the sick side as in the other one; and once he feels he has recovered his health, Bertholucio has promised to promptly pay, upon request, the balance of the agreed-upon sum — that is, another twenty-five florins of pure gold according to standard. Furthermore, Raynerio, son of the late Jacopino de Arzellata and chaplain of Santa Maria Maggiore, has officially and solemnly declared to Master Giovanni that he received in escrow the said fifty florins from Bertholucio, and has promised to give the master the entire amount as previously established, on condition that he [Bertholucio] feels completely cured.[5]

The terms of this agreement are typical of the contracts that are found in medieval notarial archives and, in the early modern age, among the records of the Protomedicato: the promise of a cure by the healer; the promise of payment of an agreed-upon sum by the patient; a trustee designated by both parties to hold the sum in escrow; and an initial installment to be paid by the patient at the first signs of improvement, with the balance to be paid upon successful completion of the cure. Another significant feature of the agreement, as indicated in the contract between Master Giovanni de Anglio and Bertholucio, was not only that payment was contingent upon the success of the treatment but also — most important — that improvement and healing were to be determined solely by the patient's perception. In the Bolognese contract, as we can see, health is defined as a condition perceived *(salus habita et percepta)* entirely from the patient's viewpoint. Likewise, illness is described as the ailing of an affected part of the body rather than as an abstract entity. In Bertholucio's eyes, healing meant being able once more to perform his daily tasks — getting dressed, putting on his shoes, washing his hands — with that part of his body which was now paralyzed. In the agreement, illness was defined entirely according to the patient's bodily self-perception. Even physicians were apt to define disease in the same manner. A fifteenth-century doctor, for instance, in describing the course of his own illness, focused on that body part which was ailing: "that part over which I had no power; and which seemed to me to be dead and estranged."[6]

Such a patient-centered description of illness and recovery is typical of the medieval agreements between patients and healers. Another example is the contract undersigned in 1244 by Rogerio de Bruch of Bergamo and Bosso the wool carder in Genoa:

> In the name of the Lord, amen.
>
> I, Rogerio de Bruch of Bergamo, promise and agree with you, Bosso the wool carder, to return you to health and to make you improve from the illness that you have in your person, that is in your hand, foot, and mouth, in good faith, with the help of God, within the next month and a half, in such a way that you will be able to feed yourself with your hand and cut bread and wear shoes and walk and speak much better than you do now. I shall take care of all the expenses that will be necessary for this; and at that time, you shall pay me seven Genoese lire; and you shall not eat any fruit, beef, pasta — whether boiled or dry — or cabbage. If I do not keep my promises to you, you will not have to give me anything. And I, the aforementioned Bosso, promise to you, Rogerio, to pay you seven Genoese lire within three days after my recovery and improvement.[7]

Who has never thought of recovery in these very same terms — to be able to do things just as one had done them before falling sick — slicing bread and eating, walking and talking normally? The patient's personal experience of illness comes to the foreground in these documents. In sharp contrast to modern medicine, illness and recovery were defined not by the physician but by the sick, who had an active role. The terms of agreements were formulated by both parties, and both voices could be heard in the contracts, as in the Genoese case cited above.

Cure agreements between patients and healers have been found scattered among medieval notarial records from all over Europe: we know, for instance, of cases from Crete (1348, 1361), Zara (1377, 1385, 1398, 1484), Ferrara (1403), Avignon (1477), Messina (1484), Hildesheim (1531), Dubrovnik (1546, 1559), and Poitiers (1620).[8] Furthermore, early modern forensic medicine indicates that the custom of stipulating contracts for a cure was widespread in Spain, France, and Germany, as well as in Italy.[9] In Norwich, England, the "Mayor's Book of the Poor" and municipal court proceedings from the late sixteenth century record a large number of agreements between healers and patients, so that Margaret Pelling, in examining these documents, noted that "much regulation of practice is better seen as legal investigation of claims against contracts."[10] The same can be said of Bologna, where the Protomedicato acted as a court in cases involving breach of contract by one of the parties: whether healers pursuing their clients for non-payment, or patients arguing that they had not been perfectly cured.

In places and times far apart from each other, the cure contracts were drawn up following the same basic pattern. Here is another example from Messina, in 1484 (a document that the Sicilian folklorist Giuseppe Pitré discussed in the 1920s as a mere curiosity):

> Master Francesco di Giovanni, who calls himself a physician from Treviso, undertakes of his own free will to treat, and with God's direction, to return to health Master Paolo Palumbo, citizen of Messina . . . and help him recover from his ailment of catarrh and chest pain [catarru pectustrictu] without asthma, in exchange for four gold Venetian ducats; which ducats Master Paolo deposited into the hands of master Pietro de La Ferra, citizen of Messina, at the time of signing this agreement. . . . so that once said Paolo is healed from his infirmity, one month from now, Master Francesco shall receive said four golden ducats; and if he [Paolo] is not healed, these four ducats will be returned to said Paolo, furthermore declaring that Master Francesco shall take upon himself the expenses of all medications.[11]

The promise of a cure is obviously the key feature of the agreement between healer and patient. It is also mentioned by medical authors as a standard aspect of the relationship of trust between healer and patient. "To the sick, who hang on your every word, thou shalt promise health, with the help of God," Archimathaeus says in *De instructione medici*—the professional etiquette manual of the collection of medical texts called the *Salernitan Collection* (twelfth century). In Lucca, in 1346, the "master surgeons" Francesco and Bonagratia delli Scolli, of Parma, advertised their services by claiming that "they shall cure anybody who will go to them . . . and they shall not receive any payment until [their patients] are free from illness and cured. They shall keep to what [was] agreed upon in their contracts, treating the rich in exchange for a sum of money depending on the nature of illness and the patients' ability to pay, and treating the poor without charge, for the love of God."[12]

Promising a cure was clearly a marketing device, a psychological trick used by the healers to win the patients' trust, as suggested by Archimathaeus.[13] Yet to see it simply as such would be misleading. It would be seeing it only from our modern perspective, which tends to privilege the viewpoint of the physician in matters of therapy. Regardless of the healer's motivations, his or her promise to effect a cure was taken very seriously by the patients, as a legally binding commitment. As indicated by the records of the Protomedicato throughout the sixteenth century, the promise of a cure was considered essential for the legal resolution of disputes between patients and healers. In fact, the promise had the official value of a contractual commitment. When filing their claims, patients had recourse to a customary norm that gave them the right not to pay for an unsuccessful treatment—releasing them, in such a case, from their pledge to the healer. In the ancien régime, therefore, the promise of a cure was not merely a marketing device of the medical practitioners; it was the mainstay—from a legal viewpoint—of the conditional contract that I have called the "contract for a cure."

It was not only the patients who thus understood the import of the deal, but also the magistrates who were called to solve disputes between the sick and their healers. This is shown by the records of several medieval municipal courts, where we find cases of healers fined for receiving payment before completing a cure, or sentenced to return advance payments after an unsuccessful treatment. In 1320 in Venice, for instance, Beatrice, a woman physician *(medica)*, was fined ten lire for accepting advance payment from a patient before restoring him to health.[14] In 1322, in the same city, the surgeon Santo da Forlì was fined for having requested five lire from a patient for his labor and medications, even though the patient was not completely cured.[15]

When a patient filed a suit for unsuccessful treatment, the judge ordered that the sick person be examined by other practitioners. In 1386 in Padua, the *medicus* Domenico da Bologna and the *medicus ciroicus* Novello de Marano were requested by a judge of the court called the Officio delle Vittuarie to visit Sir Boninsegna, who had lodged a complaint against a third physician for not having delivered the promised cure. The two examiners declared that "the infirm had not been cured properly by the physician because he did not use the proper medications." The physician was sentenced to return to Sir Boninsegna the latter's advance payment.[16] Two centuries later, in 1546, the Minor Council of the city of Dubrovnik sentenced the surgeon Giovanni Andrea to return eight gold ducats received from Sir Nicola Bazano as advance payment for treating his son Giorgio's gallstones, "because from the investigation read to this council, it clearly appears that [the physician] has not treated the patient with the necessary diligence."[17]

When there was discord over the definition of recovery, an expert was called to arbitrate in the case and sometimes to estimate the fair price of a partially successful treatment. In 1484, the doctor Bartholomeo, surgeon and town physician of the community of Zara, was summoned to settle a dispute between another surgeon, Master Francesco Stupich, of Busana, and the patient Zuanne da Modone, who was suffering from fistula:

> When questioned thoroughly by both justices . . . Bartholomeo said that, when Master Francesco went to Venice, Master Zuanne called him [Bartholomeo] to his house and showed him his affected part, saying: 'Sir, tell me whether I am cured from this illness, because Master Francesco, who has treated me, is asking for twenty-five gold ducats as payment for his services.' Bartholomeo examined the fistula, probing it with a lancet to see if it was firm, and found that the lancet entered two fingers deep, or thereabouts, into the fistula. As to whether [Zuanne] was cured, [Bartholomeo] responded that, in his opinion, he was not; and if Master Francesco had cured him, [Francesco] would have deserved more than twenty-five gold ducats; but as things stood, he only deserved ten gold ducats for his labor.[18]

When the treatment was successful, the outcome was sometimes recorded in a document that marked the end of the therapeutic transaction. Here is an example of an agreement that came to a successful conclusion. On May 16, 1414, in Bologna, "Master Pietro Bondedei, son of the late Gerolamo, received ten Bolognese lire from Ranuzzo Fantini, citizen of Bologna, as partial payment for curing an aposteme [abscess] in Ranuzzo's left hip." On June 12, according to another document, "the aforementioned Ranuzzo was requested to pay Master Pietro, surgeon, the balance of five Bolognese lire. . . . At the end of treatment, two small openings remained, to allow for the draining of the corrupt matter and a full recovery."[19] Despite the two openings, the cure was considered complete. In fact, such openings were viewed as necessary to allow the discharge of the diseased matter. This notion of healing as based upon the expulsion of corrupted humors from the body was fundamental for centuries, not only in popular culture but also among physicians. We shall see later the crucial importance of this notion in patients' perception of the healing process.[20]

The promise of a cure was accompanied by a clause, sometimes explicitly stated in the agreements, that in case of relapse patients would be treated again without charge until fully recovered. We find this clause, for instance, in a 1477 contract, signed in Avignon in the presence of a notary:

> Master Petrus de Narbona, citizen and resident of Avignon, has promised and agreed with the honest woman Guillemine Juliane, wife of the king's servant Pasquerio Auvray, a resident of Avignon, here present, to treat her, and return her to health within the next six months, from a fistula, also called *fistula lacrimosa,* that she has on her face under the left eye. This for the sum of three *scuta,* that the same Guillemine has promised and agreed to pay to Master Petrus for the aforementioned treatment and for the labor undertaken. . . . [The parties] agreed that Master Petrus de Narbona will be held responsible for restoring her completely to health and for curing said Guillemine within the said six months. In case she will not be cured, that is, restored to health, Master Petrus de Narbona will receive nothing for his work. It is also agreed that should the fistula return to affect said Guillemine, Master Pietro will be required to cure her, that is, restore her to health at his own expense, and she will not be held to pay him anything.[21]

The issue of payment to the medical practitioner in case of relapse is also mentioned in the civil law literature, where it is presented as an object of controversy among jurists. In his *Quaestiones Sabbatinae,* the late-thirteenth-century jurist Pilius ponders the following question:

> Should the physician, having received the agreed-upon payment to treat a gout that healed, be held to cure it anew in case of a relapse?
>
> A patient affected by gout hired a physician to cure him of this illness in exchange for a sum of money; he healed, but after a period of time had a relapse. Now he plans to sue the physician, asking to be treated again at no extra charge. Does he have the legal right to do this?

The jurist's response is that "in this case, one must determine whether the relapse was caused by the same humors or by different ones. If it was caused by the same humors, the physician is held responsible for curing the illness anew without charge; if the opposite is true, the physician is not responsible . . . ; and if by chance the relapse is the patient's fault because he did not abstain from banquets, the physician is not responsible to treat him again; but [the physician] is responsible, however, if the patient has no fault."[22] In case of relapse, the physician had the obligation to treat a patient without charge because he had already been paid, not for a temporary treatment but for full recovery. This opinion of the medieval jurists would be repeated over and over again in the following centuries, up to the 1600s, by the learned interpreters of the civil and the canon law.[23] We can thus say that the notion according to which the physician's fee was conditional on the patient's full recovery was not only widespread in popular culture but was also accepted by the jurists, who endorsed it as legitimate and equitable.

To protect the healer in case the relapse was caused by the patient's negligence, the cure agreements often mentioned the rules to be followed by the sick person, as we saw in the contract between Rogerio de Bruch and Bosso the wool carder. Such were also the terms between the shoemaker Buctico and the barber Giovanni da Menania, in 1398. The patient was requested "to stay on a diet and obey the orders given by Master Giovanni; if he does not obey and keep to the prescribed regimen, said Master Giovanni will not be responsible to continue with the cure, and said Buctico will be anyhow obliged to pay the balance of three ducats, whether recovered or not."[24] Healers, be they physicians, surgeons, or simply barbers, did not simply prescribe a treatment, they also gave their patients a general "rule of life." In 1291, Gerardo, a Venetian surgeon, related how he had started to treat a wounded peasant. When visiting him, "he found the man in an uncovered gondola, naked from the waist up, and it was windy weather. He told the injured man: 'Brother, you are making a mistake, because if you don't feel sick now, you will soon; you could catch a bad illness and die from it.' Then he renewed the bandage on the wound, and told the patient to stay indoors, in a warm place, and to protect himself from the wind and the cold weather, or he would catch his death."[25]

II

Historians have considered the "contracts for a cure" which I have described so far as medical oddities of little or no significance. I believe instead that they reveal an important and hitherto ignored fact in the history of the patient-healer relationship. For many centuries in European history, there was no shared consensus around a basic principle of the modern practice of medicine — the principle, that is, that medical service should be remunerated regardless of its outcome, as a service performed by a professional. Well into the early modern age, even academically trained physicians accepted to some extent the principle that remuneration for medical labor should be at least partly tied to the successful completion of treatment.

Gian Filippo Ingrassia, a renowned physician appointed as protomedico of Sicily in 1563, declared that he had to attend to "disputes, brawls, and a great deal of confusion on the issue of physicians' fees." Like his Bolognese colleagues, the Sicilian protomedico was also in charge of settling disputes between healers and patients.[26] Ingrassia decided to establish standard fees throughout the kingdom, with the following guidelines: First of all, one ought to distinguish among the different kinds of practitioners, establishing whether the healer was "a physician, with a doctorate in arts and medicine" *(medicus artium et medicinae doctor),* "a semi-physician, with a doctorate only in medicine or surgery" *(semidoctor, hoc est medicinae tantum, aut chirugiae doctor),* or a mere practitioner licensed by the Protomedicato *(licentiatus).* It was also necessary to consider the time of the visit (day or night), the social condition of the patient, the distance to the patient's house, the gravity of the illness, and the duration and outcome of the cure. According to Ingrassia, a physician should not receive a fee proportional to the length of the treatment — in fact, the faster the recovery, the more the physician should be paid. Otherwise, patients would end up rewarding an ignorant physician who took longer to achieve results, and penalizing a good physician who promptly prescribed the right treatment.[27] The physician's fee, furthermore, should be based on the success or failure of therapy. In establishing fees for surgical procedures, Ingrassia took into account the success or failure of the procedure. "For every drilling into the skull, if the patient recovers, the surgeon shall receive a Sicilian *oncia* in addition to his fee for each day of treatment. . . . If the patient dies, the surgeon shall not receive any amount beyond his daily fee." For treating an injury to the chest or the lower abdomen, the surgeon can expect an *oncia* but only if the wounded person recovers ("siquidem sanetur aegrotans").[28] Ingrassia's guidelines clearly implied that practitioners should be paid for every visit, regardless of the outcome, but that a successful treatment should be additionally remunerated. Thus, he approved of the custom according to which the physician was entitled to a bonus on the last day of treatment, when the patient was pronounced cured. "Undoubtedly," noted the protomedico, "the physician deserves some remuneration, or rather a gift *[strena],* for the good news he gives to his patient on that occasion."[29]

Pondering in puzzlement upon these guidelines, the early-twentieth-century historian, folklorist, and physician Giuseppe Pitré noted "the odd notion of not paying the healer in case of unsuccessful treatment," which he straightforwardly called "a legalized injustice."[30] Here Pitré spoke as a modern doctor rather than as a historian of popular culture. To a modern doctor, the principle that payment be bound to the patient's recovery can only seem unfair and, indeed, preposterous. The cure agreement seems a puzzling paradox to modern minds. What is most disconcerting is the fact that payment for a professional service should be contingent upon such a risky, uncertain criterion as recovery. How can this fact be explained?

First of all, we should remember that, in the late medieval period, medical service was only partly commercialized and was still anchored to considerations of moral order. There was an ethical and religious reluctance to view the healer-patient relationship as a transaction to be solely mediated by the cash nexus. This is clearly indicated by the treatises on medical ethics that, as late as the early 1600s, discussed and refuted the idea that the physician, when accepting a fee, was selling something spiritual and thus committing the sin of simony.[31] Saint Antonino, a fifteenth-century bishop of Florence, had already tried to keep the shadow of simony from darkening the reputation of Christian physicians: "For the fact that the physician asks for and receives a salary, one should not say that he sells his science or health, which are spiritual things; but one should say that he rents his service and asks to be paid for the work he has performed, as a physician now and formerly as a student."

Antonino added, somewhat contradictorily: "However, it is true that the holy physicians Cosmas and Damian took no fee when they cured the sick, but they did so because they did not want to seem to be selling the gift of health."[32] In the early seventeenth century, Paolo Zacchia, the first physician to the pope and the author of the very influential *Quaestiones medicolegales,* again discussed the issue: "One cannot sell spiritual things without committing the sin of simony: but medicine, that is, the gift of healing, is a spiritual thing; it seems, therefore, that one cannot be paid for it without sinning." But Zacchia argued against this view, stating that the opposite opinion—namely, that physicians may legitimately receive payment from their patients—is "the most common opinion, and the true one."[33]

On this issue, however, the views of the common people were probably less unanimous and clear than those of the learned doctors—physicians, theologians, and jurists—whose works Zacchia summarized. An apothecary from Bologna called Il Pastarino, in a religious treatise published in 1577, again intimated that physicians who took fees were guilty of simony: "Medicine is a divine thing, thus created by God's benign and powerful hand. Therefore every day we see physicians who do not charge a fee for their services, contrarily to the practice of other tradesmen (although to heal is a trade). By contrast, they accept the gift they are given without asking for anything else, almost as if they did not dare to do otherwise, for fear of being justly called simoniac or sacrilegious, as sellers of the holy gift of Medicine."[34]

Pastarino's statement was ironical, of course: physicians' practice was a far cry from this description. Nevertheless, the common people staunchly believed that a healer's advice (that is, his knowledge) should be freely given. In the hiring contracts of town doctors, especially in the earliest examples of such documents, it was often stated that the physician could request payment from citizens for specific treatments but not for his advice, which was to be offered without charge.[35] We can hear an echo of this notion in charlatans' custom of pretending to charge patients only for medicines or their ingredients, offering advice for free — probably a way of catering to a public that frowned upon a healer who tried to make money from his or her knowledge and expertise.[36]

Thus, at the beginning of the early modern age, medical services were still separated from the cash nexus, at least in part. They were associated instead with a noncommercial form of exchange — the exchange of charity, or mutual aid. The ideal of the physician who cured without charge — like the saints Cosmas and Damian — was strongly rooted in popular culture.[37] Public physicians were held responsible for treating without charge those too poor to pay for medical care. This moral obligation was not left to the doctor's conscience but was established in the hiring contracts between municipalities and town doctors. In 1596, for example, the contract between Gio. Batta Fabi, a physician from Bologna, and the community of San Felice stated "that the physician shall be responsible for medicating the poor without charge, for the love of God."[38]

This charitable practice was sometimes used by folk healers as a way of making their way into a community. In 1657, when a barber opened his new shop in Budrio, a village in the territory of Bologna, he immediately posted a sign announcing, "All kinds of illnesses are treated here, and the poor for the love of God." He then began his practice by treating a few patients without charge.[39] In seventeenth-century Bologna, we still find popular healers whose practice remained within the realm of the mutual exchange of charity. This was the case, for instance, with Andrea and Lorenzo of Norcia, a father and son practicing in Bologna in 1666 as *norcini*, or, as they called themselves, "healers of those who are broken in their bodies, men and women." The two healers honored their cure agreement with an innkeeper. Later, when they were prosecuted for unlicensed practice, the innkeeper testified in their favor: "They did not ask me any payment for their service, and I have not given them anything. They said they would do it out of charity, and that I would eventually do the same for them."[40] Some measure of deference toward this ideal of charitable practice was shown even by the medical authorities. When prosecuting someone for unlicensed practice, the Bolognese protomedici always ascertained whether the healer had requested payment for his or her services. If the healer had acted "out of charity," without requesting payment, this was considered to be an extenuating circumstance. In some places, unlicensed healers who rendered their services for free could not be prosecuted by the authorities.[41]

All of these elements show that in popular culture, medical practice still hovered on the threshold between commercial trade and charitable works. This incomplete commercialization is reflected in the terms of payment established in the cure agreements. In such contracts, as we have seen, what is exchanged for money is not the healer's service or labor, but rather the outcome of the treatment — the restoration of health.

III

What was the legal foundation of the cure contracts? On what notion of equity did they rest? Among the laws of late antiquity and the early Middle Ages, a direct mention of the custom of stipulating "contracts for a cure" can be found in barbaric legislation. The Leges Visigothorum (laws of the Visigoths) contain norms that regulate the contractual commitments between healers and patients. Let us examine these norms, which are given under the rubric "On Physicians and Patients":

Law III, Ancient:
When a physician is asked under contract [ad placitum] to treat an illness.

Should anyone request a physician to treat a disease or a wound under contract, after the physician has seen the wound or diagnosed the illness, he may begin treating the patient under the agreed-upon terms and after payment of a security.

Law IV, Ancient:
When a patient who has been treated under contract dies.

Should a physician undertake treating a patient under contract and after payment of a security, he shall restore the patient to health. Should the patient die, the physician shall not request the fee specified in the contract. Thereafter, neither party shall bring suit against the other.[42]

The patient–healer relationship prescribed in these laws seems very similar to the practice shown in the cure agreements. First of all, the relationship is defined as contractual.[43] After the physician has visited the patient and diagnosed the illness, he may choose to treat him or her under a written agreement in which his own obligation is clearly defined: to restore the sick person to health. If the patient dies, the healer cannot request the contracted fee. The fact that payment is conditional on the success of treatment is also stated in another Visigothic law:

Law V, Ancient:
When a physician removes a cataract from the eyes.

> Should a physician remove a cataract from somebody's eye and restore the patient to health, he shall receive five coins for his services.[44]

The presence of these norms in the Visigothic laws indicates that the stipulation of cure contracts was an old custom, probably dating from a period much earlier than the late Middle Ages—as early, at least, as the time when these laws were issued, between the fifth and the sixth century.[45] Promulgated toward the end of the Visigothic reign, these laws continued to be enforced in the Iberian peninsula, both in the Christian territories and in those subject to Arab domination, remaining effective even after the Frankish conquest. Their vernacular version—the so-called *Fuero Juzgo* (Forum Iudicum), which also included the norms "on doctors and patients"—laid the foundation for the Spanish legislation of the thirteenth and fourteenth centuries.[46]

Was the agreement for a cure, then, a barbaric custom, alien to Roman legal traditions? The historians who have studied the Visigothic laws "on doctors and patients" are inclined to think so, but they do not offer real evidence to support their view.[47] Can one say that the healer-patient relationship codified in Roman law differed significantly from the model we find in the laws of the Visigoths?

Since the Visigothic laws "on doctors and patients" date back to the second half of the fifth century, the contemporary Roman law code with which we can compare them is the Theodosian Code (A.D. 438). Although Visigothic law borrowed heavily from Roman law,[48] it did not include the sections of the Theodosian Code entitled "On Professors and Physicians" (bk. 13, title 3). Instead, we find laws on physicians and patients. Let us compare the two sets of norms. The Roman code contains only one direct reference to the relationship between physician and patient, in a law issued in A.D. 368:

> A town physician [archiater] should be hired for each of the city quarters (except for the area of *portus Syxti* and that of the Vestal Virgins). The town physicians should be aware that their salaries [annonaria commoda] come from the public, and in consequence they should honestly treat the poor rather than shamelessly serve the rich. They will be allowed to accept what their patients offer them once they have been cured, but not what those who are dangerously sick promise in exchange for health.[49]

The law does not concern medical practitioners in general, but only the public physicians, hired by the city neighborhoods.[50] As public servants, these physicians were warned to provide honest care to the poor, instead of serving only the rich. They could take gifts offered by their patients out of gratitude and respect, but they were not allowed to accept promises by the seriously ill. Remuneration for their services was left to the discretion of the patients.[51]

This section of the law on public physicians *(archiatri)* was passed on to the Code of Justinian (A.D. 529).[52] As part of the Corpus juris civilis, it was discussed in innumerable commentaries by European jurists in later centuries. I should say at this point that it was precisely this law that would be used later, by early modern jurists, to undermine the legal validity of the contract for a cure. This law's injunction that public physicians not request promises from the sick was seen by early modern jurists as a fundamental argument against the legitimacy of any contracts between doctors and patients. Should their interpretation be correct, one could say that the Roman and the Visigothic laws entailed widely differing views of the patient-healer relationship — the cure agreement being lawful according to the Visigothic code and unlawful under Roman law.

In fact, the interpretation of the early modern jurists (which will be discussed in detail in chapter 6) is highly questionable. First, the law pertaining to the town physicians did not concern all doctors but only those hired by the public. Its goal was to keep physicians already paid by the community from taking advantage of the sick by requesting additional fees. The law seems to acknowledge that physicians were usually promised payment by the sick during treatment. The law did not ban this practice in general, but forbade it only in the case of the town physicians, already supported by public money.[53]

The law on town physicians was one of only two places in which Roman legislation dealt with the doctor-patient relationship. The other was a section of the Digest under the rubric "De variis et extraordinariis cognitionibus." This section gave guidelines to physicians—but also to teachers of the liberal arts, rhetoricians, grammarians, geometricians, midwives, and wet-nurses—on how to file with the governor of the province a claim for their salary against delinquent clients.[54] This text also gave a definition of *physician* which is very interesting for the purpose of our discussion:

"Physicians are considered also those who promise health for a given part of the body or against some kind of pain, such as for instance an ear specialist, a healer of fistulas, or a dentist—provided they do not employ magic or exorcism (a term commonly applied to impostors). In fact, these practices do not belong to medicine, although some people may claim they have benefited from these expedients."[55]

Here the promise of health defines the physician's role. This certainly calls to mind the practice we have encountered in the cure agreements. While this Roman law does not make any statement on the lawfulness of contractual agreements between patient and healer, it suggests that such agreements were common in practice.[56] Another indication of the diffusion of this custom comes from ancient texts on medical deontology, for instance, the pseudo-Hippocratic *Parangeliai,* which disapprove of the healer who tries to make a deal with the patient before undertaking treatment.[57]

For all these reasons, I am inclined to disagree with those who argue that the contract for a cure was a barbaric practice, extraneous to Roman customs. In my opinion, Roman law and barbaric law (as expressed in Visigothic law) shared a basic element: the assumption, explicit in Visigothic law but also present in Roman legislation, of the purely contractual nature of the relationship between healer and patient.[58] This relationship was left entirely to a private agreement. There was no public licensing system, no state regulation of medical practice, no distinction between legal and illegal practitioners. Neither Roman nor Visigothic law specified that only those licensed to practice were physicians. Visigothic law was silent on this issue, while Roman law simply discriminated against those who used magic for healing purposes. This discrimination had important consequences, for it forbade these practitioners to take delinquent clients to court and thus stripped them of their right to a fee. With the exception of this clause, Roman law opened the practice of medicine to everyone. In Rome, a physician was whoever practiced the art of healing—whether a man or a woman, a freeborn citizen or a slave.[59] A person was a physician not by virtue of an official license issued by the authorities but owing to a demand for his services fueled by the reports of satisfied clients. The concept of a licensed professional, as we know it, did not exist in Roman antiquity (although the exclusion of those who performed magical healing can be seen as a first step toward a licensing system). Anyone could proclaim himself or herself a physician, if the community agreed. This can be seen, for instance, in a legal case brought to the governor of Egypt in A.D. 142–43, as recorded in a papyrus from Oxyrhynchos. A local physician, Psanis, protested that he was being illegally asked to render public service, which physicians were exempted from. He stated that he had been asked to serve by some of his former patients, who should have known his status as a doctor. The governor remarked ironically that Psanis's ineffective treatments may have caused his fellow citizens to doubt his credentials; but he also suggested that Psanis again proclaim himself a practicing physician, in order to recover his exemption from public service.[60]

That Roman law did not include the concept of licensed professionals is proven also by another norm of the Digest, which established that town doctors should be appointed not by the governors of provinces, but only by municipal councils, "so that the same people who entrust their bodies and those of their children to these physicians during an illness, can choose them and be assured of their expertise and moral probity."[61] In short, a physician in Rome was anyone who credibly declared himself or herself as such. A town physician could be anyone chosen by the notables of the community that employed him; he did not have to be someone licensed by the authorities after passing an examination. In this respect, barbaric legislation and Roman law were substantially similar, since neither had a licensing system for medical practitioners.

Classical histories of medicine have stigmatized the Visigothic law on physicians and patients as a typical example of the "barbaric" decline of medical practice after the fall of the Roman Empire.[62] In my opinion, this perspective is misleading. Roman law and the Visigothic law on physicians and patients do not appear to be radically different from each other. As for the regulation of medical practice through licensing, Roman law, as we have seen, was just as "barbaric" as that of the Visigoths—it ignored the very idea of professional license. In the late medieval period, jurists had to strive hard to reconcile the lack of regulation of medical practice in Roman law with the practice of their times, which was based on licenses issued by the medical colleges, by the state, or by church authorities.[63]

In reality, only by putting aside the modern notion of professional, licensed medical practice can we understand the meaning of the contracts for a cure. In the absence of licensing, it makes sense to pay for treatment only in case of success. It allows the community to distinguish effectively between good and bad healers. Significantly, the custom of paying a healer according to results can still be found today in non-European cultures that do not have an official licensing system, or where a modern medical establishment exists side by side with a strong remnant of folk medicine.[64] Furthermore, the agreement for a cure responded to an ideal of equality and fairness between healers and patients. Only to modern eyes could such a contract appear as "a legalized injustice"—because we take for granted that the conditions of the therapeutic transaction should be dictated mainly by the therapist and not by the patient. In the cure agreements, however, the terms were decided jointly by the two parties. These agreements represented a compromise between the interests of the healer and those of the patient. Their aim was to redress the imbalance in the patient-healer relationship which resulted from the healer's superior knowledge and expertise. Paying on the basis of results gave the patient some leverage in the transaction. In this manner, the agreement served as an instrument to minimize the patient's disadvantage (due to lack of medical knowledge) and to restore some measure of equality between the transacting parties.

IV

In addition to linking payment to results, the cure agreement also favored the patient by fixing a deadline for his or her recovery. The healer was bound to restore the patient to his former health within a fixed period of time. If treatment was not successful within this period, the patient was released from the obligation to pay. A time constraint was thus imposed on the healer, while at the same time the sick person got a common-sense yardstick by which to evaluate the efficacy of treatment. The deadline for recovery was constantly emphasized in cure agreements, as in, for instance, the one drawn up by the healer Antonio Mondini and Pietro Pecoroni, on October 3, 1698, in Bologna: "Having seen the disease affecting Pietro Giuseppe Pecoroni's left side, especially on his face, I hereby declare that it is my duty to cure him of the aforementioned disease by this coming Christmas without requesting payment now. Once said disease or sickness is cured, said Pecoroni will be responsible for giving me a gift of one hundred lire."

After undersigning this document, the healer added, near his signature,

"I agree to the aforementioned terms, but not to the time, as twenty more days will be needed."[65] In May of the following year, long after the terms of the agreement had expired, Pietro Pecoroni denounced Mondini to the Protomedicato. His charge allows us to see once more what was probably the typical pattern of the negotiation between healer and patient:

> Your Honor, I want you to know that I was troubled by scrofula; and while speaking about my disease with Don Giobatta Sgargi, last October, I was told of an Antonio Mondini of Santa Maria Maggiore, who had cured one of his servants of a sore on the leg that no one had ever been able to cure; and he told me that the man [Mondini] had many medical secrets. Right away I went to see Mondini and showed him my illness; and after he saw it, he assured me that he would cure me, and I would not have to pay him before the end of treatment except to reimburse him for the price of ointments; and that he wanted ten *doppie*. I told him that was too much, but I would discuss the issue with Don Giobatta Sgargi; and we did so, and having agreed on one hundred lire, we put everything in writing.

The patient was now asking that part of the money he had already paid to Mondini be returned to him. For these payments he had a receipt, signed by Mondini, in which the healer promised to return the deposit if the treatment did not work, or to treat him without charge in the case of relapse ("if the scrofula returns to his face before next August, I will be responsible for treating him at my own expense").[66]

From the point of view of the Protomedicato, Mondini was only a marginal healer, and illegal at that, since he did not have a license to practice. By trade he was a seller of used furniture. As a healer, however, he acknowledged the responsibility to cure his patient without charge in the event of a relapse — a duty sanctioned in the medieval juridical literature, as we know.[67] By 1698, only a nonprofessional healer such as Mondini would have offered a patient such a guarantee, applying a norm that professional practitioners such as physicians and surgeons had abandoned a long time back. Nevertheless, traces of the ancient principle binding the payment of the healer to the patient's complete recovery — rather than to the work performed and the duration of the treatment — still existed at the end of the seventeenth century, albeit only among nonprofessional healers. The healer's commitment to treat the patient without charge in case of relapse clearly contrasts with another prerequisite of professional medical practice — that is, the idea that a medical practitioner should be paid for his time, because time is money.

Like the commercialization of medical practices, the idea of measuring the value of treatment by the amount of time spent by the practitioner also encountered resistance. We have already seen the opinion of Protomedico Ingrassia in 1563 on this issue: the value of a physician's services, he had argued, cannot be measured by the duration of treatment, because that would paradoxically and unjustly reward inept physicians who drag out their curative measures, while penalizing those capable of curing their patients in a short time. The fear that a dishonest physician could prolong treatment for mercenary reasons was widespread,[68] and it sometimes surfaced in clauses added to cure agreements in order to prevent this abuse. In a contract between the community of Volterra and Master Filippo, son of Taddeo from San Miniato, a doctor of medicine hired in 1369 as the town physician, the parties agreed that the physician would be paid by his patients in this manner: ten soldi per day if the illness lasted not more than fifteen days; six soldi per day if the illness ended within thirty days; and a flat fee of four gold florins if the infirmity lasted more than thirty days.[69] The longer the treatment, the lower the payment to the physician, who would have to accept a lump sum in cases requiring unusually lengthy therapies. Under these conditions, the doctor had no incentive to drag out the treatment.

A sign of the widespread unwillingness to pay physicians at each visit was the belief, sanctioned by medieval jurists, that doctors should be paid not during treatment but, rather, at the completion of treatment. The issue of when to pay the physician—whether at the beginning of, during, or at the end of the cure—was discussed by civil law experts from the Middle Ages to the seventeenth century. The medieval glossators had stated that payment was due only when the cure was completed.[70] Early modern jurisprudence held different views on this issue. Here is how the jurist Speckham summarized the question in 1611:

> When should a patient pay the salary of the physician: at the beginning, during, or at the end of treatment? On this issue the interpreters of law are not in agreement. Yet it seems to be common opinion that the physician who is not a public employee cannot ask for a salary or any other compensation before the patient is cured, i.e., once treatment has been completed—and not at the beginning or in the middle. . . . Although this is the common opinion, it is derided by Zasius . . . who says that, if this were true, physicians could not go about splendidly dressed in purple clothes, as they do; and the same author adds that whether their patients die or are cured, physicians come out winners.[71]

Reporting this ironic comment, the jurist seems to suggest that the medieval doctrine, although still hailed as "the common opinion," had become anachronistic on this point. While the jurists disagreed, physicians and the sick, in contrast, had always held very clear opinions on this matter. As Francesco Ripa stated in his medical-juridical treatise *On Plagues:* "Physicians say that they must receive payment at the beginning of treatment . . . while the sick say they want to pay at the end."[72] The juridical tradition on this issue (just as on the occurrence of a relapse, as we have seen) tended to favor the sick. Gradually, however, a new opinion came to prevail, favoring the physicians and eroding the traditional principles of equity between patient and healer. In the centuries from the Middle Ages to the early modern age, medical practitioners made great progress in what the surgeon Henry de Mondeville once described as "the art and science of making people pay."[73] In the Middle Ages, physicians reacted to the constraints imposed by custom (and by the law) by requesting from the patients a lien, or pledge, as a warranty for future payment.[74] Hence the aphorism "While the patient is in pain, the doctor should firmly ask for a lien."[75] The problems encountered by physicians in collecting their fees after a cure are clearly the motivation behind a rule established in an early-fifteenth-century version of the statutes of the Medical College of Bologna: "In order to avoid the ingratitude of the populace, who would rather forget the services rendered by physicians, we request that, should a doctor in our college treat somebody without being properly paid, and should this person or anybody from his family later become ill, no member of the college shall visit him or give him advice . . . until he pays his debt in full toward the first doctor."[76]

Thus, doctors needed to band together in order to make their patients pay. In the early modern period, the statutes of several medical colleges stated that a physician should be paid according to the number of visits he made, and independently of results. Fees could vary according to whether the visit was in the city or in the countryside, but not according to whether or not the patient recovered.[77] As we shall see in more detail when examining the cases from Bologna, this form of payment prevailed in the seventeenth century, altering the balance of power between patients and healers. As medical practice became more and more professionalized, people came to accept the notion that doctors should be paid depending on the number and length of visits, regardless of results. In the cure agreements we examined above, time favored the patients, setting a deadline for the healer's performance. When medical practice is professionalized, the passing of time benefits the physician: the longer the treatment, the higher the fee.

V

The cure agreements made sense within a culture that considered medicine as the art of healing rather than a professional practice. In fact, these
agreements denied two basic tenets of medical professionalism: first, that
medical practitioners deserve to be paid because they are licensed members
of the profession, and second, that payment does not depend on the patient's
satisfaction. As medical ethics became increasingly shaped by the principles
of professionalism, negotiating with patients was rejected by physicians as demeaning and unprofessional.

Traditional medical ethics had urged healers not to exploit patients'
fears by charging exorbitant fees. "When the fate of a patient is uncertain, it
is criminal to charge a high fee for treatment," the physician Alessandro
Benedetti wrote in the fifteenth century.[78] This view was restated two hundred years later by another doctor, Ludovico Settala: "It is cruel to bargain for
fees during a serious illness. It is not only always unworthy of this noble art
[of medicine], but also cruel: while the patient considers the fee, the right
moment to treat him might be lost. Thus valuable moments may be wasted,
and once gone, the patient will worsen or die."[79]

Settala's statement indicates a new notion: discussing fees during treatment was unacceptable not only because it was unethical but also because it
was undecorous, unworthy of the noble art of medicine. According to Paolo
Zacchia, a fee negotiated by a physician lost its dignified status as an *honorarium* and became instead like the vulgar wages of a servant. "Bargaining for
money should be left to the vile mechanics," that is, to lesser practitioners
such as surgeons, because "their work is, in fact, servile."[80] The new belief
that negotiating with patients was incompatible with the dignity of the medical profession was supported by the idea that such negotiation was at odds
with the Hippocratic oath.[81] While the medieval statutes of the medical colleges had not mentioned this aspect of the doctor-patient relationship, sixteenth-century statutes often prohibited doctors from negotiating with their
patients and making agreements with them.[82]

We shall see how the custom of making agreements for a cure progressively declined and disappeared in the early modern period. In the Middle
Ages, such contracts, drawn up in the presence of a notary, were recognized
as "public documents" and undersigned even by renowned physicians such as
Bartolomeo da Varignana, Guglielmo da Saliceto, and Taddeo Alderotti.[83] By
1600, in contrast, an agreement like the one cited above between Antonio
Mondini and Pietro Pecoroni was acceptable only to marginal, unlicensed

healers, certainly not to professionals. The court cases filed by patients in seventeenth-century Bologna indicate that, by that time, only lesser practitioners, such as barber-surgeons or unlicensed healers, accepted the terms of the cure contracts. Regular physicians never did.

Yet the contractual nature of the healer-patient relationship was so entrenched in traditional medical practice that even doctors came to terms by contract — with a community if not with an individual patient. In fact, there is widespread evidence that a large number of physicians worked on retainer, for a yearly salary, with groups such as families, convents, parishes, hospitals, and confraternities.[84] The agreements they signed in this case were similar to the so-called *patti di condotta,* the hiring terms set down by contract when a municipality secured the services of a town doctor. Significantly, the statutes of some medical colleges in the early modern period prohibited their members from making cure agreements with individuals but allowed them to contract for a retainer's remuneration with the representatives of communities or groups, such as heads of families and public officers.[85]

The medieval system of town doctors, which was probably already widespread in ancient Italy,[86] can be better understood in this context. Originally, the contract between a town doctor and a community may have developed out of the practice of single individuals or groups keeping a doctor on retainer. Here is a record of a doctor being hired as a personal physician — what we may call a medieval example of private medical insurance — in a document from Siena, dating from 1233:

> I, the priest Dietaviva, rector of the church of San Paolo, solemnly and legitimately promise you, Sir Bonifacio, physician, son of the late physician Niccolo, that at the end of every January each year I shall give you forty Sienese coins, as long as I live, in exchange for your medical advice and care [*pro via et consilio meae personae*] . . . ; and I take this responsibility upon myself and my heirs, pledging my property and the property of the church, as equity to you and your heirs . . . ; and I promise that neither I nor my heirs will file any claim against you if you are away from Siena or become ill.[87]

A *patto di condotta* established similar terms on a public level. The whole community committed itself to retain a doctor on a yearly salary in exchange for his being permanently on call. Having a doctor regularly employed by the public gave both practitioners and patients advantages that were not offered by individual cure agreements. From the doctor's viewpoint, a reliable salary received under a retainer arrangement provided an attractive financial cushion against the uncertainty of the payment to be earned from the cure agreements. Payment on retainer, of course, was not conditional upon results. In fact, by practicing only privately, without having stable arrangements with communities, physicians simply could not make a living.[88]

From the patients' viewpoint, having a town doctor offered the advantage of price control, since the hiring contract (patto di condotta) established the maximum amount the doctor could ask for a single cure. Significantly, the earliest medieval examples of such contracts testify to such a price-fixing clause. Consider, for example, the hiring agreement drawn in 1214 between Ugo da Lucca, *medicus,* and the municipality of Bologna. For himself and his heirs—that is, his legitimate male descendants who might also become physicians in the service of the city—Ugo requested an income of six hundred Bolognese lire "in feudum." In exchange, he promised to serve the city by living there for six consecutive months, each year, and "to treat and cure all citizens of Bologna . . . and their families who live in the city, and all the inhabitants of the countryside who may be wounded or suffering from hernia." He also promised "not to negotiate cure agreements with any citizen, except with the people from the countryside, from whom he will be allowed to ask for payment for a cure only to the following amount: nothing from the poor; no more than a cart of wood from those who are serfs; and from the rich only up to a maximum of twenty *solidi* or a cart of hay."[89]

With this contract, the community of Bologna limited the fee that the physician could request from patients living outside the city, and ensured that he did not charge city residents for curing them. In other words, the contract allowed the city to regulate the price of medical service in a way that private agreements between healers and single patients could not.

The same terms can be seen, several centuries later, in a contract of 1527 between the community of Pieve di San Stefano (in the territory of Arezzo) and Master Bernardino di Francesco Rinaldi da Pisa, the town doctor. For six ducats a month, the doctor was requested to "treat all people affected by plague in the area, with ointments and remedies to be purchased by the community or by the patients." As for Master Bernardino, "he promised to treat all residents of said community without charging other fees and without advancing any other requests; although he can accept the gifts that his patients, out of courtesy or kindness, wish to present him." This agreement, however, "does not include what was promised to him for the cure of Madonna Crisostoma, wife of the late Fazino."[90] By signing this contract as town doctor, Master Bernardino renounced any cure agreements with individual patients. Presumably, since his agreement with Madonna Crisostoma

predated the hiring contract, he was allowed to collect the agreed-upon fee
for this case only. He was also given permission to accept any gifts offered by
his patients. Such gifts could add significantly to the income of a town doctor. A seventeenth-century physician, Giuseppe Giuli, carefully noted in his
journal all the gifts received from grateful patients.[91]

It is important to emphasize that, like the agreements for a cure, the
contracts to hire town doctors imposed on the healer some conditions that
were clearly in favor of the patients. One of the most common was the residency requirement, which prohibited the physician from leaving town without permission from the authorities and, at times, even from the patients un-
dergoing treatment.[92] This requirement indicates once more the importance
given to the final results of treatment—results that could not be ascertained
if treatment were interrupted. It was an ethical principle, acknowledged by
all categories of healers, including physicians, that patients should not be
"abandoned" before the end of the cure. In the legal cases discussed before
the Bolognese Protomedicato, some patients refused to pay for treatment on
the grounds that their physicians or surgeons had "abandoned" them.[93]

Although physicians gradually rejected the terms of the cure agreements, finding them demeaning and unprofessional, they were often bound
nevertheless to the ethical and legal obligations stipulated in the contracts for
town doctors—obligations that also tried to redress some inequalities of the
doctor-patient relationship. However, the contradiction with the principles
of medical professionalism was much more marked in cure agreements than
in contracts for town doctors. In addition to the principle of payment by result, another unprofessional feature of the agreements was the common-sense
definition of recovery on which they were based. How was recovery defined, and who could determine if it had indeed been attained? When the
parties disagreed, they turned for arbitration to a judge of the guild. Typically, this happened only as a last resort. On a daily basis, the rule adopted in
the cure agreements was that the patients were the ones to decide if they
were healed. Such a rule clearly contradicted professional principles, according to which not lay opinion but only medical experts can pass final judg-
ments on the results of medical care. But the reality is that healers are always
judged from below as well as from above: by the patients, who base their
judgment on the effectiveness of care; and by the medical authorities, who
use professional standards, including adherence to medical orthodoxy. The
first professional duty of a doctor, then as now, is to follow the established, or
canonical procedure; in other words: "traiter méthodiquement, et dans toutes
les régularités de l'art" ("to treat according to standard and by the rules of the

art"), as a physician says in Molière's *Monsieur de Pourceaugnac,* "and never ever, for all the gold in the world, cure anybody with remedies not approved by the medical School."[94]

In contrast, by emphasizing results, the cure agreement allowed patients the upper hand in evaluating the effectiveness of treatment. We should remember that, at the time, even learned medicine was largely based on symptoms, on the patient's own subjective perception of illness. It is not so strange, therefore, for the healing process to be mostly understood in terms of common experience rather than in terms of specialized medical knowledge.

More evidence of the diffusion of such a nonprofessional definition of recovery comes from the documents called *fedi di guarigione*—testimonials in which sick persons declared themselves to be cured of specific illnesses. These are fascinating documents that can be used to reconstruct the perception of illness by common people. Their function was to legitimize practitioners by publicly recognizing their healing skills. The testimonials were given to common healers as well as to holy ones, as proven by the votive offerings in the sanctuary of Saint Marcoul in Corbeny, mentioned by Marc Bloch in *The Royal Touch.*[95]

These testimonials were often presented by folk healers when petitioning the protomedici for a permit to practice. In 1613, when applying for a license to sell a balsam of his own making, Josepho Scarpetta attached this document to his request: "I, Tomaso, tenant farmer of the Dainessi, hereby declare that for the past year, having an intolerable pain in one knee, I applied Ser Ioseffo Scharpetta's balsam and, through the grace of God, I recovered; in this year I used the same balsam to medicate a friend of mine who was on his death bed for a pain in his body and stomach; and with my own hand I applied it and, through the grace of God, he healed . . . and in witness thereof I have made my mark below."[96]

In 1689 a healer, Francesco Nannini, was granted a license by the Bolognese Protomedicato on the basis of several testimonials from patients who had been cured by him "with the help of God . . . of an incurable illness called the scrofula."[97]

The custom of presenting such testimonials was not limited to folk healers. Letters of reference from patients were also included in the certificates of "diligent practice" that the physicians were requested to file with the college. These documents, often accompanied by recommendations from noble and influential patrons, stated that the undersigned had been "perfectly restored to health" and that they had been "treated diligently and canonically."[98] We find patients' testimonials printed in the little book published by an unlicensed healer, Costantino Saccardino, as well as in the autobiography of an illustrious physician such as Gerolamo Cardano.[99] In both cases, the testimonials served to advertise the healer's good reputation.

For the most part, however, testimonials of successful cures were used by the folk healers, who were excluded from the three primary groups of medical professionals (physicians, apothecaries, and barber-surgeons). For the professionals, the source of legitimization was the license granted by the medical authorities. For the folk healers, the source of legitimization was the testimonials of cured patients. We can thus speak of the coexistence of two sources of legitimization for medical practice—the medical authorities, above, and the patients, below.

The coexistence of these two sources of legitimization was not without conflict. An interesting case in point can be found in the municipal records of the city of Lille, France. In 1697, thanks to a number of patients' testimonials, a woman healer, Marie-Jeanne Dassonville, obtained permission from the city council to treat hemorrhoids. Folk healers often treated only one illness, or a group of symptomatically related complaints. The surgeons' guild opposed the license, on the ground that only their designated officials were authorized to grant permits to treat this disease—which required surgical skill because it was considered "external" and curable by "topical" or local remedies. Furthermore, the surgeons questioned the validity of the testimonials, which they considered "private documents" of no legal value.[100] The debate reflected a disagreement between municipal and professional authorities not only over who should grant licenses but also over the credibility of the patients' testimonials.[101] Who should evaluate a healer's performance: the patients or the healer's professional peers? The magistrates in Lille ruled that "testimonials by patients proved that Dassonville's remedies should be made available to the public." As "fathers of the town of Lille, responsible for doing what was best for the residents," they granted the license, stating that "this woman and her remedies are a treasure to the public."[102] This case clearly shows that the city authorities acknowledged the patients' testimonials as one source of legitimization for medical practice, next to licensing by the medical authorities.

VI

These two sources of legitimization for medical practice and the need for mediating between them had to be acknowledged also by the Protomedicato of Bologna. In Bologna, unlike Lille, the Protomedicato's role as supreme medical authority was never questioned by the city authorities. We have already seen that the Protomedicato granted licenses on the basis of patients' testimonials, thus accepting to some extent the legitimization of folk healers from below. Let us now see what happened at the door of the Studio on a Thursday in 1588, when the protomedici were leaving the building after their weekly session. The hearing had concerned Gio. Battista Cani, a healer from Milan, who had requested a license to treat "very serious illnesses with some of his remedies." When examined, the appellant "did not respond wisely, but ignorantly." The license was denied also on the ground of a previous complaint filed against Cani by a patient whom he had failed to cure. The healer was ordered to return his payment to this patient, or have his property confiscated.

While the protomedici lingered at the door, a man named Costantino Chiarlino approached them, pleading that Cani be allowed to continue treating his wife. At this point, the doctors decided to let the healer "treat the woman without the customary fine — for practicing without a license — upon request by said Costantino."[103] This case shows apparently contradictory behavior — a healer who had been denied a license after an examination proved him incompetent was immediately afterward allowed to treat a patient because of a client's intercession. The contradiction clearly has to do with the coexistence of the two sources of legitimization for healers — an official one (from the medical authorities) and an unofficial one (from the patients). It also indicates that in the late sixteenth century, the unofficial source of legitimization was still strong enough to be accepted by the protomedici and to interfere with the official licensing rule, according to which only the medical authorities could pass judgment on a healer's skills. The protomedici's behavior toward Gio. Battista Cani, moreover, shows that they felt that they should not meddle with the trust relationship between healer and patient unless that trust had been broken, when the healer had not fulfilled his promise of a cure.

At the end of the sixteenth century, therefore, the behavior of the medical authorities did not yet show unmitigated adherence to purely professional criteria for the regulation of medical practice. Even the protomedici had to accommodate their conduct to the traditional customs that guaranteed the sick an equitable relationship with their healers. This model of equity was expressed in the agreement for a cure, which represented a mediation between the interests of the sick and those of the healer. While the protomedici considered cure agreements to be beneath the dignity of the medical profession (and certainly would not have undersigned such agreements in the course of their professional practice), nevertheless, in their role as magistrates, they recognized such agreements as legally binding, at least for lower-rank practitioners, such as the surgeons.

This is shown by a lawsuit of 1574 in which the city authorities appointed the protomedici as competent judges to settle a dispute between the surgeon Ulisse Parmi and the nobleman Paolo Vitali. In dispute was the payment requested by the surgeon for curing his patient of a hernia. While the surgeon claimed that the treatment had been successful, the patient refused to pay, stating, "I am not healed, and if you will prove to me that, in fact, I am, I offer to pay immediately what is fair." Asked to establish whether the patient had recovered, the protomedici examined the scar, found it to be "firm, solid, and callused" ("firma, solida et callosa"), and ruled unanimously that the patient was completely cured. They also established the "fair price" owed by the patient. Since the surgeon "had fulfilled his promise of a cure" and had visited his patient up to three times a day for forty days, he was to receive fifteen gold Bolognese coins. As for the patient, he was reminded that people recovering from hernia were supposed to wear a bandage for at least four months, while he had admitted to wearing it for only one month. With this admonition, the protomedici seemed to imply that the patient had only himself to blame for his dissatisfaction with the surgeon's treatment.[104]

The protomedici considered their verdict in this case important enough that they decided to advertise it in print with a flyer.[105] Why? What they wanted to publicize was their newly obtained authority to settle disputes between healers and patients. Traditionally, the ordinary courts had been the judicial setting for such cases;[106] in fact the Vitali versus Parmi lawsuit had initially been brought to the ordinary court, but the judges had deferred it to the college. This marked an important shift: the medical college received from the city magistrates the judicial authority to decide civil suits on medical matters. Thus, by the end of the sixteenth century, the Protomedicato had acquired jurisdiction over all such cases, as well as the power to enforce sentences by confiscating the property of delinquent patients and of those healers who failed to return payments for unsuccessful treatment.[107]

Most significantly, in the case of Parmi versus Vitali the college doctors recognized that the surgeon's right to his fee was contingent upon establishing that the patient had been perfectly cured. Thus, the protomedici endorsed the terms set by the agreements for a cure, including the principle of payment according to results. In determining the fair amount of payment due the surgeon, they considered not only the services rendered but also the outcome of treatment. Thus, in another case brought to the Protomedicato, in 1583, in which a surgeon asked for the remainder of the agreed-upon fee, the protomedici granted it "above all, since the patient is cured thanks to his [the surgeon's] labor and industry."[108] Also in this case, however, the protomedici felt the need to investigate the patient's behavior during treatment, in order to establish whether he might be deemed responsible for jeopardizing the success of the treatment.[109]

At the end of the sixteenth century, the protomedici acted as magistrates in charge of implementing the terms of the agreements for a cure, by ordering practitioners to refund money to patients who had not been healed, or, conversely, by charging patients to pay healers who had successfully treated them. We also find the college doctors in the role of mediators between the parties who had undersigned a cure agreement. In 1586, for instance, the protomedici were called to witness a cure contract between some patients and an itinerant healer, Stefano da Capua. The sum agreed upon as payment for Stefano's services was deposited in the hands of the protomedici, who would give it to him after the successful completion of treatment. For his part, Stefano assured the protomedici under oath "that he would not leave Bologna for one month," which was the duration of treatment set in the contract.[110] By means of their intervention or mediation, the medical authorities protected the patients against the chance of abandonment before the end of the cure and also safeguarded the healer against the risk that his patients would be unwilling to pay.

Such a direct involvement of the protomedici in the drawing up of cure agreements, however, was already rare at the end of the sixteenth century and became even more so from then on. Starting around this period, we notice a dramatic shift in the medical authorities' attitude toward cure agreements. As we shall see in detail in chapter 6, such agreements were increasingly frowned upon by the medical authorities and rejected as incompatible with the professional definition of medical practice. This change of attitude would have important consequences for the relationship between patient and healer. Cure agreements implied the presence of a magistrate who endorsed them as legally binding. When no longer sanctioned by the medical authorities, as we shall see, such agreements would slowly disappear.

The judicial records of the Protomedicato display an intricate pattern of shifting rules and relationships. As will become clear when we analyze the patients' claims and the court's response, there was a complex interaction between different perspectives: what the patients denounced as a broken promise of a cure, the protomedici redefined throughout the seventeenth century as illegal medical practice—as a violation of professional norms rather than as a betrayal of the patient's trust. Throughout this process, the relationship between practitioners and patients changed dramatically. This change can be partly related to the pressure that each party in the medical system exerted on the others. There was, first of all, the mutual pressure between healers and patients, which had reached a sort of equilibrium point in the balance of power expressed by the cure agreement. Pressure on the healers was exerted not only from below, by the patients, but also from above, by the medical authorities, who set the rules for orthodox medical practice. Thus, the healers had to meet two different sets of expectations — those of the patients, who expected treatment to be effective, and those of the medical authorities, who expected it to be orthodox. At the top of the medical system, the protomedici themselves were not exempt from pressure, and they also had to respond to two different sets of expectations. It was incumbent upon them, as supreme medical authorities, to protect the professional interests of the various groups of medical practitioners, who shared common goals despite their intraprofessional rivalries. However, as public magistrates, the protomedici were supposed to defend the patients' right to equity in the therapeutic transaction. It was their difficult task, therefore, to represent both professional interests and patients' rights — a task particularly difficult at the end of the sixteenth century, when patients' rights were still based on the nonprofessional model of the cure agreement.

Chapter 3

THE MEDICAL SYSTEM AS SEEN
BY THE DOCTORS

I. A THREE-LEVEL HIERARCHY

We wish the physician would act as a physician, the surgeon as a surgeon,
and the apothecary as an apothecary.
—From a letter sent by the community of Castel San Pietro
to the Protomedicato, 1699

The time has now come to take a stroll along the streets of early modern Bologna, looking for signboards pointing out the shops of the health-related trades. How numerous were the medical practitioners in the city? What kinds of clients did they serve?

At the beginning of the seventeenth century, Bologna was definitely a city of doctors. In the year 1600, forty-three academically trained physicians were licensed to practice in Bolognese territory. One could easily recognize them by the large-sleeved garb that it was their privilege to wear—a privilege jealously guarded by the protomedici, who threatened with legal action "whoever dared to address a crowd in doctoral garb, thus dishonoring and ridiculing the real Doctors."[1] In the early seventeenth century, Bologna had thirty-nine apothecary shops,[2] identified by their multicolored signboards: a 1568 list included the signs of the Moon, the Cedar, the Doctor, the Swordsman, Saint George, the Star, the Angel, and the Saints Cosmas and Damian; a 1667 list, which showed an increase in religious symbols, included the signs of the Bunch of Grapes, the Golden Apple, the Melon, the Cross, Saint Peter, the Annunciation, Saint Matthew, Saint Hyacinth, Saint Catherine, the Pope, Saint Martin on Horseback, and the Madonna of the Rosary.[3]

For the passer-by, the practitioners' shops were indicated by signboards, which could be posted only with the Protomedicato's leave: three crosses for midwives,[4] an arm with a lancet for barber-surgeons. Sometimes, a placard tacked on the door of the workplace described the range of a practitioner's activities, as in this notice hung up by a barber in 1637: "Here is a steam bath, licensed to administer guaiac, sarsaparilla, and chinaroot, apply mercury ointments, and prepare all kinds of potions, as ordered by the Most Excellent Doctors."[5]

In 1630, the year of the plague, there were in Bologna 42 doctors, 44 master apothecaries, and 155 barber-surgeons (masters and apprentices included): 241 medical practitioners in all, not counting apothecaries' apprentices and unlicensed healers (see table 5). Thus, a city of slightly more than 60,000 residents had roughly one practitioner for every 250 people. Margaret Pelling found a similar ratio in the city of Norwich, but her figures included unlicensed healers.[6]

By 1727, when the sources also listed midwives and apothecaries' apprentices, the number of medical practitioners had almost doubled, with roughly one healer for every 150 people. We find the same ratio throughout the eighteenth century (see table 5).[7] It should be noted, however, that the rolls of licensed healers on which these figures are based were supposed to include those practicing in the countryside. These figures thus may overestimate the density of medical practitioners in the city, although undoubtedly most healers were concentrated there.[8] Furthermore, these figures do not take into account those healers who were on the fringes of the official medical system, such as charlatans holding a temporary permit to practice, or the unlicensed healers who offered an alternative source of medical care. In any case, it is important to emphasize that the number of medical practitioners in early modern Bologna was much greater than one might expect.[9] Even considering only the official medical establishment, it is clear that the city offered a rich and diverse pool of therapeutic resources, with numerous licensed healers, often employed by associations such as confraternities and parishes to provide medical care to their members.[10]

Nor should we forget that the people of this Catholic city also had supernatural medical resources. The sick of Bologna often turned to their saints, hoping that they would grant a miraculous cure. The belief in the healing power of holy men and women had a long history in Bologna. In the early seventeenth century, the church of Santo Stefano still housed a twelfth-century epitaph, commissioned by a doctor for his daughter: "Here rests Nonacrina, daughter of Grillo, the doctor. May the Heavenly Physician give her what her father was unable to give. May she, who could not be saved by her father's medicine, be healed by the Heavenly Doctor."[11] These words testify to the close association of health and salvation which was at the core of

Table 5.   DOCTORS, APOTHECARIES, BARBER-SURGEONS, AND MIDWIVES LICENSED TO
PRACTICE IN BOLOGNESE TERRITORY

	Doctors			Apothecaries		
Year	Category	N	Per 1,000[b]	Category	N	Per 1,000
1630		42	0.68	m.	44	0.71
1659	coll.	15		m.	41	0.66
	noncoll.	49				
	total	64	1.03			
1683	coll.	13		—		—
	noncoll.	69				
	total	82	1.26			
1698	coll.	18		—		—
	noncoll.	87				
	total	105	1.66			
1727	coll.	15		m.	83	
	noncoll.	78		a.	89	
	total	93	1.41	total	172	2.61
1744	coll.	19		m.	85	
	noncoll.	81		a.	107	
	total	100	1.55	total	192	2.98
1772	coll.	17		m.	67	
	noncoll.	124		a.	30	
	total	141	2.04	total	97	1.40

Table 5 *(continued)*

| Year | Barber-Surgeons[a] | | | Midwives | |
	Category	N	Per 1,000	N	Per 1,000
1630	m.	83		—	—
	a.	72			
	total	155	2.52		
1659	m.	67	1.08	—	—
1683	III	47		50	0.77
	II	14			
	I	30			
	total	91	1.40		
1698	III	49		23	0.36
	II	18			
	I	9			
	total	76	1.20		
1727	III	76		60	0.91
	II	14			
	I	16			
	total	106	1.61		
1744	III	124		35	0.54
	II	5			
	I	18			
	total	147	2.28		
1772	II	146		76	1.10
	I	25			
	total	171	2.47		

Sources: A.S.B., Coll. Med., bb. 235, 236, 342.

Abbreviations: coll. = collegiate doctors; noncoll. = noncollegiate doctors; m. = masters; a. = apprentices. Dashes indicate data missing from the sources.

a. Barber-surgeons were divided into three classes (I, II, and III) until 1744, and afterward into two (I and II).

b. Ratios (per thousand) were calculated using the population of the city as given by A. Bellettini, *La popolazione di Bologna dal secolo XV all'unificazione italiana,* (Bologna, 1961), table 1, pp. 25–28.

the fascinating Christian belief in healing miracles. In eighteenth-century Bologna, the advance of "medicalization" had not yet destroyed this belief. Hospitals, for instance, while witnessing momentous change in medical praxis, could still occasionally be the site of miraculous healing.[12] They kept the aura of sacred places, thus revealing the twofold character of therapeutic expectations—medical and religious, natural and supernatural, earthly and heavenly—deeply rooted in this culture.

Let us first examine how the various healing trades were defined and regulated by the medical authorities. The college envisioned and tried to fashion the field of medical practice as a hierarchy of professionals with mutually complementary roles: physicians, apothecaries, and barber-surgeons. This division of medical labor was meant to correspond to the Galenic tripartition of therapy into diet, pharmacy, and surgery.[13] The three aspects of therapy, and the corresponding roles, were all seen as important and necessary, but not equally so. Their hierarchical order was supposed to reflect their different degrees of universality and effectiveness. While drugs and surgical procedures were considered "local" remedies, used only for treating specific parts of the body, diet was the "universal" treatment, directed at the entire human frame. The ancient Greek meaning of diet, in fact, was much wider than ours: it implied regulating not only food and drink but life in general— the balance between sleep and activity, rest and exercise, and *excreta et retenta* (what entered and what came out of the body), as well as control of the emotions and passions that affect physical health.[14] Diet was seen therefore as the fundamental remedy, the cornerstone of all therapies. Prescribing a diet in this sense was the exclusive competence of the physician, and just as diet was the mother of all therapies, so was the physician at the top of the hierarchy of the healing tasks. Only the doctor was supposed to oversee the treatment of the entire body. His role was prescriptive, rather than executive—he was responsible not only for prescribing the diet but also for deciding when to use the lesser remedies, such as pharmacy and surgery. He and only he could tell the apothecary or the surgeon what to do.

The ranking of therapeutic tasks was also based on a crucial distinction between the inner and the outer body. A basic classification of diseases in early modern medicine was the distinction between internal and external illnesses. On this distinction was based, in turn, the division between physical medicine and surgery: the physician dealt with internal illnesses and remedies, and the surgeon with external ones. Only the physician could treat the inner body and prescribe drugs to be taken orally; only he controlled access to the body through the mouth. If there is a fundamental rule in the set of medical regulations enforced by the Protomedicato, it is the prohibition on the administration of oral drugs by practitioners other than physicians. This rule was constantly repeated for two hundred years, in decrees and public notifications on medical practice, as well as in each license granted by the protomedici to surgeons and barber-surgeons, midwives and charlatans: "Let he or she give nothing by mouth."[15] The prohibition was an obvious attempt to protect the physicians' own turf from the intrusion of all other practitioners.

While the hierarchical and yet complementary relationship between medicine and surgery was based on the distinction between the inner and outer body,[16] the interdependence between doctors and apothecaries was founded on the hierarchical partnership between prescribing *(regola)* and dispensing *(ministerio)*. As stated in the preface to the Agreements of 1606 between the College of Medicine and the company of the apothecaries, "without the help of the apothecary the physician cannot attain his goal; without the physician's rule, the apothecary cannot practice his healing trade."[17] The hierarchy of therapeutic skills thus implied a distinction between prescriptive and executive roles, seen as noble and as menial, respectively. From the perspective of the medical elite, there was a huge gap between physicians, on the one hand, and apothecaries and surgeons, on the other. Paolo Zacchia, the author of the most important medico-legal treatise of the seventeenth century, made this point succinctly by saying that the physician "treats the body by using his intellect, not his body." By contrast, he added, apothecaries and surgeons use their hands rather than their minds; they cure the body with the body, and their work is therefore seen as resembling the work of servants.[18]

In Bologna, the medical college undertook the task of policing the boundaries between the three health trades. This was the Protomedicato's main effort from the end of the sixteenth century to the end of the eighteenth, and it was not a small one. While the three-level hierarchy was an ideal cherished by the medical elite, probably since antiquity, it hardly ever corresponded to reality. In spite of Galen's endorsement of the tripartition of medicine into diet, pharmacy, and surgery, medical practice in Galen's own times did not adopt the corresponding division of labor among practitioners. Ancient epigraphic sources clearly indicate that medicine and surgery were commonly practiced by the same individual, who was called *medicus chirurgus* (physician and surgeon). In all likelihood, it is wrong to claim, as some historians have done, that medicine and surgery already were of separate and unequal status in ancient culture.[19] In the Middle Ages, medical practice was also far from the ideal of the three-level hierarchy. Medieval documents from Bologna show that the term *medicus* was not reserved for physicians but was also given to surgeons, barbers, and even women (the word *medica,* or female doctor, was also used to indicate women healers in the thirteenth and fourteenth centuries in other European contexts).[20] At the beginning of the sixteenth century in Bologna, the statutes of the medical college allowed surgeons to receive the doctoral degree.[21] Surgery, therefore, was not yet seen as an inferior practice, one with which the highest ranks of the medical profession would not condescend to meddle.

Things had certainly changed at the end of the sixteenth century. By then, conflicts and contrary opinions notwithstanding, the College of Medicine of Bologna had managed to implement the tripartition of therapeutic roles and to enforce its own authority upon the lower-rank healers. This is even more significant when one considers that elsewhere — in London, for instance — the three-level ideal pursued by the medical elite was never fully achieved, even on paper.[22] By contrast, such a hierarchy became a reality in Bologna, where the medical system largely corresponded to the one envisioned by the college doctors. For two centuries, most of the Protomedicato's activity was directed at zealously watching over the division of roles and the hierarchical ordering of practitioners.

Why such a systematic, meticulous effort? For the medical elite, the three-level hierarchy in which they held the top position clearly had a deep meaning — a meaning that we can at least partly surmise by investigating the origins of this ideal in European culture. As Benveniste pointed out, the tripartition of therapeutic tasks was based on an extremely ancient model.[23] He argued that the Galenic ranking of surgery, pharmacy, and diet derived from a much more ancient, Indo-European tripartition of therapy into healing with plants, healing with the knife, and healing with sacred spells. For the Indo-Europeans, these different forms of healing corresponded to the three main social classes: healing with plants to the peasants, healing with the knife to the warriors, and healing with words to the priests. Bruce Lincoln has suggested that this tripartition underwent an important change in the Hippocratic Corpus: healing by spells was cast out of the medical art, which was purified of its ancient magical component.[24] In Galenic medicine, diet replaced magic as the highest form of healing but retained its priestly associations. When he prescribed a diet, the doctor was seen as taking over a sacred role — supervising the whole of a human life.[25] Through diet, therefore, the learned physician acquired an almost priestlike social status. As we shall see, the doctors of Bologna were strongly attached to this religious definition of their role.

Let us look in greater detail at the division of therapeutic skills, as envisioned by the medical college. The relationship between physicians and apothecaries was symmetrical: apothecaries could not intrude in the physician's proper domain, but neither could the physician cross over into the apothecary's territory—by law, "no doctor could sell medicines, on his own or through others."[26] It was different in the case of surgeons. Whereas no surgeon could medicate as a physician, the college doctors were automatically included, by statutory rule, in the list of "perfect surgeons," without having to take any examination.[27] In practice, the separation of physic and surgery was complied with, especially for those surgical tasks that the physicians considered beneath their dignity. In 1749, the Medical Faculty of Paris wrote to the College of Medicine of Bologna inquiring about the relationship between physicians and surgeons in the city. The college replied that "those physicians who also work as surgeons do abstain from menial surgical procedures for which they use the surgeons as assistants."[28]

The boundaries between the three health professions were also stressed by ceremony and ritual. Each of the three groups had its own festivities, churches, and patron saints. For instance, both physicians and barber-surgeons venerated the healing saints Cosmas and Damian, yet they celebrated the saints' day (September 27) separately—the barbers' guild in the Church of the Saints Cosmas and Damian, and the College of Medicine in Saint Peter's Cathedral. The cathedral was also the place where the solemn graduation ceremony was held. Significantly, licensing examinations for surgeons could not take place there, according to the medieval statutes of the college. This was obviously aimed at avoiding any blurring of the symbolic boundary between surgical licenses and medical degrees.[29]

In order to institutionalize the three-level hierarchy, the college progressively took over the jurisdiction of the company of barber-surgeons and that of the apothecaries, taking away their privilege of issuing licenses for the trade. The college's control over the licensing of apothecaries was already a fact by the end of the sixteenth century, while its right to examine and license barbers was established later, in the first half of the following century. In 1616, the Protomedicato decreed that those wishing to draw blood—the barbers' main therapeutic task—were not only to be licensed by the guild but also to be approved by the college. In 1638, however, the licenses granted by the guild were declared "void and invalid," and the guild was prohibited from issuing more in the future. The college rejected the guild's request that its representatives be present during the licensing examination. Starting in 1645, the licensing examinations taken by the barber-surgeons were regularly recorded in the proceedings of the Protomedicato, just as the examinations of apprentices and apothecaries had been since the beginning of the century.[30] Midwives were the last group to be brought under the supervision of the college. Beginning in 1686, they, too, were required to pass the Protomedicato's examination and, just like the other lower-rank practitioners, to take an oath never to draw blood or to administer oral remedies.[31]

Some barbers tried to escape the Protomedicato's control by claiming to be "simple barbers." Such statements, however, were checked by the Protomedicato's constable, who regularly inspected the barber's shops. In 1683 Sebastiano Barbetta, who styled himself "captain of the honorable protomedici" but was called "Sebastiano the henchman" by the populace, related how he had visited the shop of the barber Sebastiano Bacchelli and asked to see his license to draw blood: "Said Bacchelli insisted that he didn't draw blood and didn't medicate; but I looked in his satchel, and I found five lancets for drawing blood. As a consequence, I seized some of his property: two walnut cabinets, four walnut chairs . . . a tin basin, a small copper can."[32] Beginning in the second half of the seventeenth century, the Protomedicato frequently meted out punitive confiscations and fines to barber-surgeons caught practicing without a license.

Of the three official groups of healing practitioners, the barber-surgeons were definitely those most in demand by lower-class patients. What did they do? The medieval (1320) and early modern (1557) statutes of the guild of the barber-surgeons of Bologna state that "a barber's practice does not merely imply shaving, washing, and cutting hair, but also pulling teeth, and drawing blood from men in whatever way and from any body part, as well as applying leeches." In his *Piazza universale di tutte le professioni del mondo,* Tomaso Garzoni stated that the goal of the barbers' trade was the "cleansing" of the body, adding that "barbers are also useful for drawing blood from the sick, and for applying leeches, medicating wounds, applying bandages, pulling decaying teeth and such things, so that their craft . . . is subordinated to the science of medicine."[33] In fact, barbers not only drew blood and pulled teeth but often performed surgical procedures. In 1596 a barber from the community of Sant'Agostino, in the countryside of Bologna, certified that he had "medicated wounds and serious fractures of bones caused by gunshots . . . accurately fixed broken and sprained ankles . . . , treated and cured bunions, carbuncles, and gangrene."[34]

Barbers' surgical practice was regulated by the Protomedicato through a multilevel licensing system. In the second half of the seventeenth century, a three-degree system was established. Barbers of the first degree — the lowest — were allowed only to draw blood and to apply related remedies, such as leeches, under a physician's supervision. Barbers of the second degree could in addition treat wounds, always under a physician's direction. Barbers of the third, and highest, degree could practice general surgery, treating all sorts of "external" diseases. Without a physician's supervision, however, they could not treat "complex and deep" wounds and ulcers, especially those affecting the male urinary tract. Here again, the hierarchical ordering of skills depended on the fact that the inner body was considered more important than the outer. The further the surgical procedures went beyond the body surface, the more restricted they were to the highest-rank healers.

There is plenty of evidence that daily cooperation between physicians and barbers was the norm in early modern Bologna. When pursuing their clients in court for nonpayment, for instance, barbers often summoned physicians as witnesses of their performance. In their testimonies, patients often indicated that they had been referred by a barber to a physician for advice or treatment. "Together they often came back to me for advice," the doctor Galerati said in 1665 about the barber Bossi and a patient, Pellegrino Atti, affected by "Gallic ulcerations of the male member."[35] Acting as mediators between doctors and patients, barbers were often very useful to a physician starting a new practice. At the same time, the barber's subordinate rank was never questioned. For instance, the rule forbidding barbers to draw blood without a doctor's order seems to have been generally respected. Several patients' testimonies suggest that such was the case. In 1593, for instance, Orsolina Capelli declared to the protomedici:

> I went to Josepho Monaro's mill to take care of his mother, who was not well; this was on a Saturday night, and as soon as I arrived at said mill I also got sick and went to bed. I then sent for a daughter of mine, so that she would go and call a barber, as I wanted to be bled. My daughter went to San Gioanni and called on Messer Giorgio the barber, so that he would come and draw my blood; but Messer Giorgio, my daughter told me, refused to come unless Josepho Monaro did say a word to Messer the physician; in which case, having received permission, he would do as ordered.[36]

In this case, as in many others, the barber refused to draw blood without a physician's leave, whereas the patient had decided to be bled on her own initiative. In the seventeenth and eighteenth centuries, bloodletting was a remedy to which people often resorted without consulting a doctor.

As already stated, the cooperation between doctor and barber was based on the complementary of inner and outer body, and internal and ex-

ternal remedies. The barber was responsible for the outside of the body—
and was correspondingly located at the borderline of the official medical system, on the boundary between legal and illegal practice, and on that between
learned and popular medicine. Not surprisingly, barbers were given the task
of dealing with contagious diseases; they were dispatched by the Senate to
"go and check, and come back and report" on every "suspected case of contagion."[37] At the end of the eighteenth century, the smallpox vaccination was
considered to be "low-degree surgery" and was entrusted to lower-rank surgeons. In fact, contact with contagious diseases meant contact with impurity
and danger or, symbolically, as Mary Douglas has argued, with that which
defies social classifications. On a deep cultural level, the barber's liminal position was probably due to his contact with blood.[38] In the hierarchy of medical skills, drawing blood was the lowest of all tasks, located at the outer
boundary of official therapeutic practices. Just like sweat and excrement,
blood overflows from the body's boundaries; bleeding was used therapeutically as a way to expel corrupted humors. Sweating was also used for healing
purposes. In addition to the barber-surgeon, there was the steam bath attendant *(stufarolo),* who treated the sick with hot baths and steam. Just like cutting nails and hair, a periodic bloodletting helped to keep the body in good
shape—preserving its "cleanliness," to employ the term used by Garzoni, a
word implying the double meaning of clean and "polite," that is, well-
groomed and socially acceptable. By drawing blood, therefore, the barber
performed a role that was perceived as analogous to the excretory function of
the body. And just like the excretory function, the barber's role was considered indispensable, certainly, but nonetheless coarse and low—and somehow
tainted with impurity.

Yet, as menial as the barber's role was, it was absolutely indispensable.
Bloodletting was not only an important aspect of Galenic therapy; it was
probably the remedy most frequently requested by patients. For the majority
of the people, barber-surgeons were the most important healers in the
Bolognese medical system. After the reform of surgical practice in 1742, they
were still recognized as licensed practitioners but were divided into two
ranks: those licensed in the first degree could only perform their traditional
tasks of drawing blood and administering plasters and ointments, massages,
baths, and hot vapors *(stufe);* second-degree barber-surgeons were allowed to
perform more complex surgical procedures.[39]

Controlling barber-surgeons was not a major issue for the Protomedicato, since this group never truly threatened the college's authority—not
even in the mid–eighteenth century, when all over Europe surgery moved

decisively upward from trade to profession. In order to increase their status, surgeons distanced themselves from the barbers' guilds and formed colleges of their own, independent of and often opposed to the medical colleges. This happened in Paris, for instance, where the Académie Royale de Chirurgie was founded in 1731 despite harsh opposition by the Faculty of Medicine. The separation of French surgeons from barbers was made effective in 1743 by royal decree. It was otherwise in Bologna. In 1749 the Paris Medical Faculty wrote to the Bolognese medical college asking about the status of surgeons in the city. The college answered that "[in Bologna] the surgeons do not have a college or even an association, but form only a mere informal group."[40] As a matter of fact, the surgeons of Bologna could not identify themselves with the only organization actually available to them, the company of barbers, which bound them to a humiliating partnership with the lower strata of the profession. In Bologna, the separation between barbers and surgeons, which elsewhere involved the surgeons' challenge to the supremacy of the medical authorities, happened entirely under the control of the medical college. As such, it was a reform from above, rather than a rebellion from below initiated autonomously by the surgeons.[41]

The Bolognese barber-surgeons' subordination to the medical college was never questioned. The college had more problems controlling the apothecaries, whose guild was richer and more influential than the barbers' guild. Within the Protomedicato's measures to control licensed healers, trials of apothecaries were much more frequent than those of barbers. The college's supervision of apothecaries started in the second half of the sixteenth century and was a consequence of the Protomedicato's public responsibility to check the quality and fair price of medicines. The first Index (Tassa)—or list of essential drugs that every apothecary was requested to keep in his store—was issued by the college in 1563. The first official pharmacopoeia prepared by the college's protomedici was dated 1574. Both were constantly updated and reissued in the seventeenth and eighteenth centuries. In 1555, the apothecaries' guild was still responsible for establishing the official prices of medicines—which were supposed to vary "according to price fluctuation" but always remain within the boundary of "fair price." In 1568 this authority passed over to the Protomedicato.[42]

The protomedici also oversaw the opening of new apothecary shops, and only they could authorize the buying and selling of a shop's stock of drugs, after inspection of their quality. In 1568 the minutes of the Protomedicato's sessions began to record inspections of apothecary shops and the measures (such as the seizure of mortars) taken against those found out of compliance. For more than two hundred years, the Protomedicato's notary wrote regular reports on these inspections.[43] The inspections took place quarterly in the city and twice a year — in May and September — in the villages of the countryside. Each of the major villages, such as Castel San Pietro, Budrio, Crevalcore, Molinella, and San Giovanni in Persiceto, had its own apothecary shop (by 1614, Budrio had two) and town physician. Aspiring apothecaries and barber-surgeons from the countryside would come to Bologna to take the Protomedicato's licensing examination. In the villages, authority over lesser practitioners was given to the town physician, who starting in 1638 could be given the title of "viceprotomedico." This usage was discontinued in 1697, probably because it put collegiates and village doctors on the same level; country practitioners, who had often graduated from foreign universities, were considered inferior by the college.[44]

Inspections of apothecary shops usually resulted in the discovery and seizure of stale or poor-quality medicines. In 1605, for instance, the apothecary at the Sign of the Sun had to appear in the Protomedicato to explain why his store was so defective. In the country, the apothecary of Castel San Pietro was fined in 1607 for not having any guaiac in stock; in 1610 his theriac was thrown away because of its poor quality. The stale medicines seized from the shops were sometimes donated to the hospitals of San Giobbe and Sant'Orsola, for use by the poor.

As we may expect, the apothecaries did not welcome this control. In 1617, when the protomedici criticized a syrup at an apothecary shop known as The Stairs, its owner proclaimed, "I won't allow even the pope to throw it away." His offensive words were reported to the college: "[He said that] the Doctors were despots, and that he was damned if he didn't manage to get out of their tyranny, and that said college was full of very ignorant and mean men — rogues, who presumed to know medicines better than the apothecaries, . . . and that they should not presume to be the owners of Bologna, . . . because he . . . was every bit as much a citizen as they were."[45]

The history of the Protomedicato was marked by constant tensions with the apothecaries. Within the apothecaries' guild — which also included practitioners of lower-ranking trades, such as grocers, candlemakers, brewers, charlatans, tobacconists, ragmen, papermakers, and paint sellers — the apothecaries were the ruling elite, with total control over the council that was the guild's governing body. They also had social and intellectual ambitions. As we have seen in chapter 1, they did manage occasionally to have their sons graduate in medicine and even enter the medical college. In 1647, a group of apothecaries formed a scientific academy to discuss issues of medical chemistry. While the handicraft nature of the trade could not be denied, in 1648 the new statutes of the guild redefined "the hand of the apothecary" as "imbued with learning."[46]

In fact, the conflict between physicians and apothecaries also had intellectual grounds. It is well known that Galenic medicine was challenged in the seventeenth century by remedies of chemical origin. (Medicines made of minerals were marginal in the official Galenic pharmacology, which was based primarily on vegetal or animal ingredients.) In mid-seventeenth-century London, the medical chemists and followers of Paracelsus attacked the Galenic pharmacopoeia, which symbolized, in their eyes, the power of the Royal College of Physicians and the medical hierarchy that the college was trying to impose.[47] In seventeenth-century Bologna, several of the healers prosecuted by the college for illegal practice were chemists *(spagirici)* who promoted the new theories in medical chemistry (iatrochemistry). One of them, Vincenzo Canobio, was reported in 1693 by a doctor because "he was spreading rumors about us physicians in the apothecary shops, and wanted himself to act as a physician, by ordering medicines and drawing blood, and treating this and that patient . . . while bandying about the word that Doctors don't know what they are talking about."[48]

On this front, however, the college also managed to maintain its hegemony; chemical remedies were incorporated into the official pharmacopoeia extremely slowly.[49] In practice, the apothecaries' subordination to the authority of the Protomedicato and the college remained unshaken—even in 1766, when the guild took on the more prestigious title of Noble College of the Apothecaries. The medical college tolerated this new title for a few decades, until 1792, when it challenged it publicly and acrimoniously, viewing it as an attempt "to rise to a higher status, and throw off the yoke of subordination [to the college]."[50]

This brief survey is far from an adequate history of interprofessional rivalries in the medical system of early modern Bologna. My object is simply to show how the medical college managed to keep its supremacy over the other groups of health practitioners throughout the seventeenth and eighteenth centuries, despite the tensions caused by the upward mobility of surgeons and apothecaries.

In the second half of the eighteenth century, however, the three-level hierarchy underwent an irreparable crisis, in spite of all the Protomedicato's efforts. This was especially evident in the villages around Bologna, where, during this period, the protomedici were called increasingly often to mediate heated disputes between the town physicians, on the one side, and apothecaries or barber-surgeons, on the other. These were the most serious cases of interprofessional conflict that the Protomedicato was called upon to solve. Charges by physicians against lesser practitioners—rare until the end of the seventeenth century[51]—gradually increased to peak numbers in the second half of the eighteenth century. What had happened?

The traditional stratification of the medical profession, with its three-level ranking, was no longer heeded. By the late 1700s, physicians often stooped to performing surgical procedures, including menial ones such as drawing blood—a fact that surgeons, resentful of this unfair competition, loudly denounced in their complaints to the Protomedicato.[52] The highest medical ranks were invading the realm of the lower ones, and vice versa. Complaints were filed not only by practitioners but also by communities, which were affected by the divisiveness of these conflicts and wished for a return to the traditional medical order. "We wish the physician would act as a physician, the surgeon as a surgeon, and the apothecary as an apothecary," the community of Castel San Pietro pleaded with the Protomedicato in 1699.[53]

The Protomedicato reacted by reaffirming the traditional rules, but without much conviction. During this period, the sentences inflicted on lower-rank practitioners were, for the most part, mere reprimands—not even fines. Gerolamo Lodi, a surgeon practicing in Crevalcore, denounced by a doctor, Pigozzi, in 1766 for ignoring the physician's authority, was simply admonished to remain "within the boundaries of his limited profession and simple office" and to show proper respect to the town physician.[54] Others who got away unscathed, having received similar reprimands, included Alessio Porta, apothecary of Molinella, reported in 1745 by the doctor Luatti; Simone Gordini, surgeon of Castel San Pietro, denounced by the doctor Fracassi in 1759; and Francesco Cossarini, surgeon in San Pietro in Casale. In Cossarini's case, the community splintered into factions, one hostile to the surgeon and one favorable to him. The splintering reflected the viewpoints of different social classes. The complaint against the surgeon was filed by "the well-off among the citizens and residents of San Pietro in Casale," who denounced Cossarini as "an insolent and fanatical imposter" who "continually scorned the authority and rights of the village's doctor, whom they [the well-to-do villagers] have hired and are resolved to keep." The poor, however, were on Cossarini's side. In his defense, the surgeon presented statements by several local priests, arguing that "the poor villagers and sharecroppers of these communities are too poor to afford using the doctor."[55]

Significantly, in these cases it was often the community, rather than the Protomedicato, that finally settled the controversy. In 1702 the people of

Castel San Pietro, having tried several times, to no avail, to prevent the barber Taddeo Azzoguidi from "drawing blood or administering oral medicines without a doctor's order," finally fired him, "aware that said barber was incorrigible." In fact, Azzoguidi had already been tried and reprimanded one year earlier by the Protomedicato.[56] In these cases, the key factor working against the lower-rank practitioners was the balance of power within the community, with the well-off residents regularly siding with the town physician. The Protomedicato proved more impartial, as if trying to show an even-handed attitude toward the different groups of professionals.[57] This is evident, for instance, in the handling of a complaint filed by the township of Crevalcore against a surgeon, Domenico Bazzani, in 1781. The community —or, rather, the local officials—sided with the physician in taking action against the surgeon. The charges were the usual ones: Bazzani had "exceeded the limits of his profession, openly acting as a physician." He was also accused of treating the doctors with disrespect, telling his patients not to seek their advice, and of having once drawn blood from a pregnant woman "who needed care, but certainly not bleeding." Also mentioned were several patients who had died in suspicious circumstances after being treated "by him alone."[58]

Summoned by the Protomedicato, Bazzani defended himself energetically: First of all, a good number of the local officials who had reported him were relatives or friends of the town doctor, so they were clearly biased. He had prescribed oral medicines only to help "poor people, who could not afford a physician." As for drawing blood from the pregnant woman, it had been necessary. The surgeon openly criticized the doctor's diagnosis in that case: the woman had not died of weakness, as proved by "the strong fever and the inflammation of the lower abdomen affecting her." Bloodletting, therefore, had been therapeutically appropriate.

The times had indeed changed. This surgeon's behavior was clearly unprecedented in the history of the Protomedicato. He did not merely defend himself against the accusations, or prove that they were false; he also questioned the doctor's clinical judgment, pitting against it his own independent opinion on matters of diagnosis and therapy. Surprisingly, the Protomedicato ruled in favor of Bazzani, who was acquitted of "exceeding the limits of his profession," even though he had admitted administering oral medicines and behaving disrespectfully toward the town physician.[59]

As this case shows, the Protomedicato did not always side with the town physicians, as one might have expected. How can we explain this? In part, it was a matter of professional rank: the college doctors, proud members of Bologna's medical elite, did not choose to identify themselves with mere country doctors, such as the town physicians. Also, by proving sensitive to the new claims of rising professionals such as the surgeons, the protomedici were trying to present themselves as impartial and fair judges and thus to bolster their image as supreme medical authority, at a time when that image was challenged. Shortly before the final collapse of the old medical regime, the college doctors strove to hold on fast to their magisterial role as the most precious core of their social identity—for which it was sometimes even worth sacrificing the interests of the professional group to which they themselves belonged.

II. Licenses and Prohibitions: Controlling Popular Medicine

We have seen, above, how the Protomedicato managed to control apothecaries and barber-surgeons. Now we shall examine the Protomedicato's attitude toward popular healers, that motley group of practitioners—charlatans, *norcini,* herbalists, distillers, and women—who worked beyond the pale of the official medical system. The Protomedicato's basic rule in regulating these healers was the same as the rule applied to medical practitioners in general: those wishing to practice any branch of medicine needed to be licensed by the college. The Protomedicato, therefore, sorted out popular healers into those who should be prevented from practicing, and those who could be granted a limited license. It is important to emphasize that all unlicensed healers—whether they were barber-surgeons not approved by the college or charlatans—were equally liable to prosecution in the eyes of the Protomedicato. So was any practitioner who overstepped the limits set down in his license. A barber who prescribed oral medications was just as punishable as the charlatan whose practice extended beyond selling the medical "secret" he had been allowed to supply to the public.

The proceedings of the Protomedicato from 1605 to 1776 include 195 criminal cases against such illegal healers (not including apothecaries and third-degree surgeons) (see table 6), plus 131 civil suits that were filed regarding matters of payment.[60] At first sight, therefore, the activity of the doctors' tribunal seems to have been mostly repressive. How harsh was this repression, and which groups were its main target?

As one can see, the charlatans were the main group to be subject to the Protomedicato's control. Through the court records, we can have a close en-

Table 6.   CRIMINAL PROCEEDINGS AGAINST POPULAR HEALERS IN THE
BOLOGNESE PROTOMEDICATO, 1605–1776

Popular Healer	N	%
Charlatans	75	38.5
Barbers	54	27.7
Women	23	11.8
Grocers	13	6.7
Distillers *(spagirici)*	8	4.1
Herbalists *(simplicisti)*	5	2.6
Priests	3	1.5
Friars	1	0.5
Unspecified	13	6.7
Total	195	

Sources: Data compiled from A.S.B., Coll. Med.

counter with one of them. In July 1689, Francesco Sangalli from Verona addressed the crowd in the public square of Bologna, offering a balsam, a "preserve" against toothache, and a "chemical stone" of proven efficacy in case of scabies — all of this for a reasonable sum. Yet Sebastiano Barbetta, the Protomedicato's constable, was in the square at the same time. Barbetta first seized the charlatan's horse and then apprehended the man himself. Searching Sangalli's room at the inn, Barbetta also confiscated (as he later reported) "an unsealed box with a few glass containers of oil, a can of electuary, three bags of powdered or chopped herbs, another big box with four living vipers, an ordinary pot filled almost to the brim with some kind of black stuff, much the same as the electuary, a smaller one containing some red stuff, and many printed recipes." And here is Francesco Sangalli's self-defense in court:

> My trade is to sell and supply oils, balsams, and chemical stones against scabies, which things have been taken away from me by some ruffians. . . . The preserve [that] I prepare against toothache, and that I sell in cans, is made of powder from the roots of oyster plant, carolina, aromatic calamus, ginger, and suchlike herbs that I find on the mountains around Modena and Parma, and that I grind to powder, adding honey and a little Roman vitriol for color's sake. The balsam I administer helps against aches, bruises, and wounds, as per the recipe. I make it with common oil, rosemary, sage, wormwood, pinerose [*rosa di pino*], Greek tar, rose water, and virgin wax; and I boil everything, re-

ducing it to a thick substance. To make the chemical stone I used limestone, *zenabro,* quicksilver, and gold dust. The stone helps cure scabies, if one washes himself with water in which the stone has been immersed.

Francesco Sangalli owned many printed "recipes"—the broadsheets distributed by charlatans, giving information on the efficacy and use of their remedies. Yet he confessed that he did not know how to read or write. When the judges asked him whether he knew the "virtues" of the ingredients he used for his compounds, he answered: "As for the limestone, I don't know exactly its virtue; the quicksilver is silver that walks by itself, so that it makes scabies go away; but the gold dust is an ointment sold by apothecaries, like the *zenabro,* a coloring substance also sold by apothecaries. I don't know the virtues of these things, since I did not study. . . . I learned to make this stone from the people who walk around the world, and especially the charlatan Andrea Gobbi was the one who taught me."[61]

Although Francesco Sangalli used these ingredients without knowing their "virtues," he was well aware of their social value because he had purchased them from apothecaries—the official representatives of the learned pharmacopoeia. In his view, therefore, such ingredients had primarily a social and symbolic value, just like the printed recipes that he could not read but that he knew full well would attract the public because, being printed, they had the appeal of that which is precious and rare. Distributed to people most of whom could not read, the broadsheet was an appropriate medium for dispensing "medical secrets" whose main characteristic was mysteriousness. The broadsheet was, so to speak, part of the medical secret's symbolic aura. It was a decorative element that the charlatan knew how to use in marketing, just as he knew how to manipulate the color of his compounds. In this sense, the broadsheet was part and parcel of the charlatan's merchandise, just as plastic containers and advertising props are an integral part of the products we buy today. And like the advertisements for today's products, the broadsheet had an almost magical value. Medical authorities were well aware of this: "And since many others, who sell simple or compound remedies belonging to medicine, try to add value to their stuff not only with magic words but also with printed recipes vainly promising impossible things; and write many lies, cheating simple people . . . we order that no one should dare to print booklets, recipes, or other sheets describing said virtues . . . unless they have been approved and undersigned by us."[62]

Francesco Sangalli was one of "the people who walk around the world," the varied group of itinerant healers which included, among others, semi-professionals such as the norcini, who were in high repute with their contemporaries.[63] The norcini, who specialized in lithotomy and the cure of hernias, did not use quack remedies but used well-tested, empirically ac-quired surgical skills. The trade was transmitted from father to son in a par-ticular geographic region, the area around Borgo alle Preci and Norcia—hence the name *norcini*. The case of the norcini suggests that the transmission of popular medical lore could be rooted in specific local cultures. This is also suggested by the manuals for barber-surgeons, which mention a variety of "bloodletting schools": blood, apparently, could be drawn in different ways—for instance, the Neapolitan, the Calabrese, and the Sicilian way—depending on the area where the barber had been trained. And while study-ing French surgeons in the eighteenth century, Toby Gelfand came across the very interesting fact that most of them came from one region—Gascony.[64]

Lorenzo and Andrea Adriani, father and son, were working in Bologna as norcini in 1666. Arrested for illegal practice, they were soon released with-out fine or other sanction, probably because their patients testified in their fa-vor. When describing to the protomedici the operation he had performed on an innkeeper suffering from hernia, Lorenzo emphasized that, being an hon-est surgeon, he did not give any oral medication to his patient but only pre-scribed a proper diet for the period following surgery: "In such cases we usu-ally give a remedy to keep the body regular, and a rule for living, such as, at first, some bread with a little oil and butter; tomorrow we'll start him on some chicken or capon broth, and in this way we will gradually bring the cure to completion."[65] In this healer's words we perceive a very different de-meanor from the self-touting attitude displayed by the charlatan Sangalli. Quietly proud of his skills, Lorenzo appears deeply dedicated to his calling and to the well-being of his patients.

Similar undertones can be heard in the voices of some barbers prose-cuted by the Protomedicato for practicing without a license. We meet one of them in the records of the protomedici's inspection in the countryside in 1657. In the public square of the village of Budrio, the protomedici find an unpleasant surprise: a signboard above a door stating, "All kinds of illnesses are treated here, and the poor for the love of God." As the residents tell the protomedici, the shop belongs to a barber, Antonio the Roman; he is im-mediately arrested and interrogated. "I work as a surgeon," he says, "med-icating wounds, ulcers, bones, and fractures." When the protomedici ask him if he is certified, he answers that he got a license in Rome but has now lost it, and that in Bologna "although I took the exam, I wasn't licensed." His practice seems to flourish despite being illegal. After spending only one

month in Budrio, Antonio already has a long list of cures to relate proudly
to the protomedici:

> I treated a woman, for the love of God, suffering from a pain in her arm, and
> a pain caused by a catarrh of the liver or the stomach. She was fifty years old,
> I don't know if she was married or not, she couldn't stand heat or cold. I ap-
> plied a poultice made with blued water, broad-bean flour, and rose oil. . . . I
> also treated a man from Budrio, whose name I don't know, on his private parts
> with the Egyptian ointment . . . and I cured him . . . nor did he require any
> other treatment, for his were simple ulcerations. I also cured many for pains in
> the legs . . . , as well as a man with a head injury on the temporal muscle, a
> simple wound without broken bones. . . . I cured a man from Molinella who
> had a salty humor in one leg and many ulcers on both legs; I treated him with
> a potion of plantain, black grass, bay oil, pinerose [rosa di pino], and yellow
> wax. After decocting these herbs, one should mix them with a little cow fat
> and verdigris.[66]

Antonio seems to be a very ordinary representative of the barbers'
craft, profession, or trade. The remedies he prepares with his own hands are
made of vegetal or animal ingredients that are easily found (unlike those of
the charlatan Sangalli, which were rare chemical substances sold by the
apothecaries). Antonio's remedies are typical of popular medicine. Made of
common, easily available ingredients, they met basic needs, such as stopping
bleeding and preventing and relieving the inflammation of wounds.[67] Barbers
were experts in external remedies such as ointments and balsams. In 1685 a
barber from Bologna, Paolo Marchesini, asked the Protomedicato's leave to
sell a balsam of his own making, which he had been using for more than
forty-eight years. This "ointment-like compound" could be applied with
butter on wounds, used with "egg whites and tow" to stop bleeding and treat
the swelling caused by "transveined" blood, or administered with "cabbage
and chard leaves" on burns.[68] Cabbage and chard leaves, egg whites, tow, and
butter: coupled with these homely accompaniments, this barber's balsam was
obviously not a "medical secret," like those dispensed by the charlatans. It belonged to a popular lore on ointments and washes which was part of a barber's equipment just as much as the lancet was his main tool—a lore probably drawn from a knowledge of herbal remedies which was widespread
among the common people.

Antonio the Roman did have this knowledge, but what mattered to
the protomedici was the fact that he did not have a license. His being a for-

eigner (Roman licenses were not accepted in Bologna) probably also weighed against him. In any event, the protomedici allowed him to practice first-degree surgery (limited to drawing blood) for just one more month, after which he had to leave the territory of Bologna.

The third group targeted by the Protomedicato's control were women healers. Some of them were midwives, whose trade had a semiprofessional character. Bologna's midwives, however, did not belong to a socially recognized trade association. Excluded from the guild system, women — unlike barbers and apothecaries, who were backed by their guilds' political and social clout — had no public voice. Midwives were not included in the three-level medical hierarchy, although in the second half of the seventeenth century their names started to appear on the published rolls of licensed practitioners — a sign that they were recognized as part of the official medical system.

Women's healing practice seems to be circumscribed by the constraints set by their gender. Beyond assisting during childbirth, a midwife's tasks extended to all aspects of female sexuality. In 1642, for instance, Angela Righetti was sentenced to pay a fine of twenty-five lire and to forfeit the drug she "made and sold for women's purgation," that is, for menstruation.[69] When Virginia Calegari was in danger of miscarrying in her second month of pregnancy, in 1717, her mother called on a certain "Angela midwife." "Said midwife," the woman testified, "took me to the apothecary, and there she ordered some [drug] to eat . . . and I gave this to the patient." Virginia died a few days later at the Hospital of Santa Maria Maddalena, where her husband had brought her. It was her husband, Lazzaro Calegari, who filed charges against the midwife Angela Nannini: from the man's deposition, we learn that Virginia had also been treated by a doctor and that the decision to call the midwife had been taken solely by Virginia's mother. Angela Nannini was reprimanded by the Protomedicato and was ordered to stop prescribing oral medicines.[70] In such cases, the protomedici reaffirmed the prohibition on administration of oral drugs, but they never questioned midwives' expertise with regard to the female reproductive system and its ailments.[71]

Itinerant women healers also seem to have limited their practice to female diseases. A Frenchwoman, Giovanna Dupont, who was visiting Bologna in 1709, distributed a broadsheet describing her ability to heal "all those women or girls whose uterus came out of place" by means of "a marvelous medical secret of her own."[72] The restriction of women's practice to the treatment of female diseases was not just a consequence of the Protomedicato's control. It was also prompted by cultural norms that heavily limited women's activities. In 1687, Caterina Cattani Greca asked the Protomedicato to let her post above her door "a signboard listing the diseases that she cures with her remedies, offering assurance that they do not go beyond external use." She could not sell her drugs in the public square like a mountebank — she argued in her request — "because she was a well-born woman,"[73] and honest women had no place in public. In 1698, Ancella Ferrari, denounced by the husband of a patient whom she had treated for an eye disease with a potion and bloodletting, ran away from home, "fearing prison." She begged the medical authorities to believe "that she had treated only her children, and only by using external and female medications."[74]

External and female medications: with these words, Ancella Ferrari pinpointed exactly the restrictions that women practitioners had to face. Not only were they to use external remedies, like all inferior practitioners; being women, they also had to limit their practice to female patients or to the members of their own families (as suggested by Ancella's attempt to convince the protomedici that she had medicated only her children). Women could occasionally go beyond the sphere of "female medications," but only if they were under direct male supervision. For instance, Lavinia Olimpi was mentioned as the co-holder of a license that had been issued in 1638 to her husband, Domenico, for "treating, with external medications, several kinds of diseases affecting the exterior of the body."[75] Because of her experience with these medications, Lavinia was authorized to apply them on patients even in her husband's absence.

Yet these institutional and social restrictions did not totally suppress women's medical practice, which has left many traces. In eighteenth-century Bologna there were women such as Maria Comper, known as Maria La Romana, who enjoyed a reputation, in 1763, for being "very knowledgeable about medical things."[76] Her fame spread even in the countryside. She cured of sciatica the wife of Antonio Baiesi, from the village of San Martino da Bertalia, in the environs of Bologna. Having heard from Baiesi of Maria's skills, a woman from Bertalia went to Bologna and asked Maria to come and visit her husband, who was "sick with a chronic illness, for which he had been unsuccessfully advised by the honorable doctors Pozzi, Molinelli, and Tacconi." With her practice, Maria la Romana supported herself and her family, even vying against Bologna's most prestigious doctors: it is perhaps worth mentioning that Molinelli was the very same man for whom Pope Benedict XIV created the first chair of surgery at the University of Bologna. A renowned practitioner, Molinelli symbolized the academic and social rise of Bologna's surgeons in the eighteenth century[77] — and yet, as we can see, his fame was overshadowed in this case by a woman healer. Charges against

Maria la Romana were filed by Baiesi over a disagreement about payment: the man argued that he had fully paid what was due for his wife's treatment by providing Maria and her family with room and board for eight days, in addition to giving her twenty-three lire and some hemp; but the healer demanded ten more lire, threatening to foreclose on the man's property for that amount. Maria was definitely an exception, as a lucrative medical practice was rare among women. Actually, one of the reasons why there are relatively fewer traces of women healers in the records of Bologna's Protomedicato may well be that their fees were rarely substantial enough to warrant a legal proceeding. In all likelihood, women healers most often treated their patients for very little compensation.

While it is clear that women were excluded from the professional practice of medicine,[78] it should be noted that several female figures were prominent among the saints to whom the citizens of Bologna appealed in their pressing need. In addition to the Virgin Mary, whose cult left a long record of healing miracles in sixteenth- and seventeenth-century Bologna,[79] other women saints were paramount among the city's supernatural healers. The most important among them was probably Caterina Vigri, a fifteenth-century nun whose canonization proceedings were started in 1669. During these proceedings, a witness testified that "there isn't one sick person in this city who doesn't resort to her."[80] Contact with Caterina's "holy body," as well as her apparition in dreams, were believed to have led to many healing miracles.[81] Other holy women who were reputed to have thaumaturgical powers included Diana degli Andalò and Paola Mezzavacca, in the Middle Ages; Prudenziana Zagnotti, in the seventeenth century; and Anna Callegari Zucchini and Sister Rosa Torregiani, in the eighteenth century.[82]

In a more earthly sphere, women, despite their marginal role in professional practice, were constantly present at the bedside of those who were ill. In the Protomedicato's trials, the voices testifying about the illness and the treatment of relatives or neighbors were primarily those of women. Women were the ones who provided daily care for the sick. Catta Diolaiti, of Bertalia, tells, for instance, about Domenico Guarlandi, a shoemaker of her village, who became sick in 1697: "He, being a single person, sent for me through Bertalia's parish priest. I went to his house, and faithfully assisted him during his illness, doing what was prescribed for him and what he needed."[83] Catta had been called to the witness stand by a barber, to testify about his treatment of Domenico. Women and barbers often met at the bedside of patients. When Stefano Golinelli broke his leg in Budrio, in 1700, his servant declared that "a woman called Madonna Virginia Nicolai Giovanini . . . gave him first aid; and afterward she was joined by a barber of Budrio named Sebastiano Atti, and together they did perform the required tasks."[84]

Women and barbers, therefore, worked side by side: in the menial, daily chores of the treatment, they were the ones who actually took care of the sick body. Indeed, they were caregivers, not just healers. The barber's role, as we know, included a general responsibility for the "cleanliness" of the body; and the midwife's tasks included washing and dressing the dead, in preparation for burial.[85] Theirs were hands that touched the body without repulsion, caring for it in any condition—whether alive or dead, dirty or covered by sores.

How strict was the Protomedicato's control over healers such as the charlatan Sangalli, the barber Antonio, and Maria la Romana? The Protomedicato's justice was not harsh. Criminal proceedings against popular healers almost always resulted only in the seizure of unlicensed medications, mild reprimands, and low fines (which were often further reduced on appeal). For barber-surgeons overstepping the limits of their trade, the harshest punishment was temporary suspension from practice. Only repeat offenders were jailed, for a short term, and the heaviest penalty—banishment from the territory of Bologna—was inflicted only in exceptional cases. Over the Protomedicato's two centuries of activity, only three people were condemned to exile: in 1614, Rodolfo Vacchettoni, a norcino who had been convicted of prescribing oral medications and extorting money from several patients and whose medications had allegedly killed a man affected by "a light case of scabies";[86] in 1689, Gio. Batta Terrarossa, a surgeon who, in spite of several reprimands, had obstinately persisted in practicing as a physician;[87] and, in 1730, Sebastiano Poggi, a surgeon who falsely claimed to hold a doctoral degree.[88] It is worth looking closely at Poggi's case because it shows the conditions under which the protomedici felt bound to punish with utmost severity the illegal practice of medicine.

In 1719 Poggi, a thirty-three-year-old resident of Bologna who claimed to have studied surgery in Florence, Rome, and Montpellier and to have practiced for twelve years in the territory of Spoleto, requested from the protomedici a license to practice surgery in the city. He was granted a license to practice as a third-degree surgeon. One year later, Poggi was accused by several patients of prescribing oral medications and was subsequently tried in the Protomedicato. Under interrogation he admitted knowing that his license to practice as a surgeon allowed him only "to apply external remedies, not internal ones; and that I couldn't treat, for instance, a case of ulcerated lungs, because it's a disease one can't see, and I have no leave to treat such diseases." He was sentenced to pay a fine and was suspended from practicing for a period. But in 1725 he was prosecuted again, on the same charges. This time, however, he claimed he had the right to prescribe oral medications, having been awarded the doctoral degree at the castle of Dozza.

Poggi's doctoral title had been granted by means of the so-called *privilegio in camera,* the privilege that gave the Palatine counts the right to confer at will doctoral degrees in medicine. In Bologna, the noble families Campeggi and Malvezzi had this privilege and awarded the degree from their castle in Dozza.[89] The candidate had only to present himself at the castle with a certificate proving that he had discussed the Hippocratic aphorisms with a doctor of medicine.[90] The granting of degrees *in camera* by aristocratic patrons was very irksome to the Protomedicato, since it contravened the college's exclusive right to bestow the title of medical doctor. Like the cardinal legate's habit of issuing permits to charlatans,[91] this custom was one more reminder of how the professional licensing system had originally been connected to aristocratic patronage. However, the licenses granted to charlatans were one thing, and doctoral degrees were quite another. On this last issue, the college was inflexible. In 1604 it obtained from the legate a decree forbidding holders of *in camera* doctorates to practice in the territory of Bologna.[92] Subsequent decrees by the Protomedicato reinforced this norm. Nevertheless, doctoral degrees *in camera* kept being awarded even into the first half of the eighteenth century, as indicated by the Poggi case.

The protomedici asked Poggi to explain to the court how he had obtained his doctoral degree. He described, to their chagrin, a ceremony that was a close parody of the one described in the college statutes.[93] The procedure, Poggi stated, was simple. It sufficed to find two (not overly scrupulous) doctors willing to interrogate the candidate and to release a document certifying his medical expertise. The graduation ceremony followed at the castle of Dozza. Poggi's examiners had been the doctors Bonaveri and Taruffi, who had asked him to elaborate on Hippocrates's first and thirty-seventh aphorisms and on two philosophical arguments. As for issues pertaining to medical practice, they had asked him to discuss a case of angina and the proper treatment for pleuritis.

In turn, the protomedici asked Poggi to give a written answer, in Latin, to the following question: by whose authority did he practice as a physician? In sham Latin, which recalls to our minds the famous scene of the oath at the end of Molière's *Malade imaginaire,* Poggi answered: "Habeo in virtute Privilegi otenere Domu Campeggi sub seque qualiter remedie ego prescriptit pro cura pleura vel inflamatio ala polmone nel esame facto pro conseguedo talis Privilegi."

In his first trial, Poggi got away with a reprimand: he was simply warned not to prescribe oral medications any more, and to limit his practice to surgery. His "misdeeds," however, were reported to the two patrons he had mobilized in his support, the Bologna legate and the landgrave of Hesse. When informed by the protomedici of the trespasses of his protegé, the latter, who had sent a dispatch from Mantua on Poggi's behalf, wrote back: "I will take care henceforth to keep Poggi in his place, since he is taking undue advantage of my protection." Poggi was admonished a second time in 1728, after several patients accused him of prescribing oral treatments for various illnesses. He was also charged with publicly laying claim to the title of "doctor" and—an act of outrageous impudence in the eyes of the protomedici—with distributing in Bologna a broadsheet with his own portrait in doctoral garb, and the inscription "Sebastiano Poggi, excellent physician and surgeon."[94] The Protomedicato sentenced him to exile in 1730, after a new trial in which he was convicted of prescribing an oral medicine to a woman who died suddenly after taking it. Apparently, the sentence was not enforced, as Poggi remained in Bologna undisturbed. He was tried again in 1734, this time in the Archdiocesan Court, on charges of having "assisted prostitutes during delivery without reporting their pregnancy to the Ospedale dei Bastardini (the Foundling Hospital) and [of] having helped them to abandon their infants." He was sentenced to ten years in jail, but the penalty was waived by the pope's pardon. Poggi continued to practice in Bologna, challenging the Protomedicato, which again brought him to trial in 1744. He was once more sentenced to exile, and this time the verdict seems to have been implemented, because I cannot find any more traces of Poggi among the Protomedicato's records after this date.

Poggi's arrogance had finally overstepped the protomedici's long-tried forbearance. The college doctors, at first tolerant of his trespasses—probably thanks also to the intercession of the man's aristocratic patrons[95]—did finally retaliate against this prolonged challenge to their exclusive control over medical degrees. The verdict in Poggi's first trial (which concluded in 1730 with a sentence of exile) may have been influenced by his involvement in the sudden death of a patient. Ultimately, however, what sealed the fate of this would-be doctor, with his fake Latin and his unscrupulous use of powerful patrons, was his brazen and obdurate defiance of the college's authority.

The practice of charlatans who did not lay claim to a doctoral title was not nearly so threatening to the college, and as a consequence, these healers usually received milder sentences, such as reprimands and fines. It is important to notice that charlatans also were granted special licenses to practice in Bolognese territory. For two hundred years, the granting of such licenses was one of the Protomedicato's regular activities, as important as examining barbers, midwives, and apothecaries. Licenses for charlatans, distillers, norcini, and women healers were usually given for a limited time and were restricted to specific therapies or illnesses. For example, the license granted in 1647 to Caterina Panzacchia specified that she was allowed to treat "headaches, ringworms and scrofula, eye diseases, scabies, leprosy, rashes, herpes, and ulcers on the legs" by external methods.[96] Like the licenses of barbers and midwives, these licenses contained a warning against prescribing oral medications and the requirement that the licensee practice under a physician's supervision. Thus, in 1616 the norcino Marino Marini was allowed "to castrate, remove cataracts, and extract gallstones" as long as he worked—the license specified—under the direction of a certified physician.[97]

These licenses were clearly used to integrate popular medicine, at least in part, into the official medical system. The Protomedicato's attitude toward popular healers had a punitive side (the enforcing of disciplinary actions) but also a permissive one (the issuing of licenses). These two aspects of the protomedici's activity should be examined together—particularly because they were often directed toward the same healer. Take, for instance, the case of a woman healer, Anna Beloi, charged (probably by one of her patients), arrested, and tried by the protomedici in 1697. The woman was sentenced to pay a fine of thirty lire plus trial expenses. The medicines that she used were confiscated, and she was ordered to abstain in the future from medical practice of all kinds. This happened on October 30. On November 17 of the same year, she was granted a license to treat "hemorrhoids, herpes, ringworm, ulcerations on the legs," with the usual restrictions.[98] This was not the only instance in which a healer was granted a license after having been prosecuted for illegal practice. In 1623, for instance, the Protomedicato ordered the confiscation of the medications that Michele Zanardi, of Ferrara, was selling in Bologna's public square. Zanardi was also fined four lire. Shortly afterward, the protomedici analyzed his compounds and granted him a one-month license to sell a remedy called "Artificial Balsam."[99] Another, similar case is that of a father and son named Baccolini, from Tolè, who were reported for illegal practice by the town physician of Vergato and were convicted by the protomedici in 1750. After one month in jail, they were released and granted a license to practice as first-degree surgeons.[100]

The interconnection between the Protomedicato's punitive actions and its permissive ones was even clearer in the case of barbers and midwives. In 1697—to mention just one case of many—the barber Antonio Masina was fined fifteen lire for carrying surgical instruments without being certified as a surgeon. Afterward, he sat for the examination and was approved as a third-degree surgeon (the highest rank in the profession).[101] Likewise, in 1744 the surgeon Matteo Toni, found practicing without a license, was ordered to abstain from practice and to take the examination within a month.[102] The same happened in 1746 to the midwife Diamante Merli, of Castagnolo, who was officially granted a license one month after receiving a warning not to practice.[103]

Clearly, healers were punished not for being unskilled but simply for not having a license, as indicated by the short interval between prosecution and certification: a healer's skills could not dramatically improve within such a brief period. Likewise, the seizure of medicines from illegal healers was not motivated by concerns about safety; in fact, the drugs thus confiscated were usually given to local hospitals—the Ospedale di Sant'Orsola or the Ospedale di San Giobbe, a hospital for syphilitics—as a charitable gift. The same happened to the surgical tools confiscated from unlicensed barbers, and to defective medications found during the inspections of apothecary shops.[104]

If we look at the graph of the Protomedicato's actions in issuing licenses for and prohibitions against medical practice (see the figure), we can see that both showed parallel trends over time. The correlation was stronger in the first half of the seventeenth century, when the number of licenses exceeded the number of interdictions. This pattern was reversed in the next half century, with a sharp increase in the number of punitive measures. This was also the period when the college reformed surgical practice—the first step in a process that would eventually lead to a radical transformation of the medical hierarchy. The licensing of charlatans and other popular healers, although decreasing, continued even in this period. As late as 1747, a few years after the reform of surgery, the protomedici, faced with the problem of controlling the illegal practice of dentists, hernia specialists, steam bath attendants, charlatans, and the like, had recourse once again to the granting of licenses following examination.[105] The issuing of such licenses for what was called (with open disdain) "petty practice" was continued, in fact, until the early nineteenth century.[106]

This uninterrupted flow of licenses indicates that the medical authorities were relatively tolerant of marginal healers. To a certain extent, the official medical system tried to accommodate even the practice of charlatans.

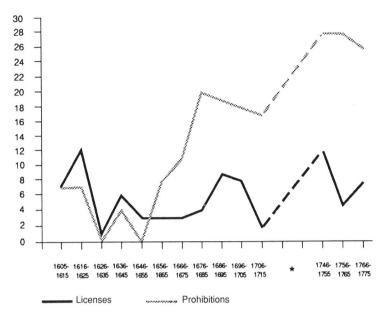

Licenses for medical practice granted by the Protomedicato to popular healers and prohibitions against medical practice addressed by the Protomedicato to popular healers, 1605–1776. *Black line*: licenses; *gray line:* prohibitions. The data for 1716–46 are incomplete because some of the Protomedicato's records are missing.
Data compiled from A.S.B., Coll. Med.

The Protomedicato's control over popular medicine was not rigid and unswerving. On the contrary, in the protomedici's hands, licensing was a flexible procedure, which they could tailor to each individual case. A few rules, including the prohibition against prescribing oral medications, were imposed on all nonphysicians, but each license was nevertheless unique, so that the protomedici were able to gauge and adjust their control over each individual healer, as occasion required.

Take, for instance, the case of Colomba Consolini, a midwife from the village of Budrio. After attending the regular classes in surgery at one of Bologna's chief hospitals, the Ospedale della Vita, in 1750, she applied to the Protomedicato for a license to practice as a first-degree surgeon (with authority to draw blood, apply poultices and ointments, and administer rubs and enemas). Her case was obviously odd and disconcerting for the protomedici: here was a woman who was not content with the only role officially allowed to women healers but who wished to practice surgery, a field from which women had been excluded for centuries in Bologna.[107] The protomedici chose to compromise, using the flexibility inherent in their licensing system. Officially they did not grant a first-degree license (Consolini's name does not appear on the roll of certified barber-surgeons). At the same time, they did not exclude her from the surgical profession, nor did they ask her to limit her practice to midwifery. Instead, they issued a special one-year license allowing her to apply leeches and ointments (including mercury-based ones) under the direction of a physician, and to administer enemas (but only to women). Colomba could also draw blood from the hands, arms, and legs of both women and men. One year later, her license was renewed, with an additional restriction: she could still draw blood from men and women "indiscriminately" but was to perform all other operations on women only.[108]

In this way, Colomba Consolini's surgical practice was restricted but not completely suppressed. Half a century later, after the Napoleonic reform of the medical system, this kind of flexible, individual licensing would no longer be possible. By then, the medical authorities had grown much more intolerant of popular healers, women in particular.[109] Medical licensing in the ancien régime was somewhat discretional and arbitrary, but also relatively flexible and tolerant. Thanks to this flexibility, the medical system was able to incorporate some popular healers, both men and women, albeit in clearly subordinated positions.

III. The Aura of the "Medical Secret"

Many licenses issued by the Protomedicato during its two hundred years of activity concerned the sale of "medical secrets," or patent medicines. One such "secret," for instance, was the "remedial compound against live and dead poisons," created by Martino Grimaldi the Neapolitan. As explained in its attendant broadsheet, this "electuary" was to be used against all kinds of poisoning "from the bite of rabid dogs and poisonous snakes . . . [and] against worms, small and large, . . . colic pains and wind in the stomach, the illness of women, young and old, tertian and quartan fevers, . . . chest pain, injured ribs, . . . pestiferous and malignant fevers, . . . and to protect oneself from the plague."[110] We find traces of the popularity of the Grimaldi electuary throughout the history of the Protomedicato, as the medication's sale license was renewed for more than a century and a half. The patent was originally granted in 1617 to Martino Grimaldi himself (although two years earlier he had been forbidden to practice medicine). Martino left his "medical secret" to his brother-in-law, Gio. Batta Galvani, who bequeathed it to his wife, Isabella Fontana, "who always had a major role in preparing said electuary." Isabella's last will and testament passed it on to her servant, Fulvio Baroncini, "known as Brighella." He handed it down to his widow, Bernardina Guidotti, who in turn gave it to her heir, Margherita Luppi Bettini; Margherita left it to her great-grandson, Domenico Maria Galeazzi, who signed it over to his widow, Bianca Bulbarini Galeazzi, who finally gave it to her nephew, Giuseppe Moreschi, in the year 1755.[111] Not surprisingly, when applying to renew the license, the heirs asked for a re-issue of the "Grimaldi privilege," as if this were a special benefit granted exclusively to their family.

The Grimaldi were not the only dynasty of "professors of medical secrets" in Bologna in the seventeenth and eighteenth centuries, nor were they the only ones to receive the Protomedicato's stamp of approval. In 1649, Giovanni Garofalo obtained "permission from the authorities" to print a broadsheet explaining the "virtue" of the Garofalo electuary—a potion he had inherited from his father, Gioseffo Garofalo, who had been first interdicted from practice and later licensed by the protomedici. The Garofalo electuary, too, was a cure for all ills, guaranteed to "counteract any poison, bring about vomiting, make the body regular, promote urination, vivify the heart, and purify the blood."[112]

How are we to understand the medical authorities' tolerance of "medical secrets"? At the beginning of the seventeenth century, Paolo Zacchia lamented that the popularity of such secrets was spreading, even among doctors: "Good God, how vain is this belief in medical secrets! Yet it is widespread not only among the common people but among all kinds of men—even among the physicians."[113]

Men of learning and illiterate charlatans alike seem to have shared a keen interest in medical secrets. Although seventeenth-century medical ethics deplored their use,[114] doctors kept avidly collecting them, in that century as well as in the next. For instance, a "Codex medicinae faciendae," compiled in 1734 as a commonplace book by a Bolognese doctor, listed "several ways to administer chinaroot, how to apply a mercury-based ointment the way it is done in Naples"; "a medical secret against fistula"; and a "specific remedy against bleeding."[115]

Describing the manuscripts of Giovanni Meli, a physician and man of letters of the eighteenth century, the historian and folklorist Giuseppe Pitré noted that they contain a large number of medical secrets, with the names of the people who had recommended them ("medical secret by the priest-schoolmaster," "dye tried by the waitress at the Lion's, who had learned it from a monk," etc.).[116] According to Pitré, the interest in folk remedies that was displayed by a man of learning such as Meli underscores eighteenth-century medical culture's empiricism and its receptiveness toward popular wisdom. Pitré's view of Meli coincides with the conventional image of early modern science: a science based on experiment and observation, and therefore open to the contribution of popular empiricism. Although much can be said in support of this view, I doubt that it really applies to medical secrets such as those licensed by the Protomedicato. As described by the charlatans who applied for a permit, these potions don't seem to be based on much empirical testing, nor did the protomedici's procedure in examining them include close scrutiny and experimentation. I also doubt that the notion of "medical secret" is really an autonomous expression of popular culture. Rather, it seems to me to be a projection onto popular culture, through the mediation of the charlatans, of an upper-class notion — the idea that the value of a medication is enhanced by its rarity, by its being a privilege of the few.

This notion is clearly visible in the Protomedicato's vision of pharmacopoeia: remedies were classified either as "noble" and "rare," or as "humble" and "common," appropriate for the populace. As we already know, poor-quality medicines confiscated from delinquent apothecaries were donated by the Protomedicato to the hospitals, to be used for the poor. This classification of medicines along social lines is vividly described in the protomedici's reports on their inspections of apothecary shops. In 1669, for instance, during their rounds in the countryside, the protomedici visited the shop of the fortress at Castelfranco and found that "there were no noble medicines for the soldiers." They were somewhat reassured, however, by finding that "for the officers there were *confettioni giacintine* [a superior medicine]," and that, as the apothecary had pointed out, "ordinary medicines were sufficient for the sick soldiers." The protomedici decided that it was unnecessary to reprimand the apothecary "simply for charitable reasons, prompted by the soldiers' complaints," and happily proceeded to Crevalcore. They bypassed the village of Sant'Agata because "it is known that there is no apothecary shop or town physician there, and that the apothecary is rather a mere grocer." For similar reasons they skipped San Pietro in Casale. The inspection ended at the two apothecary shops of San Giovanni in Persiceto. One of them, furnished with "a rich and clean set of fine majolica vases," was praised by the protomedici in preference to the other, which was certainly well stocked but whose jars were just "old earthenware, gloomy-looking."[117]

Fine and coarse vases: they stand as an apt symbol for the contrast between noble remedies and common ones. Ordinary remedies were adequate for the soldiers, while the officers needed more precious medications such as the *confettioni giacintine*. Just as the medical establishment was hierarchically divided into those who performed noble tasks (such as administering oral medications) and those who performed menial ones (such as drawing blood), remedies were also divided into the precious and the ordinary. The latter, applied by barbers, were made of low-priced, easily available ingredients (such as herbs, animal fat, and egg whites). Medications prescribed by a physician, in contrast, needed precious and carefully selected ingredients. This is shown by the great care paid by the protomedici year after year, from the end of the sixteenth century to the end of the eighteenth, to the selection of the forty-one ingredients of theriac. Theriac was the most noble and precious of medicaments, the very symbol of the official pharmacopoeia. Its recipe dated back to Galen, and the protomedici were meticulous in choosing the most precious and genuine ingredients, as close as possible to those used in antiquity. Honey was to be "of the purest kind," while the ancient wine, Falerno, could be replaced by modern Malmsey, but only if it was "extremely pure, not subjected to the corruptions of acidity, because it must perfectly combine the thick juices, and the gums, that go into theriac, and preserve the unadulterated qualities of all the ingredients of such an important medicine."[118]

The importance of theriac in the origins and development of the Protomedicato has already been mentioned,[119] but perhaps it has not yet been clarified why this drug became a symbol of the official pharmacopoeia all over Europe. Indeed, from the Renaissance on, theriac was prepared with solemn public ceremonies in Bologna as well as in Venice, Milan, Genoa, Padua, Byzantium, and Cairo.[120] The records of the Bolognese Protomedicato document the high value attributed to theriac by registering, year by year, the protomedici's careful inspections of the drug's ingredients. The protomedici personally oversaw the killing and skinning of vipers (whose meat was the drug's main component);[121] the exact weight of the compound; its solemn distribution to apothecary shops; and the expenses for the ceremony, including a fee for the priest who was engaged to invoke God's blessing over the drug.[122] In 1756, the cost of making theriac was 704 lire, including "the apparatus of refreshments, dinners, and related items."[123] Theriac was dropped from London's pharmacopoeia in 1788 and from Edinburgh's in 1756—although the *Encyclopédie* still recommended its use.[124] In Bologna it was made until the end of the eighteenth century, and the Protomedicato continued to preside over the solemn ritual of its preparation.

What was the therapeutic function of theriac? Basically it was an antipoison drug, just like the "medical secrets" sold by Martino Grimaldi and Gioseffo Garofalo, the wondrous effects of which were mentioned earlier in this chapter. According to a learned medical tradition, theriac generated heat in the body, thus counteracting the action of poisons, which were believed to kill by their coldness.[125] The range of theriac's applications was truly impressive. An official broadsheet on the "main virtues and powers of theriac," released in Bologna in 1692, listed forty-eight possible uses, ranging from "protecting oneself against the plague," to counteracting "the bite of poisonous animals," "ingested poisons," "vertigo," "paralysis," "falling sickness," and "male impotence" (if taken with some wine). It could also be used as a remedy for "the stoppage of women's menstruation (when taken with red chickpea broth)," to "extract, or pull out a dead fetus from its mother's womb," and to treat "the French disease." It also helped "keep the body in good health for a longer time, if it is taken once or twice a month with a little wine; it gives immunity from illness by evacuating all the useless excrements; it purifies the blood, and prolongs life."[126]

As we can see, here is a promise of a universal cure, quite up to the standard set by the grand claims made in the charlatans' broadsheets. Actually, if we compare this official eulogy of theriac with the boasts in a broadsheet written in 1675 by a charlatan, Antonio Bortolotti, to advertise the virtues of his "theriacal gentian," we find that the mountebank's claim was less inflated: "Said compound — says Bortolotti's handwritten broadsheet — takes away all the body's aches, but especially poisons and cold fevers." Moreover, the instructions for the use of Bortolotti's theriacal gentian contained a modicum of sound empiricism. In fact, the broadsheet recommended, when applying the drug to a viper's or dog's bite, that one "cauterize said bites twice or three times, particularly the ones caused by rabid dogs."[127]

In concocting their medical secrets, charlatans such as Antonio Bortolotti combined a model derived from learned medicine (theriac, the prodigious and rare drug) with a genuinely popular element (the use of herbal remedies). Interestingly, the recipes that the charlatans submitted to the protomedici when applying for the licensing of their "secrets" often listed the same two basic ingredients: herbs and theriac.[128] This seems to suggest that these "secrets" represented a mediation between the popular knowledge of herbal remedies and the official pharmacopoeia. It is not surprising, therefore, that the protomedici approved and licensed their sale. Because of their combination of a noble drug (theriac) with a common one (herbs), they must have appeared to the medical elite as a humbler, diluted form of theriac, suitable for the lower classes. And actually, in 1726 the Protomedicato sent to the apothecaries instructions on how to prepare a cheap "theriacal water" for the poor, made of herbs and theriac just like the patent medicines of the charlatans.[129]

As mentioned above, theriac was basically an antipoison drug. Its appeal depended on the widespread assumption that illness was due to a poison entering the body from the outside, especially through food. Thus, theriac was the drug par excellence in a society that was deeply afraid of poisoning. It is on the common ground of this diffused fear that learned and quack medicine met and competed against each other. There are numerous indications of the popularity of theriac. Many patients interrogated by the protomedici had experienced its bitter taste. And the records of the Protomedicato include several petitions from grocers wishing to keep it in their stores "because very often people ask for it."[130] (Only apothecaries were allowed to sell theriac.) Charlatans tried to meet this high demand by supplying a cheaper, lower-quality imitation of the official drug. In this way, they came to compete with physicians and apothecaries—the official distributors of the drug, who must have resented this unfair competition. The proliferation of medical secrets and the physicians' interest in them can be seen as a reaction by the medical profession to the charlatans' challenge.[131] In Molière's *Amour médecin,* we see Sganarello, bewildered by the physicians' contradictory opinions, turning to a quack selling the Orvietan—a powerful medical secret supposedly capable of curing "la gale, la rogne, la tigne, la fièvre, la peste, la goutte, vérole, descente, rougeole."[132] Likewise, in Bologna too, as we shall see in more detail in chapter 5, learned physicians and charlatans often met at the bedside of the same patients. In order to compete with the quacks, the doctors also needed the powerful aura that surrounded the possessors of medical secrets.

One purpose of the grand theriac-making ceremony was certainly self-promotion by the official medical establishment.[133] The marketing techniques adopted by charlatans could be just as aggressive, and these healers' egos were sometimes as large, as those of the doctors. In 1771, a full-sized portrait was posted in the public square of Bologna; it was an advertisement for Filippo Vitali, a charlatan licensed by the protomedici to practice dentistry. The poster was removed several times by order of the Protomedicato—but an obstinate Vitali kept re-posting it on "the right-hand pillar at the head of the street called Le Chiavature" (a street that at one time ran between two leading hospitals).[134]

The fashion of medical secrets can be understood in the context of this rivalry between charlatans and the medical establishment. Both offered basically the same merchandise (theriac) and used the same self-touting technique, claiming that their stock in trade was more amazing than the competition's. In such conditions, the offer of medical remedies was subject to the dictates of fashion. "It is a peculiar characteristic of fashion — to use the words of sociologist Georg Simmel — that it renders possible a social obedience, which at the same time is a form of individual differentiation."[135] In order to compete with the official pharmacopoeia, the charlatans' offer needed to look different from it, but only superficially different. Medical secrets were all different and similar at the same time: they all contained theriac, and they all repeated the same formula, each promising to be more powerful than the others. Just like fashion, they represented "a form of individual differentiation" that nevertheless was based on social conformity. The charlatans' secrets did not represent a form of alternative medicine but were, in fact, a mimicry of the official pharmacopoeia.

The advertising of medical secrets used what Mikhail Bakhtin has called "the language of the marketplace": "Let us stress that popular spectacles and popular medicine, herbalists and druggists, hawkers of magic unguents and quacks, could be seen side by side. There was an ancient connection between the forms of medicine and folk art which explains the combination in one person of actor and druggist."[136] Such was the case in the Middle Ages and in the Renaissance. In early modern Bologna, however, the public square was no longer — to use Bakhtin's words —"the center of all that was unofficial." It no longer "enjoyed a certain extraterritoriality in a world of official order and official ideology." While the "language of the marketplace" in the Renaissance was centered on the joyous celebration of bodily functions — eating, drinking, healing, impregnating, and giving birth[137] — the broadsheets of the charlatans who were licensed by the Protomedicato were pervaded instead by a very different motif — a body afraid of poisoning. The dominant body image was no longer the "grotesque body," joyously open to the world, but a body whose orifices — especially the mouth — were dangerous areas to be jealously guarded and protected.

This was, in fact, the image of the body which the medical establishment projected by insistently forbidding lesser healers to administer oral medications. The protomedici took upon themselves the fundamental role of guarding the mouth: the tasks of regulating diet, the cornerstone of all therapies, and of distributing theriac — the cure against all poisons — to the city were exclusively theirs.

One more detail should be added to complete our description of the official medical system in early modern Bologna. I have already mentioned how the Protomedicato and sometimes the entire college were asked to give medical advice to the community in the case of epidemics. Their advice was also requested on a more frequent basis. In fact, the Protomedicato was expected regularly to inspect the quality of food brought into the city. During the plague of 1630, for instance, while public measures against the epidemic were undertaken by the Assunteria di Sanità, the Protomedicato was asked by the Tribunes of the Plebs to examine all the meat and wheat imported into the city.[138] As the reader may remember, the tribunes were the magistrates in charge of overseeing the city markets and controlling the price and quality of bread and other staples.[139] I stressed in chapter 1 the way in which the tribunes and the Protomedicato were kindred institutions: their membership overlapped, as the college doctors were often appointed as tribunes by the Senate. More important, the two magistracies had similar functions: the tribunes were entrusted with protecting the people from food frauds, while the protomedici were supposed to guard them from medical abuses. From the viewpoint of the medical authorities, food and medicine were closely associated:[140] as we know, prescribing and controlling diet was a physician's foremost therapeutic task. The tribunes, responsible for the good quality of foods sold on the market, regularly requested the protomedici's opinion concerning the edibility of fish, fruit, and wheat imported into the city.[141] Nor did the protomedici consider it beneath their status to perform these inspections, which were a regular part of their duties throughout two centuries. As late as 1775, for instance, the protomedici were requested by the Tribunes of the Plebs to inspect "several kinds of groceries" seized at the border by customs officials because of their dubious quality. Faithful to their role as guardians of the mouth, they went and examined barrels of tuna, caviar, and stockfish, testing them with fire to establish whether they were still edible. Some, they declared, were "not acceptable for sale without danger to the public health," while others they judged to be too "spicy, almost caustic, which could damage most stomachs" or "hurt the most delicate ones."[142]

Why did the protomedici accept the role of food inspectors—a role that today seems so menial and inappropriate for the supreme medical authorities? In order to understand this, we should remember that the medical elite saw itself as, and in fact was, an integral part of the urban ruling class. A major aspect of the legitimization of political power in the old regime was the set of reciprocal expectations between aristocracy and common people, which E. P. Thompson called the "moral economy."[143] At the core of the moral economy was the people's idea that the governing class should be held responsible for guaranteeing the supply, quality, and fair price of necessities such as bread. The authorities, in turn, were willing to legitimize their rule by adopting a paternalistic attitude and posturing as protectors of basic needs. In the specific case of Bologna, historians have shown the importance attributed by the ruling class to control of the quality and price of bread, as a way to attain social consensus.[144] No doubt the authorities viewed all of this not as a popular right but as their gift to the people—a view that was expressed through rituals such as the throwing of food to the crowd during the inauguration ceremony for every new *gonfaloniere di giustizia,* the judicial figurehead with largely ceremonial powers who was chosen every two months by the Senate.[145] The people, however, believed that they had a customary right to press for control over the quality of bread, and they were at times sustained in this belief by the authorities, who occasionally ordered the destruction of poor-quality wheat.

The social role of the Protomedicato was also related to this moral economy. In old-regime Bologna we find, in addition to a moral economy of bread, a moral economy of medicine.[146] Just as the Tribunes of the Plebs were supposed to guarantee the supply, quality, and fair price of bread, so the Protomedicato was expected to ensure the supply, quality, and fair price of medicines. And as the tribunes sometimes ordered the destruction of low-quality wheat, so the protomedici directed the disposal of low-quality drugs. In their role as guardians of the mouth, the college doctors were part of the political structure that ensured the legitimization of Bologna's ruling class.

Chapter 4

PATIENTS' RIGHTS AND THE
DOCTORS' PRESTIGE

I. THE "FAIR PRICE" OF MEDICAL SERVICE

Thus far, we have examined the Protomedicato's criminal proceedings against popular healers. We shall now look into the civil suits brought to the court during the same period, from the early seventeenth century to the end of the eighteenth. The Protomedicato's civil jurisdiction officially started in 1581, when Cardinal Legate Cesi conferred upon "the illustrious doctors of the college, its deans and protomedici" the power "to settle and arbitrate any lawsuits and litigations that may arise between doctors and patients."[1] Previously, disputes between patients and healers over payment had been settled by the ordinary courts, with the college doctors summoned occasionally to give their opinion as experts.[2] Despite occasional conflicts with other courts, the Protomedicato was to maintain jurisdiction over civil cases until its demise at the end of the eighteenth century.

Civil lawsuits filed with the Protomedicato most often involved disputes over the payment of fees to physicians and barber-surgeons, or the payment of apothecaries' bills for medicines. The litigants expected the protomedici to establish a fair price for medical services and for medicines. Physicians and barber-surgeons appealing to the protomedici to obtain payment from dilatory patients were required to present evidence and witnesses of the services rendered and to swear to the truthfulness of what was stated in their bills. Having heard both parties, and after verifying the circumstances of the case, the protomedici established the fair price of treatment, which was sometimes at variance from what had been requested by the practitioner himself. Patients had to pay within a specified time; if they refused, the protomedici ordered seizure of a quantity of the patient's property worth the amount due.

The Protomedicato's hearings in these cases were "summary," that is, swift and informal, consistent with the tradition of mercantile courts and with what was prescribed by jurisprudence on the issue of disputes over payment of medical services.[3] As a consequence, most healers and patients presented their own case instead of hiring an attorney,[4] and trial costs were thereby contained.

Usually the protomedici first made an attempt to bring about an out-of-court settlement between the parties. In fact, a large number of these cases were solved in this manner, as we can infer from the fact that many filed charges never resulted in a trial.[5]

As we might expect, most of these lawsuits were filed by licensed practitioners (see table 7). In contrast, unlicensed healers were almost never plaintiffs, and for very good reasons. In the first half of the seventeenth century, they realized that they had no right to payment and that by appealing to the Protomedicato they risked being charged with illicit practice. I will discuss these few cases filed by unlicensed healers in chapter 6, when describing the disappearance of the agreement for a cure. Not surprisingly, the issue of payment for medical services is closely related to the history of the agreement for a cure. As we have seen, by the end of the sixteenth century it was commonly acknowledged that patients who had contracted such an agreement should pay only if the treatment had been successful. But whereas the patients supported this principle wholeheartedly, healers and medical authorities had strong misgivings about it. The Protomedicato's lawsuits allow us to examine these viewpoints — the practitioners' expectations on matters of payment, and the criteria used by the protomedici to establish a fair fee.

The Protomedicato's records of these cases clearly indicate that medical practitioners tried to avoid the terms of the agreement for a cure by asking to be paid for each visit, no longer considering results but only the services

Table 7.   LAWSUITS IN THE BOLOGNESE PROTOMEDICATO TO REQUEST PAYMENT FOR MEDICAL SERVICES OR MEDICINES, 1605–1776

Filed by	N	%
Barber-surgeons	73	56
Physicians	20	15
Patients	18	14
Apothecaries	9	7
Unlicensed healers	3	2
Unspecified	8	6
Total	131	

Sources: Data compiled from A.S.B., Coll. Med.

rendered and the distance traveled to visit a patient. As Carlo, barber of Sant'Agata, told the protomedici in 1664 when suing a patient for nonpayment: "For my labor I ask one *testone* [one lira and a half] per visit."[6] Paying for each visit—a custom that had long coexisted with the agreement for a cure—became the general rule in the second half of the seventeenth century, supplanting other forms of payment. During this period, claims filed with the protomedici to request payment no longer included a description of a whole course of treatment but listed instead the number of procedures performed—enumerating the bloodlettings, leech applications, enemas, and the like performed by barber-surgeons, or the total number of visits made by physicians.[7] The main consideration in establishing the amount due for medical services, therefore, was no longer an appraisal of the whole course of treatment and its results. The key factor was now the number of specific services rendered, regardless of their outcome.

This new rule, obviously favoring the practitioner, was not readily accepted by the public. The custom of paying only a deposit during treatment, with the balance due at the end, as in the agreement for a cure, was still alive in the second half of the seventeenth century.[8] As late as the early eighteenth century, either one of the two forms of payment could be optional, as indicated by the choice offered in 1701 by the barber-surgeon Sebastiano Atti to Carlo Ragazzi, who had asked the barber to treat his wounded niece. The barber—as Ragazzi testified in his complaint to the protomedici—had callously requested him to pay "either twenty soldi per visit plus travel expenses, or forty lire at the end of treatment; otherwise I should find somebody else willing to treat her for less."[9]

The very existence of these legal cases is proof that barber-surgeons and physicians had considerable trouble getting paid for each visit and often had to put up with working on credit. In 1664, the barber-surgeon Antonio Bossi began treating on credit Peregrino Atti, a vintner affected by "malignant and callous ulcerations of the virile member and testicles, and other Gallic wounds around the waist." The treatment lasted fourteen months. When Atti suddenly died, the barber had no choice but to bring an action in the Protomedicato against Atti's heir for nonpayment.[10] Dr. Gallerati, a member of the college who testified on behalf of the plaintiff, mentioned having told the barber several times "that he should learn not to work on credit in his profession."[11] Apparently it was not easy for a barber-surgeon to follow this advice. Working on credit was so common that in 1760, after the surgeon Carlo Bartolotti died, his father and heir had to sue thirty-four ex-patients before the Protomedicato for nonpayment.[12]

Physicians often found themselves in a similar predicament. In their case, the pressure to treat patients on credit derived from the custom of working on retainer — usually a yearly salary — for the regular care of a family. The physicians' complaints to the Protomedicato indicate that this salary often went unpaid.

"Most Illustrious Doctors, I have no words to describe the ungratefulness of those who refuse to pay their physicians . . . , a common fault in Italy, and one that the illustrious Scipione Mercuri so justly censured," Dr. Vincenzo Gotti of Budrio wrote the Protomedicato in 1684. In a letter laden with learned quotations from Seneca, Saint Bernard, the Code of Justinian, the jurist Baldo, Ecclesiastes, and whatnot, he proceeded to rail against the "sin against divine and human laws" committed by one Paulo Sgargi, who refused to acknowledge by proper payment "the efforts and labor this writer went through while treating Sgargi himself and his numerous family for over seven years."

Apparently Gotti had begun working for Sgargi while still a medical student, when his predecessor, Dr. Carradori, "had chosen him, as his own pupil, to work as his substitute in Sgargi's household, just as other major physicians used to do in Bologna . . . with many families and monasteries." The Protomedicato sentenced Sgargi to pay Gotti the same amount (twenty Bolognese lire per year) that he had paid for the services of Gotti's predecessor.[13]

Such a dispute was far from unique. In 1706, Dr. Vanini sued the Alimanni family, claiming that he had treated several family members over a ten-year period without being paid for his labor.[14] In 1746, Dr. De Buono sued the widow Bertuccini, on the grounds that he had visited her late husband two hundred times between 1733 and 1744 without receiving any payment.[15]

Obviously, physicians and barber-surgeons based their claims on the idea that treatment should be paid for regardless of its outcome. And yet the old notion of payment by results had not disappeared: practitioners did sometimes mention the patient's full recovery as grounds for advancing their claim to a fee. Statements such as "I treated her day and night, until she healed," and "I cured and restored the patient to health in a period of three months," can be found among the claims for payment filed with the Protomedicato.[16] Nevertheless, by the mid–seventeenth century the outcome of treatment had become a marginal consideration in the minds of the practitioners; what was paramount now was the number of visits or procedures performed. The protomedici fully concurred with this view. From the early eighteenth century on, they routinely asked barber-surgeons and physicians suing for nonpayment to present a detailed list of visits made or services rendered. Only on the basis of such a list would they proceed to establish the fair price of treatment.

What do the Protomedicato records tell us about the amounts charged by medical practitioners for their services? Unfortunately, not all lawsuits provide this information. Often, barber-surgeons and physicians, while describing the number and type of services rendered, did not specify the requested fee, leaving it to be determined by the protomedici. In 1687, for instance, the surgeon Gioseffo Arzelli of Mirandola asked the protomedici to establish a fair fee for his successful treatment of a tumor, as the patient refused to pay "unless they [the protomedici] decided how much was due."[17] Only in some cases did the medical practitioners explicitly state the fee requested for each visit or procedure. This happened increasingly often in the early eighteenth century, when it became common practice to break down the description of treatment into items, that is, the procedures performed. In the period from 1700 to 1776, barber-surgeons requested fees ranging from 1 lira per visit—the most common request—up to 5 lire, an exceptionally high fee, charged in only one case. In 1719, the barber-surgeons' fee for treating patients outside Bologna was 2 lire per visit plus "the cost of hiring a horse . . . , which is to be provided by the person who comes to pick us up . . . and an extra charge in case of bad weather."[18] During the same period, physicians' fees varied from 15 soldi (0.75 lira) to 5 lire per visit. For physicians, also, 1 lira per visit was the most frequent fee. Thus, the rank of the practitioner does not seem to have affected fees: regardless of their different professional standing, physicians and surgeons charged the same amount for the same procedure. It should be noted that physicians' requests for payment in these lawsuits primarily involved surgical procedures. As a matter of fact, physicians practicing surgery became increasingly common in the eighteenth century. By this time, doctors and surgeons often billed patients for similar services rather than distinct and complementary ones, as had been the rule in the past.[19] Clearly, the doctors who stooped to performing a surgeon's task had to put up with the current market price for surgical procedures.[20]

There was often a gap between the fee requested by practitioners and the amount they were ultimately awarded by the Protomedicato. We can see this by comparing the practitioners' requests with the fees set by the protomedici. Such a comparison can be drawn only in 30 percent of these cases (40 out of 131)—that is, only in those cases in which barber-surgeons or physicians declared the monetary value they set on their own work rather than simply deferring to the Protomedicato's evaluation. For example, in 1701 the barber-surgeon Cattani, while relying "on the sum decided by the illustrious dean and protomedici of Bologna," nevertheless specified a fee of one hundred lire for treating Francesca Calegari for three months.[21] He was granted sixty lire—40 percent less than he had requested. Such a reduction was common—interestingly, the fees granted by the protomedici were lower than what was asked by the practitioners in 31 cases out of 40. Of the 31 cases, 20 concerned barber-surgeons; 8, apothecaries; and 3, physicians. Reductions were not applied equally to the three groups. Barber-surgeons were the least well supported by the court, as their requests were reduced, on average, 45 percent. Apothecaries demanding payment for medicines were the least affected, with an average reduction of 21 percent. Only a few physicians filed requests, but those who did also saw their claims dramatically lowered by the Protomedicato, with an average reduction of 32 percent. For example, when Dr. Garani sued Geminiano Pagliani's widow in 1707, demanding fifty lire for treating her husband in a terminal illness, the protomedici ruled that he was owed much less and granted him only twenty lire.[22]

How can we explain these reductions? First, we need to examine the guidelines adopted by the court in establishing the fair price of medical services. As the protomedici declared on one occasion: since in Bologna medical fees were not fixed directly by the law, the Protomedicato had to take into account and evaluate "the kind of patient, the kind of illness, and the kind of healer" involved in each case.[23] These same criteria had traditionally been adopted by Christian authors writing on medical ethics. GianBattista Codronchi, for instance, had stated in the sixteenth century: "A doctor's fair and proper salary should be reckoned considering the kind of treatment, the physician's labor and effort, the patient's financial status, as well as local customs."[24]

How much weight did each of these criteria carry with the Protomedicato? The kind of illness, which implied a qualitative assessment of the difficulties of treatment, as in the old-fashioned agreement for a cure, played only a marginal role in the court's decisions.[25] In 1670, the protomedici discussed the fee due to Dr. Bottoni for treating a terminally ill woman throughout a nine-month period. After the patient's death, the widower had refused to pay the physician.[26] It is noteworthy that in this case the protomedici expressly debated the incurability of the disease. Traditionally, medical ethics had prohibited practitioners from undertaking treatment, and from charging a fee, when the disease was plainly past hope and medication useless.[27] By the late seventeenth century, however, this traditional notion was somewhat in abeyance: the protomedici acknowledged Dr. Bottoni's right to a fee, although they granted him only fifteen lire — a very small sum for more than nine months of treatment.

In contrast, the kind of healer had greater weight in the protomedici's mind. In establishing a fair price for treatment, the protomedici attempted to bolster the hierarchical ranking of the medical professions, especially the difference between physicians and barber-surgeons, which was no longer reflected in the market price of their services. The fees requested by barber-surgeons were more severely adjusted by the protomedici than those of other practitioners.

And yet it would be wrong to conclude, on the basis of these decisions, that the protomedici's main object was to protect the physicians' professional interests. If that had been the case, they would have honored the fees requested by the doctors who appealed to the court. As we know, they didn't; the doctors' requests were also dramatically lowered by the protomedici. The fact is that the Protomedicato took into account yet a third element in establishing fair medical fees: the economic and social status of the patient. In 1672, for instance, the barber-surgeon Gio. Battista Cavazza claimed payment for treating Barbara Gotti for gangrene and curing her. The treatment had lasted two and a half months. The Protomedicato decided that Cavazza deserved thirty lire, "notwithstanding he was the parish's barber, because the cure had been of outstanding merit."[28] But after a plea by the patient's husband, who lamented his poverty, the protomedici lowered the fee to ten lire.[29] In many other cases, the poverty of a patient was a major consideration that led to lowering a practitioner's fee. In a case heard in 1747, the surgeon Lodi's request for one lira per visit was cut in half "because the patient is poor." The protomedici further met the patient's financial needs by ruling that he could pay half of the amount within fifteen days, and the balance within three months.[30]

The patient's poverty was a very important consideration, as we may expect, especially in those cases filed by the patients themselves. In 1710, Antonio Bosi, a peasant, appealed to the Protomedicato to "moderate the demands of Messer Pier Paolo, who asks for ten paoli per visit."[31] Messer Pier Paolo, a barber-surgeon from Bologna, had rendered his services in the country and was now requesting five lire per visit, an exorbitant fee for a surgeon. The Protomedicato reduced it to one lira and eighteen soldi — a decrease of more than 60 percent of the practitioner's initial request.[32]

Medical men were aware of the importance of a patient's financial status in the Protomedicato's eyes, so much so that in their pleadings they often mentioned a patient's ability to pay. When Dr. Bertocchi sued the widow Ranuzzi in 1699, he attached to his bill a note from the parish priest asserting that the woman "owned a well-furnished apartment with household goods, clothes, jewelry, and linens, and that the apartment undoubtedly belonged to her as her own dowry."[33]

By considering the patient's financial status, the protomedici clearly distanced themselves from the economic interests of practicing physicians and surgeons. In 1719, the barber-surgeons of Bologna wrote to the protomedici to inform them of their official fees, asserting that whenever they were called out of town "to treat all sorts of external diseases among peasants, even poor ones," they always charged the same sum: two lire per visit, plus travel expenses.[34] They clearly implied that the price of treatment should be one and the same for all, rich or poor. The protomedici, however, were of a different mind; they thought that a patient's social condition should make a difference when medical fees were concerned. In this respect, their view was certainly at odds with the practitioners' economic interest. In 1747, the barber-surgeon Lodi treated Domenico Malvasi for a wound. When the patient refused to pay, the surgeon sued him in the Protomedicato and was awarded forty lire. Confiscation of Malvasi's property was ordered. On appeal, however, Malvasi argued that the surgeon's fee should be paid by the person who had wounded him, one Agostino Masi, since the law stated that medical expenses incurred by the victim of an assault should be paid by the person who had inflicted the injury. The Protomedicato revised the fee, bringing it down from forty lire to twenty-five, in view of Masi's more limited financial means.[35]

Such episodes clearly show that the protomedici's notion of a fair fee could conflict with the financial interests of the practitioners. A significant case in this respect was a suit that was filed in 1719 with the Protomedicato and was settled on appeal by the college two years later.[36] The parties were Dr. Landi, a public lecturer in medicine (but not a member of the college),[37] and the brothers Michele and Sebastiano Costa, of a family of sharecroppers. In 1718, Sebastiano fell sick with "a malignant fever, with decubitus ulcers and gangrene." Dr. Landi was called, and after forty-two days during which the doctor visited his patient daily, the latter healed. On a trip to Bologna to buy medicines for his brother, Michele Costa was warned by the apothecary that the services of a public lecturer would be expensive and was advised to find a hospital bed for his brother. Proudly, Michele answered that "he did not want to send his brother to the hospital, and that he had enough to pay Dr. Landi his due, since he owned his own cattle and barn, plus some farmer's stock."[38] As he himself testified in court, "I told the apothecary that I owned a couple of oxen which I would sell, and since the price of meat was rising at the time, that I was going to sell said oxen for a better price, and that with the money . . . I would pay Dr. Landi — but only as suitable to my social standing [secondo il mio stato]."

By the end of the treatment, however, the doctor requested five lire per visit, a much larger fee than expected. Moreover, the Costas' good fortune took a turn for the worse, "for their cattle died," as the parish priest testified on their behalf. Michele Costa tried to come to an amicable settlement with the doctor. "Instead of money, he seemed willing to accept a portion of my crops plus some hemp seeds and fodder."[39] The agreement, however, did not work out, and Landi summoned the Costa brothers before the Protomedicato, demanding payment of five lire per visit.

The debate over the Costas' finances was crucial for the outcome of the case in court. Dr. Landi's lawyer argued that their claim of poverty was unsubstantiated and that the doctor fully deserved the requested fee, considering that barber-surgeons were currently charging two lire per visit in the countryside. Dr. Landi, after all, was capable of serving at the same time as physician as well as surgeon. As for the Costa brothers, they proudly stated over and over again that they did not consider themselves poor, but they petitioned to pay "according to their social condition and financial situation." In order to verify the latter, the protomedici carefully examined the sharecropping contract between the Costas and the Countess Malvasia; the will of their paternal uncle, which had left them some property in equal shares and co-ownership (in comunione); and even the notarized statements of their wives' dowries.[40]

When, finally, the Protomedicato established Dr. Landi's fee at three lire and five soldi per visit (a reduction of 35% from his original request), the physician appealed to the cardinal legate, who returned the case to the medical college. In 1721, the college upheld the Protomedicato's sentence.

Posed between a physician and public lecturer on the one hand and a family of sharecroppers on the other, the college doctors — contrary to what one might expect — did not side with their professional colleague. With their sentence they seemed rather to strive for some measure of equity and fairness. Taking into consideration the Costas' financial and social status, they put limits on Landi's demands. At the same time, they upheld the medical hierarchy by granting the physician a slightly higher fee than the two lire per visit usually awarded to third-degree surgeons.[41] Their decision in this case, therefore, derived from the consideration of the two items most relevant to the fair price of medical service: the practitioner's rank and the patient's social condition.

All of this suggests that the Protomedicato's intent in handling these cases was not merely to protect the self-interest of the medical men. By lowering the practitioners' fees, the protomedici obviously tried to acknowledge the interests of patients and to grant them some equity in medical transactions. This is confirmed by their settlements of disputes over bills for medicines due to the apothecaries. As we saw in chapter 1, charges for drugs had to conform to the official prices of medicines which were periodically revised and published by the Protomedicato together with the apothecaries' guild.[42] An officer of the guild, known as the *tassatore,* was responsible for ascertaining that sale prices conformed to this list, but in case of disagreement both customers and apothecaries could turn to the Protomedicato as a court of appeals.

For the protomedici, this provided an opportunity to ensure that apothecaries observed the regulations established by the medical college for the preparation of drugs. In fact, apothecaries were entitled to be paid for medicines only if they had prepared them in accordance with a prescription signed by a physician. Payment could be withheld if the medication varied from the recipe prescribed in the pharmacopoeia—that is, customers did not have to pay unless it was proven that the remedy had been made according to standards.[43] In this way, the protomedici simultaneously protected the rights of the sick as consumers of medicines and enforced their own view of the medical hierarchy.

As I have already mentioned, the apothecaries' bills challenged by patients in court were significantly reduced (21% on average) by the protomedici from the sums previously established by the tassatore of the apothecaries' guild.[44] The protomedici, therefore, seem to have been stricter guardians of the "fair price" of medicines than were the officers of the apothecaries' guild. Here, also, their conduct seems to have been prompted by a spirit of fairness and nonpartisanship, rather than by the self-interest of the medical establishment.

Thus, when ruling on medical fees, the Protomedicato seemed to be more sensitive to the interests of the sick than to those of medical professionals, including physicians (as shown by the case of Landi versus Costa). How can this be explained? The behavior of the medical elite seems to conform not so much to the principles of economic or professional ethos (the defense of the self-interest of a professional group) but rather to what Norbert Elias called "estate-ethos": "Of every fairly stable elite group, caste or social stratum that is exposed to pressure from below and often from above as well, it can be said . . . that, to the people comprising it, their mere existence as members of an elite social unit is, partly or absolutely, a value and end in itself. The maintenance of distance thus becomes a decisive motor or matrix of their behaviour. . . . The symbols or ideas in which such social units express the goals or motivations of their behaviour therefore always have the character of prestige-fetishes."[45] The fetish of prestige certainly influenced the behavior of Bologna's medical college: the annals of the college record meticulously, for more than two centuries, the collegiates' fastidious, almost obsessive, observance of the rules of precedence and rank for doctors in theology, law, and medicine during public ceremonies.[46] We should recall here what I stressed in chapter 1: the medical college was not a professional association but rather an elite inaccessible to most physicians. When I analyzed the social composition of the college, I pointed out that the majority of its members came from the patrician-mercantile upper class that controlled the city's public offices. The doctors of the college did not identify with other physicians. They felt themselves to be above any professional group, part of the oligarchy governing the city. This may help us to understand why the protomedici's behavior was prompted by their estate-ethos rather than by the self-interest of the medical profession.

In order to understand the protomedici's conduct, one should also take into account the role played by Christian values in medical ethics. In their effort to mediate between the interests of sick persons and those of medical practitioners, the protomedici were influenced by a notion of Christian charity strongly redolent of aristocratic patronage. Charity, in this view, implied a paradoxical reversal of roles between the strong and the weak, so that the weak actually derived strength from their weakness. The strength of the weak, in the eyes of the upper classes, was based on their right to protection —a right supported by the mandates of Christian ethics as well as by the aristocratic dictum "noblesse oblige." The obligation to protect the weak was a typical trait of ancien régime political culture, in which paternalism was rampant and the powerful often legitimized their rule by posing as protectors of the poor. The Christian obligation of charity, perceived through the lens of paternalism, smoothly merged with the cult of prestige associated with the estate-ethos. It is in this framework that we can understand the medical college's attitude toward the sick. The protomedici's attitude clearly paralleled the paternalism of the urban ruling classes. They did not see the sick from the modern viewpoint, as clients dealing with professionals, but rather as clients in relation to patrons, plebeians vis-à-vis patricians. Seen in this light, the patient appeared as a weak party, and as such, was entitled to protection. The aristocratic duty to protect merged with the Christian commandment of charity. What the protomedici meant to grant to the sick by warranting the fair price of medicines and medical services was not so much equity as, in fact, charity—which, as such, was properly addressed first of all to those patients who suffered the double frailty of sickness and poverty.

In Bologna, the charitable duty of protecting the sick was keenly felt by the upper classes during the Counter Reformation. The city's social framework was made up of groups that acknowledged their duty to protect the physical as well as the spiritual well-being of their members. Many Bolognese parishes retained a physician for the poor. A decree issued in 1570 by Cardinal Gabriele Paleotti mandated that each parish should hire a physician for this purpose.[47] Paleotti also formed a congregation whose goal was to visit and financially support the poor and the sick of the city.[48] Confraternities played an important role in assisting the sick, in Bologna as well as in other cities. In 1576 the Compagnia dei Poveri (Company of the Poor) was founded in Bologna. It paid a yearly salary to a physician in order to provide its members with free medical care.[49] While this company had been created by men of the lower classes, the Congregazione degli Agonizzanti, founded in 1627 in the church of Sant'Isaia, had been established instead by wealthy and aristocratic patrons. As described by Antonio Masini (author of a seventeenth-century guide to Bologna), the congregation "assigned certain citizens to each parish of the city, with the authority to distribute the congregation's help to the sick, who do not wish to go—or cannot go—to the hospitals. There are a physician and a surgeon to serve the sick, besides other medical practitioners kept by the parish and the city for the sake of the poor."[50] In 1644 a testator appointed the congregation to manage a charitable trust for the purpose of distributing medicines to the indigent, or, in the words of the donor, "to help all the sick people who are poor, provided they be born and bred in the city of Bologna, who can prove their citizenship through the baptism books, and who can testify their poverty through the reverend curate, wherever they live, by providing them with all the medicines, ointments, balsams, decoctions, plasters, and any other remedy needed to treat their illnesses, except for those medicines whose recipes include gold, pearls, or gems."[51] By the end of the seventeenth century, the congregation annually distributed medicines worth 1,436 lire to the poor.[52] A similar legacy was entrusted to the Congregazione degli Agonizzanti by a certain Balduzzi in 1706; in this case, the benefit was limited to the poor of the parishes of San Biagio and San Tommaso, and the medicines had to be purchased in a specified apothecary shop. At the end of the eighteenth century this trust was still underwriting medicines for the poor.[53]

It is noteworthy that when the Compagnia degli Agonizzanti was founded, its executive board included, in addition to several high-profile prelates and senators, six doctors of medicine, all of whom were members of the college, not least among them the well-known protomedico Ovidio Montalbani.[54] The statutes of the company stated that sick persons wishing to receive medicines should contact the company's officers directly. Thus, the company's charity was not anonymous; it was tendered by means of a personal relationship of patronage between the noble and the humble, the rich and the poor, emphasizing the paternalistic nature of their social bond.

"Charitable citizens" were also encouraged to provide financial support for the city hospitals.[55] Such patronage flaunted their munificence by turning their "charity" into a grand, carefully orchestrated public spectacle. Thus, the inauguration of a new hospital in 1725 became an occasion to celebrate the ruling classes' bounty. The sick were carried from the old building to the new Ospedale della Vita amidst festivities including "the gathering of a large crowd, windows adorned with banners, bells pealing, and an indulgence specially granted by the pope." The *Te deum* was sung "to the harmonious resounding of many drums" in the hospital's new church, and the sick, "comfortably carried by coach," were joined in a parade by the members of the hospital's archconfraternity of Santa Maria della Vita—"the majority of them Doctors and dignitaries of this city," as was noted pointedly in a contemporary chronicle.[56] This image of the city's sick and the city's notables united in a pageant clearly shows how the urban elite's charity was inseparably connected with their pursuit of prestige.

II. MALPRACTICE

Un homme mort n'est qu'un homme mort, et ne fait point de conséquence;
mais une formalité négligée porte un notable préjudice à tout le corps des médecins.
—Molière, *L'amour médecin*, act 2, scene 4

Those sick persons who were poor were acknowledged and to some extent protected. But what about the patients' peculiar vulnerability in entrusting their bodies to a healer: was it also acknowledged and protected? Let us see what happened when patients brought charges against practitioners for incompetence or negligence, that is, for malpractice. These legal cases are rare, which means that I will be able to review most of them. They involved minor practitioners such as barber-surgeons, apothecaries, and unlicensed healers, but apparently no physicians.[57]

On August 5, 1618, Ginevra Mangini — the thirty-six-year-old wife of a Bolognese notary — fell ill "with measles and *mal mazzucco,* accompanied by constant fever." Her physician prescribed an ointment of cedar-flower oil to be applied on the side of her heart to "comfort and arouse the vital and spiritual parts of the body." The women of the household applied the ointment purchased by the patient's husband at the Star, the shop owned by the apothecary Sirani. As testified by the woman's maid and by her sister-in-law:

> It seemed that the oil affected her, so that she began to rave, shouting that her heart was burning, and asking that we take away that fire as she could not endure it . . . ; but not believing that such changes were caused by the said oil, we did not heed her, and made her keep the ointment, believing we were doing the right thing. . . . And in the morning, we found that the skin where the oil had been rubbed on, and likewise the part of her shirt that had been soaked with the oil, were badly burnt.[58]

Ginevra died one day later, still screaming: "My heart is burning, my heart is burning, I'm on fire, take this fire away from me." To the priest who tried to persuade her to "confess and reconcile herself with God," she said that "she could not, and that first they should remove that fire from her body, and she beseeched me, for God's grace, to check and see myself that part that had been anointed."[59]

Because of an error — the apothecary had mistakenly switched cedar-flower oil with sulphur oil — Ginevra died with the excruciating feeling of being on fire. During the trial in the Protomedicato, where her husband brought charges immediately after the event, the doctor who had prescribed the ointment minimized the apothecary's responsibility in the woman's death: "I don't believe, however, that the death of this woman could have been caused by the sulphur oil — the heat from the oil may well have altered the course of the disease to some extent, but it could not, in and of itself, have caused her death."[60]

Not surprisingly, the apothecary fully concurred with this view, arguing that "by itself, this external ointment cannot cause alterations, or any more pain than what she already suffered." His defense was based on the premise that a medication applied externally could not be dangerous. "This oil can be given even internally to some patients, it cures them and is not such that may damage anyone when applied externally." (Yet the witnesses from Ginevra's household uniformly testified that the skin on which the oil had been rubbed was "all black and burnt" the following day.) According to the apothecary, an externally applied medication could not have caused such serious consequences. "The delirium and raving that were mentioned were brought about by the extremely serious illness that she probably had, and in fact, are accidents and effects deriving from the *mal mazzucco* and petechia by which she was affected."[61]

No other experts — neither physicians nor apothecaries — were summoned as witnesses in the case, which was concluded in a very few days. In their verdict, the protomedici called the apothecary's behavior "incautious." They declared that his error had certainly worsened the patient's condition, although nothing could be said as to the true causes of the woman's death. The apothecary was suspended from practicing and his shop was closed for an indefinite period of time. He was also fined nine lire. The verdict was issued on August 19, 1618. On August 25, the apothecary was allowed to re-open his shop, but on the condition that only his son — who had been approved by the college as an apprentice apothecary — be allowed to serve customers. When the college gathered for the celebration of Saints Cosmas and Damian, on September 27, the apothecary appealed to the protomedici's clemency, and he was reinstated into practice. Thus, the case was quickly dispatched by the Protomedicato with a very lenient verdict, soon followed by a pardon.

When passing sentence in cases involving malpractice charges against licensed practitioners, the Protomedicato was an extremely lenient court. Let us examine another case, this time involving a surgeon. In 1761, a family from Budrio filed charges in the Protomedicato against the barber Alessandro Guidetti, for having prescribed a fatal dose of jalap to be taken internally. In their opinion, without the intervention of the town's doctor the patient would have died. The entire village, they said, was clamoring about "this violent medicine, inappropriately used."[62] When examined by the protomedici, the surgeon Guidetti acknowledged his mistake: he had written *resina di gialappa* (jalap resin) instead of *radice di gialappa* (jalap root) on the prescription. He was clearly in trouble. As a barber-surgeon he had broken two basic Protomedicato rules: not only had he prescribed an oral medicine, he had even signed a prescription — something that only a physician was allowed to do. The protomedici fined him for breaking these rules, but their sentence did not mention his error or his endangering the patient's life. Unlike other surgeons who had overstepped the boundaries of their profession, Guidetti was not even suspended from practice. The fine was reduced after he pleaded that he worked "as a simple free-lancer" (without a regular contract with a community).[63] Clearly, in this case the protomedici punished the surgeon for transgressing the rules of the medical establishment, not for his negligence toward a patient.

The protomedici's rulings in these cases clearly contrast with the severe penalties established by the college laws. According to these laws, if a healer's error or incompetence endangered a patient's life, the usual fine for illicit practice (one hundred gold *scudi* for a physician, or fifty gold scudi for a surgeon) was doubled. If the patient died because of the healer's negligence, the fine rose to five hundred gold scudi, in addition to corporal punishment to be meted out by the cardinal legate.[64] These laws, however, were mere words on paper. In point of fact, they were never applied during the Protomedicato's two hundred years of activity. We saw above, when discussing control over illegal practice in chapter 3, that only rarely did the court sentence unlicensed healers to exile. Even in those cases, the Protomedicato's severity seemed aimed at chastising repeated violations of the rules of professional practice rather than misconduct toward a patient.

The Protomedicato's verdicts were very lenient even in cases of manslaughter. In 1588, Giacoma Gandolfi filed charges with the protomedici against a woman healer, Marina Rondoni, accusing her of causing the death of her daughter Angelina, a three year old affected by ringworm: "I entreat Your Honors to believe that, my little girl being sick, I was told to find this Marina, who says that she is capable of treating this disease; and I went to see her in her house on a Monday, twenty-five days ago."[65]

Giacoma vividly remembered the agreement for a cure she made with Marina. Thanks to her deposition, we can almost hear the two women talking:

> "Madonna Marina, here is my daughter, whom I would like you to cure, if you are sure you can, of the ringworm that she has on her head."
> "I will certainly cure her, and if I do, I want three lire from you in payment, but nothing if I do not cure her."
> "I will spare no expense, as long as my girl heals."
> "Fear not, that I have heart enough to heal her."

Giacoma also describes the treatment in detail.

And she [the healer] took one of her waters, and with a sponge she bathed her [the girl's] head; and that water smelled so strongly that it gave me a headache. I took my daughter home after that, and that very first night her head became swollen. I went back to the woman on the morrow, and I told her what happened, and she gave me some water, telling me to keep sponging the girl with said water. Which I did five times, and then I started anointing part of her head, as the woman had taught me. . . . But the disease did not stop . . . , and on a Friday, that will be two weeks ago from tomorrow, she died.

After hearing the healer's confession (which is not reported in the records), the protomedici ordered her to return to Giacoma the money advanced for the cure. They also reprimanded her and ordered that she stop medicating in general and prescribing both the water and the ointment (which, however, they did not confiscate or examine). The Protomedicato did not take any other action against Marina Rondoni. Yet to all appearances she was probably guilty of manslaughter (the water or ointment she had used might have contained mercury, which poisoned the little girl). Moreover, Giacoma Gandolfi had not just charged the healer with fraud or simply asked the protomedici for her money back. Her plea to the protomedici stressed the details of Angelina's death; it was clearly for this death that she sought explanation and justice: "The second evening after the ointment had been applied, stuff started to come out of her head, that is, blood and *marza* [rotten matter] . . . and after she died, [her body] got all swollen, and a large amount of black stuff came out of her mouth and nose."

Yet the protomedici did not pay attention to these details. They did not start an inquiry to establish whether the girl's death was due to poisoning. How should we interpret their behavior in this case? Obviously they did not bother to investigate in depth the healer's responsibility in the girl's death. In their eyes, this was just one of the many cases of illicit practice, to be quickly solved with a reprimand and with the restitution of the extorted money to the injured party.

An error committed by a healer against a patient's body was viewed with forbearance by the protomedici even when it clearly involved stark incompetence or ignorance — in which case, according to early modern manuals of legal medicine, a medical practitioner was clearly liable for damages. In 1739, Gioseffo Pozzi, one of Count Malvasia's sharecropping farmers, went to the Protomedicato for redress. Showing the protomedici his right arm, he asked that they proceed against barber Filippo Nanni, also known as

"Pernazza," because of his "imperizia" (lack of skill). The barber, Pozzi explained, had made a mistake when bleeding him, so that his arm had become swollen. Examining the man's arm, the protomedici diagnosed an aneurysm — a swelling caused by the puncturing of an artery or nerve, which could result in partial or total paralysis of the affected part. According to the medical knowledge of the time, occasioning an aneurysm by bloodletting was the very epitome of a barber-surgeon's blunder. It was a well-established principle that blood should be drawn not from the arteries but only from the veins. Puncturing an artery was, therefore, a major fault for a barber and was branded as such in phlebotomy handbooks.[66] Furthermore, authorities on medical law such as Zacchia itemized such an error as one of the instances in which a surgeon could be legally prosecuted for his lack of skill.[67]

When examined by the protomedici, Filippo Nanni, otherwise known as Pernazza, was found to be an unlicensed barber-surgeon, despite his twenty-five years of practice. He admitted to having bled Pozzi three months before, "from the cephalic vein," and attributed the swelling to the patient's neglect of his instructions. "The day after he was bled, Pozzi, in my presence, removed the pad *[piumazzolo]*, and with his hand pressed the lips of the cut, so that a little blood came out, nor did I notice any swelling, but I warned him against touching the wound, because of the danger which could come from it."[68] Pernazza was clearly well versed in the art of shifting the blame from himself onto others. On this very same occasion, he took the opportunity to report to the protomedici a fellow healer and rival — a Carmelite friar who claimed to be a surgeon and apothecary and prescribed bloodletting and purges. When the protomedici interrupted him to ask whether he knew that puncturing an artery may lead to an aneurysm, the man answered yes. He was admonished and warned to stop practicing surgery, because he was unlicensed, but no other measures were taken against him — not even the usual fine for practicing without a license.[69] Nor did the protomedici's ruling mention any compensation for damages to the unfortunate patient.

It definitely looks as if the protomedici were very reluctant to punish even illicit healers for medical error — very loath even to admit that a practitioner's lack of skill could lead to a patient's death or disability. Malpractice cases, unlike those concerning payment of medical fees, show the protomedici as being less sympathetic to patients' rights and more mindful of the collective interests of the medical profession. One trial, especially, suggests that the protomedici viewed with marked disfavor, and were likely to turn against, patients who accused their healers of malpractice. This case also involved an apothecary, Angelo Michele Cantoni. On July 28, 1673, a priest,

Gioseppe Padoani, filed a charge against the apothecary for administering a harmful medication which, by the apothecary's own admission, had not been prepared according to the recipe. The plaintiff testified, moreover, that as soon as the apothecary saw the bad effects of the medication, he tried to shift the blame to the physician who had prescribed it, by saying that "it was no surprise that such remedy caused such effects, because a corrosive spirit can derive from it."[70]

The physician involved in the case was a collegiate, Ippolito Poggioli, who thought it appropriate to respond to the apothecary's criticism with a printed letter of self-apology addressed ostensibly to the medical college but clearly aimed at the general public. In the letter, the doctor maintained that the remedy he had prescribed could not have caused the effects observed in the patient, had it been prepared according to the recipe. He supported his statement by citing many medical authorities, ancient and modern. The circumstances of the case seemed thus to be highly unfavorable to the apothecary, who not only had broken a crucial professional rule in disregarding the physician's recipe but had even dared to criticize a college doctor.

In spite of these circumstances, however, the protomedici's handling of the case shows a heavy bias in favor of the apothecary. They repeatedly asked witnesses whether Padoani could be considered to have been of sound mind during his illness, and whether he was a priest of good repute. In short, they questioned the truthfulness and moral character of the victim rather than those of the defendant.

Perhaps Padoani was pressured to withdraw his charges. In any case, on September 28 he returned to the Protomedicato, obviously aware of the insinuations against his good name. He protested that he had not intended to punish anyone by pressing charges but had only wished to make the truth known; that he would not stain his honor as a clergyman with a lie; and that he would leave to God the task of redressing the injury he had suffered at the apothecary's hands—although the latter's fault, he pointed out, "was clear and evident to anyone." Clearly, Padoani did not mean to retract his charges; he simply meant to let the protomedici know that he would no longer expect justice from them. The protomedici pronounced their sentence two days later, on September 30—"having only God in front of their eyes," as proclaimed in the formula prefixed to their verdicts. Like the plaintiff, they decided to leave to God the task of punishing the apothecary, and without any explanation whatsoever they acquitted him of all charges.

The sentences in these malpractice cases were always favorable to the practitioners. Did people notice this blind spot in the Protomedicato's justice?

We have already mentioned that malpractice charges were much less frequent than those filed against a healer for breaking a contract for a cure. By filing charges for breach of contract, patients could reasonably hope to regain at least part of their money. In contrast, they probably knew that they could not expect much as a result of filing a malpractice charge. This does not mean, of course, that patients were not capable of recognizing a healer's or a practitioner's incompetence or negligence. All that I can infer from the sources is that patients did not appeal to the Protomedicato for redress from malpractice injuries, although they might well have been aware of such injuries. For example, Orsola Alberici of Castel San Pietro knew very well that her son had been crippled by a doctor:

> As I was asked for the truth I can truly say that, since the second day of Lent to the present day, my son Lorenzo Alberici has been lying in bed, as Your Honor can see him, and the nature of his disease has never been understood, either by Dr. Arrighi, physician in Castello, or by the apothecary, Sig. Giuseppe Rinaldi. The doctor bled him first from his right arm three or four days after he fell sick, and a second time four days later from his left foot, but neither was beneficial. He then ordered that Sig. Giuseppe Rinaldi, apothecary, again bleed him from the same foot; and in consequence of such bleedings my son has been crippled, as Your Honor can see him, so that he can neither stand nor sit down.[71]

Orsola Alberici made this statement to the college's notary, who had been sent by the protomedici to Castel San Pietro in 1701 to investigate the conduct of the village surgeon, whom both the physician and the apothecary accused of overstepping the limits of his profession. Orsola took this opportunity to testify, instead, against the village physician, who she believed was responsible for her son's disability. She did not lodge a formal complaint against Arrighi; she simply tried to get the ear of the medical authorities about her son's misfortune—an affliction for which she probably felt there was no remedy or justice available. The protomedici, in turn, were only interested in solving a case of heated rivalry and conflict among the village practitioners and had no time for or interest in her story. Orsola's charge against the physician was totally ignored.

A considerable amount of courage was needed to formally file malpractice charges against a professional practitioner. This can be seen in the trial of a surgeon in 1770. In this case, several years passed before charges were filed by a whole village. The entire community thus sided with the victim against the practitioner. In 1770, the *massaro* of the municipality of Sant'Agostino lodged a charge against the surgeon Pietro Melloni in the Protomedicato, for an incident that had taken place three years earlier. Awareness of the grievance had grown slowly within the community:

> Your Honor should know that in the village of Sant'Agostino, people were saying that Sig. Pietro Paolo Melloni went to visit Andrea Giovannini's wife, who was sick and pregnant . . . , and gave her some mercury by mouth, although her teeth were locked and he had to force her with an iron tool or pliers . . . ; likewise, he insisted on forcibly removing the baby from her body. Although Giovannini was opposed to this treatment, Melloni said, "Let me do it, as I know what I'm doing," and the patient herself did not want this to happen and showed her unwillingness with signs; but despite it all, he insisted on forcibly removing the baby, and a few hours after the surgery, the woman died, and so did her creature, without being baptized.[72]

The woman's husband, a sawyer, confirmed this deposition. He remembered that Melloni had turned toward him and the priest, who were both in the room during the delivery, and said "that it was proper to help the woman by extracting the creature, and I told him, not even knowing what I was saying, that he should do what he thought right." Initially, he had not wanted to file charges against the surgeon, "because I didn't want to harm anyone."[73] Apparently, the community had pressured both him and the massaro to take legal action. What the villagers found unacceptable was the violent treatment of the woman in labor. As reported by the massaro: "The whole village talked of how Melloni had extracted the fetus violently against the woman's wish and her husband's will."

At the trial in the Protomedicato, Melloni denied all charges — first of all, the charge that he had given mercury by mouth (the most serious crime from the viewpoint of the medical authorities), but also the charge that he had violently extracted the fetus. He claimed that he had merely explored the uterus and that the birth had been spontaneous. (But all the witnesses' depositions were against him.) The Protomedicato's verdict followed the usual pattern: Melloni was found guilty of "overstepping the boundaries of his trade and avocation" because he had prescribed an oral medicine despite his being a simple surgeon, and was fined fifty scudi. On the count of "violent extraction of the fetus and violent administering of mercury," the protomedici ruled that the charge was not sufficiently proved, and left the case open for future retrial.[74] In other words, the protomedici found the practitioner guilty and punished him for transgressing against the official medical hierarchy but did not bother to fully investigate and prosecute the malpractice charges. And actually, by this time (the 1770s), the protomedici seemed to have lost much of the zeal with which they had previously guarded the boundaries of the three medical professions. The verdict sentencing Melloni to a fine of fifty scudi was pronounced on March 23, 1771. On March 30, only a week later, Melloni appealed to the protomedici's mercy and was granted a total pardon from the fine.[75] Melloni, who was a repeat offender (having been disciplined in 1754 and 1763 for administering internal medications),[76] ended up only paying trial expenses.

Yet there was more to this case than mere malpractice. Melloni's behavior was at odds with the principles of traditional medical ethics. By extracting the fetus against the woman's will, he had forced her to submit to a relatively new and experimental procedure. In the second half of the eighteenth century, the presence of an obstetric surgeon at delivery was still unusual in Bologna, and particularly so in the countryside. This explains why the people of Sant'Agostino cast a suspicious eye on Melloni's performance as a childbirth attendant. Furthermore, his use of violent means in inducing labor seemed unprecedented and illegitimate. In fact, Melloni's conduct violated traditional medical ethics, which firmly opposed any kind of experimentation on patients. Only those treatments and medications whose effectiveness had been proven over time were to be employed by the conscientious physician or surgeon. Debating medical men's responsibilities toward their patients, canon law jurists had advocated for centuries the concept that it is better to leave patients in God's hands than to expose them to new and uncertain medical procedures.[77] This Christian moral principle was also supported by the therapeutic conservatism of Galenic medicine, which discouraged experimentation on patients.

And yet, in spite of all this, the Protomedicato did not find Melloni's behavior objectionable. One reason for this might be that the medical college was trying in those years to support the surgeons' attempt to include obstetrics within surgical practice, taking it away from the midwives. Perhaps this extension of male professional expertise seemed to the protomedici a more compelling goal than loyalty to the principles of traditional ethics.[78] In any case, it is clear that in Melloni's trial the Protomedicato's behavior was determined by the wish to protect the surgeons' professional interests rather than by the wish to protect the patients.

In the protomedici's conduct, therefore, it is possible to notice a contrast between the sentences they delivered in the lawsuits concerning payment and those they delivered in lawsuits concerning malpractice. In the former, they complied with the Christian ideal of "fair fee" and upheld the patients' right to a fair price for medical service. In the case of malpractice suits, by contrast, they did not protect the victims and did not punish unskilled or negligent practitioners. Why?

In evaluating a judge's conduct, one ought to measure it against the laws that the judge was called upon to enforce. The judicial conduct of the protomedici, therefore, should be evaluated in the context of early modern legal norms on patients' rights. In the seventeenth century, a vast juridical literature existed which dealt specifically with the "privilegia infirmorum" (special rights of the sick). First developed in the Roman Catholic countries at the beginning of the seventeenth century and later circulated throughout Europe,[79] these treatises collected and discussed the civil and canon laws concerning the sick. The sick person, like the poor, was viewed as handicapped by his condition and consequently as requiring legal protection by means of special rights or "privileges." Thus, for example, the sick were exempt from torture and were allowed to file charges against their enemies in any court of law, regardless of jurisdictional prerogative. Furthermore, their cases were undertaken by magistrates as an obligation of the latters' office, and their last wills were free of the usual legal restrictions and encumbrances.[80] Most significantly, the privileges of the sick derived from a paternalistic view of society, according to which the social fabric was cemented by the provision of protection in exchange for dependency between superior and subordinate. For example, the fathers who denied medical treatment to their children lost their *patria potestas* (paternal power, guardianship) over them; the husband who denied medical treatment to his wife lost his right to her dowry if she died from her illness.[81] Thus, the privileges of the sick were seen as inherently linked to a state of dependency; they derived from the acknowledged duty of the powerful to succor the weak. They were meant not as rights in the modern sense but rather as a concession, a gracious gift granted from above,[82] in a vertical social compact whereby those in authority (including fathers and husbands) offered protection to those in their charge. The legal literature on the "privileges of the sick" provides further illustrations of the paternalistic stance that we have seen at work in the protomedici's conduct toward the sick. The relationship between doctor and patient was seen as similar to that between aristocratic patron and plebeian client. From this viewpoint, it is possible to understand the protomedici's handling of the lawsuits concerning payment. By protecting indigent patients from practitioners' greed, the protomedici felt that they were fulfilling their aristocratic duty to shield the weak and at the same time satisfying popular expectations. They were playing by the rules of the paternalistic "moral economy" that also bound the medical authorities, as we saw in chapter 3.

Significantly, the legal commentaries on the privileges of the sick have very little to say about patients' rights in case of malpractice. And yet a practitioner's legal responsibility for the death or disability of a patient was acknowledged by both civil and canon law.[83] It is true, however, that Roman law did not allow criminal prosecution of manslaughter by the hand of a medical practitioner. According to Roman law, a practitioner who fatally injured a patient could be prosecuted on criminal charges only if he had deliberately inflicted the injury. If the injury had been due to a lack of skill or to negligence, even if it led to the death of the patient, the practitioner could be brought to justice only with a civil suit pressing a claim for damages.[84]

Early modern jurists followed the text of the Roman law, arguing that in case of a patient's death a medical practitioner could not be criminally prosecuted on grounds of incompetence or negligence.[85] Paolo Zacchia, the foremost authority in seventeenth-century legal medicine, also shared this opinion. He modified it somewhat, however, by suggesting that unlicensed healers and those low-grade practitioners who exceeded the boundaries of their profession ought to be subject to criminal punishment in case of a patient's death.[86] This view was adopted by other jurists who also thought that empirics and charlatans should be liable to criminal, not only civil, prosecution.[87] Clearly, when seventeenth-century jurists discussed malpractice, the focus of their interest was how to penalize illegal practice, and not how to compensate the victims of a licensed practitioner's misdeeds. The possibility that a licensed practitioner might be open to malpractice charges was, in fact, never contemplated in these texts. Furthermore, and somewhat paradoxically, the legal literature on the privileges of the sick never mentioned the right of the patient to be compensated for damages caused by malpractice. In view of all this, we can say that the protomedici's attitude to malpractice was consistent with the jurisprudence of their own times. But we should not forget, however, that their behavior was at variance with the text of the law. The law explicitly recognized the rights of the victims of medical error to file a civil suit for damages.[88] The protomedici could have applied this law, but they didn't, just as the jurists ignored it in their tracts on the privileges of the sick. Why so? Perhaps because jurists and protomedici alike viewed the patient as a weak person in need of protection, rather than as a citizen with the right to claim compensation for damages. The very notion of the privileges of the sick was the reverse side of the image of the protomedici as learned and powerful protectors. It was definitely meant to enhance and not to undermine their prestige. For the protomedici to acknowledge a practitioner's liability for malpractice was too risky — it could too easily turn against them. After all, as practicing physicians, they also might be liable to an action for damages. In handling the issue of malpractice, the Protomedicato clearly revealed its ambiguous position as a professional court in which the doctors could simultaneously play the roles of defendants and judges.[89] Whereas in the lawsuits over medical fees the protomedici presented themselves as aristocratic protectors of the sick, in the case of malpractice they behaved instead as professionals bent on defending their self-interest, shielding themselves, as well as their partners in the medical trades, from the burdens and risks of liability.

Finally, we might wonder why the protomedici did not use malpractice trials to penalize unlicensed healers. Why didn't they sentence illicit healers to pay damages to their victims? Why didn't they use this occasion to discourage illegal practice? The answer is probably that, as we have seen in chapter 3, prosecuting illicit practitioners was not one of their primary goals. Nor was it their goal, as we can now see more clearly, to protect the sick from harm caused by a practitioner's mistakes. What mattered to the protomedici, in this as in other respects, was to uphold their role of control over the official medical system. Defending the medical establishment was more important to them than protecting the patients' bodies from medical error. Molière's irony caught their viewpoint exactly when he had the doctor Tomès say what the protomedici were arguing by their deeds, if not by words: "Un homme mort n'est qu'un homme mort, et ne fait point de conséquence; mais une formalité négligée porte un notable préjudice à tout le corps des médecins."[90]

Chapter 5

THE MEDICAL SYSTEM AS
SEEN BY THE SICK

I. HEALERS AND PROTECTORS

In previous chapters, we have tried to understand the behavior and ideas of the elite doctors who controlled the official medical system through the court of the Protomedicato. We now move on to examine this same system through the eyes of sick persons.[1] How did patients view the different kinds of practitioners? What did they expect from them? And first of all, how did the people of Bologna choose a healer? The most common way, apparently, was through horizontal networks of kin, friends, and neighbors. "On the Monday following Carnival Sunday, as the inflammation in my chest had gotten worse, my wife Margherita asked Mistress Virginia, wife of Messer Gerolamo, tailor, who both live next door to us, to find me a medical man, and she answered that she knew of a good doctor."[2]

Another way of finding a practitioner was to heed recommendations by former patients, who had been cured thanks to particular healers' skills. News of medical success spread quickly, as also did, no doubt, news of medical failure: several patients would often file a joint complaint against the same healer—a clear sign that the sick had their own information networks.[3] It was also common to choose a medical practitioner on the advice of a patron or friend of higher social standing, who would even, at times, provide the money to pay for treatment. Financial help in times of sickness seems to have been part of the exchange of services and favors typical of early modern patronage networks. In 1663, when Agata Aspertini was afflicted, to use her own words, by "a pain in the stomach, which kept moving around" ("male di stomaco, e revolutione di esso"), she turned for help to a lawyer's wife for whom she had occasionally worked as a servant. Not only did this lady send for a distiller she knew of but also, Agata testified, "she gave me a charitable gift of five lire, since I am a poor woman," to pay for the prescribed medicine.[4]

In 1670, Bonaventura Gammi, a tailor in the retinue of the Marchesa Lambertini, fell seriously ill. "Cheer up, Monsù Bonaventura,—announced two of the Marchesa's footmen, entering his bedroom—we've found a doctor who'll take care of your disease, and he has been sent to you by our lady the Marchesa."[5] The practitioner in this case was Gio. Batta Terrarossa, a surgeon who passed himself off as a physician and whom we shall have occasion to meet again. Unlicensed healers often exploited the prestige deriving from their contact with a noble and powerful patient to attract clients from the lower classes. Aurelio Righettini, a distiller suspended from practice in 1669 by the Protomedicato, "used to treat one Signor Gioseffo, a chamber attendant of Cardinal Carafa, the legate. This gentleman, he told me, gave him five *doppie* for his medication. He also treated an apprentice, but only with powders and pills, not with the electuary, because the boy didn't have enough money for that."[6] (Righettini had been licensed "to treat the sick" by the legate. His case indicates that political authorities were still issuing medical licenses, despite opposition from the protomedici.)

The patients who filed suits in the Protomedicato were of all social classes: nobles, priests, merchants, and peasants, with a concentration, however, of urban craftsmen and artisans, such as innkeepers, tailors, shoemakers, journeymen, and apprentices. It is interesting to notice that the clientele of licensed and illicit practitioners were not differentiated by social class. We quite often find the same practitioner—whether physician or charlatan—engaged in treating people of very different social standing. Apparently, a patient's social status was not a factor in the choice between a licensed or illicit healer. The clientele of an unlicensed practitioner, for instance, might very well include people from the upper echelons of society, while the urban middle classes, conversely, often employed regular doctors. Both the high-born and the common people were equally willing, if hard pressed by illness, to turn both to licit and to illicit practitioners until a cure could be found. For example, the wife of Andrea Bossi, a shoemaker, who suffered from swelling in her left arm, was treated first, in 1691, by Dr. Oretti, a college doctor, and later by a barber who practiced illicitly as a physician. When her condition worsened, she turned to another regular doctor.[7] Experimenting for the sake of health, a patient would often try one practitioner after another, regardless of their licensed or unlicensed status.

In 1698, the archpriest of San Giulio, Ludovico Petroni, a long-time sufferer from gallstones, was asked by the protomedici whether he remembered the names of all the medical men he had employed.

Yes, sir—the priest answered—I remember almost all the doctors who treated me. The first was Dr. Zuffi, who treated me for a month; the second was Dr. Muratori, who also treated me for about a month; and then Dr. Piella, who took care of me for a few days; and then I was advised by Don Angelo Michele Pellegrini to employ an old doctor, a foreigner whose name, I believe, is Terrarossa. He didn't visit me more than two or three times; and now I am under treatment by an empiric from Genoa, whose first or last name I don't know.[8]

This deposition was given before the Protomedicato during new criminal proceedings against Terrarossa, the surgeon and false physician whose 1670 trial I mentioned in chapter 3. In 1670, Terrarossa had been suspended from surgical practice and had left the city. Almost twenty years later, he had returned to Bologna hoping to set up shop again. The archpriest Petroni was not one of the people who had filed charges against Terrarossa initially, but as soon as he heard that the surgeon had been denounced for illicit practice, he hurried to the Protomedicato to claim restitution of his money. At the same time, the archpriest was quite ready to admit that he had sought treatment from both licensed and unlicensed healers, including the Genoese whom he declined to identify because, in all likelihood, he still wished to avail himself of his services. It should be noted that to seek treatment from illicit healers was considered a sin by Counter-Reformation religious authorities,[9] but the archpriest Petroni was clearly lax on this point. So were, in this particular instance, the protomedici, who did not bother to prosecute the Genoese empiric whose services were satisfactory to his patient, at least for the time being.

Thus, the official and the illicit realms of medical practice often shared the same patients. Licensed and unlicensed practitioners often came in and out of the same sickrooms. Far from being two separate worlds, legal and illicit practice formed, in the eyes of the sick, a single pool of medical resources, out of which one could pick and choose at will. This is shown, among other things, by the language used by the sick to describe illness. Some of the patients of illicit healers knew the learned medical term for their disease, indicating that they had probably also seen a regular doctor. In 1672, for instance, a woman who was currently being treated by an unlicensed healer described her disease as "the dropsy, which the physicians call ascites."[10] In fact, as far as diagnostic terminology goes, the language used by patients and popular healers was not very different from that employed by the representatives of the official medical system. The medical nomenclature of the times was often borrowed from common language. Even an academically trained physician was just as likely to use a popular term as the learned one in speaking of disease — for instance, using a common word such as *scolatione* (the clap) to indicate gonorrhea.[11] In society at large, the popular classification and naming of illnesses still overshadowed learned medical terminology. In the patients' self-diagnoses, the term that recurs most often is *pain (doglie)* ("a pain in the chest, and especially in the left arm," "a pain in the head," etc.). In the admission log of the Ospedale di Sant'Orsola for the years 1702–52 (written by the custodian, who probably recorded the terms used by the applicants for hospitalization), the word *doglie* occurs most often, next to other generic terms such as *sores, tumors,* and *ulcers,* which were also commonly used by surgeons.[12] When sick persons entered a hospital, therefore, their complaints were still defined in a nonspecialized manner, leaving ample room for the patient's self-diagnosis. Even the protomedici often employed the popular nomenclature of illness: for instance, in the licenses issued to popular healers (usually for the treatment of specific ailments), they regularly indicated diseases in plain language: "illnesses of the head, ringworm and scrofula, eye disease, scabies, leprosy, . . . sores, hemorrhoids, sacred fire, ulcers on the legs," and so on.[13]

Self-diagnosis still played an important role in this culture, as did self-therapy.[14] Patients used all sorts of available therapeutic resources, whether legal or illegal. If they could afford it, people called on physicians, but they were quite ready to switch to illicit healers if the official treatment did not work. As a last resort, a sick person would sometimes end up with medical self-help. "I have been aggravated by a bad disease for about three years," a woman said in 1698. "I sought treatment from several people, including a certain Anna, but later decided to stay away from her, and I went instead to the barber in San Mamolo. . . . Thereafter I have treated myself."[15] "My wife's disease, according to the doctors, is cancer in one breast," a shoemaker testified in 1663. "She has tried various medicines prescribed by Dr. Carlo Rinisi, who treated her for a long time. . . . At the present time, my wife treats herself."[16] Self-therapy was only a last resort for these people, but one that signals their sturdy self-reliance in medical matters. They definitely saw themselves as competent judges of medical success. This self-reliance led them to employ what we may call a sort of medical experimentalism, trying out several healers, both licensed and unlicensed, and even resorting to self-help, based presumably on techniques gleaned from their contact with various healers.

However, this is only part of the story. It must also be said that simultaneous contact with both official and illicit healers was at times a source of anxiety and irresolution for the sick. Let us return to the lawsuits. We know that charges would be normally filed for breach of a cure agreement — in other words, the patient would sue the practitioner when the time fixed for completing the cure had expired and the treatment had been unsuccessful. In some cases, however, healers were denounced *during* treatment, *before* the agreement's expiration date. This happened whenever something in the healer's conduct made the patient wary and distrustful. This is what happened to Ippolita Riccioli, "a poor widow with three daughters," as she described herself, who in 1672 filed charges against an unlicensed healer, the so-called "doctor Fabricio." As the woman told the protomedici, the healer had "treated her in an irregular or unorthodox manner, using powders, cumin, and pigeon dropping." She asked for a refund of the deposit she had advanced for treatment, if the protomedici could establish "in examining the medications used, that the treatment had indeed been harmful."[17] She did not ask the protomedici to enforce the terms of the cure agreement but asked them to check whether the remedies used by Fabricio were "canonical," that is, orthodox. Examined by the court, Ippolita gave a detailed account of her case:

> I suffer from dropsy, an affliction I have had now for about two years. . . . Seeing me in this condition, Sig. Zaniboni told me that he wished to send me an excellent man capable of curing me; and a few days later, indeed, he sent me a man who entered my bedroom asking about my disease. I told him that I was sick with dropsy; and he replied by requesting a gold *doppia* in exchange for curing me . . . ; and on hearing this, being anxious to get well, I told him: I'll gladly give you the money.[18]

The transaction thus began with the usual sign of mutual trust between patient and healer — an advance payment. But soon Ippolita became uneasy with Fabricio's healing methods, and especially with his insistence that she keep his remedies secret: "He brought me some powder and told me to mix it with a little wine and drink it, which I did; and he didn't want me to show this to anybody, but to drink it only in his presence." "When I asked him what remedies these were, he answered that he was not going to teach them against his own interest, since they were medical secrets of his own."[19]

This healer's secrecy clashed with popular custom. The rooms of the sick were usually open to a public of bystanders and neighbors, who came to pay a friendly call and satisfy their curiosity about medical matters.[20] Fabricio, of course, had his own reasons for secrecy; he had been tried once already by the Protomedicato and well knew he was breaking the official rules, as we learn from the high point of Ippolita Riccioli's deposition. "He told me ever so often: beware, you should never tell on me, and especially on my giving you oral remedies."[21]

This sufficed for the protomedici. Fabricio Ingegneri, "commonly called Dr. Fabricio," had violated a fundamental rule of the official medical system, and an order was issued against him *in absentia,* to be posted in public places throughout the city, prohibiting him from practicing "any branch of medicine."[22]

Only a few days later, however, Ippolita Riccioli withdrew her charges. As she explained in her statement to the protomedici, her conscience was upbraiding her for causing "Fabricio to lose his reputation and honor." The oral medications he had given her, she now claimed, had been prescribed "with the approval and assistance of a collegiate doctor." She had filed charges against Fabricio "under pressure by two malevolent people, who had made her great promises, assuring her that they would take her to other doctors . . . more knowledgeable than Fabricio. They also had scared her by saying that Fabricio would kill her."[23] Paradoxically, she now begged the protomedici to petition Fabricio on her behalf so that he would forgive her and resume treating her again "despite her faults."

Ippolita did not gain anything from her suit, because Fabricio was sentenced *in absentia* and thus could not be forced to return her money. The net result of her action was only the loss of a medical resource, the contact with a healer whose skills she had not fully put to the test because she had been frightened by his unusual methods.

Like other patients, Ippolita was caught between the desire to get well and the fear of unorthodox treatment. Her vacillating behavior exemplifies the conflicts arising from the patients' double bond with the legal and the illicit medical realms. On the one hand, the official practitioners guaranteed that medications would be "canonical," that is, according to standard; the illegal ones, on the other hand, promised a cure. But illicit medications represented a risk that the sick were not always ready to face. Hence, patients who regretted having signed a cure agreement with an illicit healer turned to the medical authorities for protection. One such patient was Angelo Ratti, a carpenter, who filed charges with the Protomedicato in 1695. For ten years, the man explained, he had been suffering from "pains" that in the last five years had become so bad that he was no longer able to work:

And I didn't fail, following the doctors' advice, to take decoctions and other medications . . . but, to tell the truth, I was almost brought to despair, since I was constantly getting worse. One day I talked to a fellow, the son-in-law of Tracchia the vintner, and to Father Fabrizio, who says mass to the Putte di S. Giuseppe, who both of them had taken mercury as a remedy for their pains . . . and they assured me that they had healed thanks to the mercury administered by a soldier of the guard named Fanti.[24]

The carpenter and Fanti signed a standard agreement for a cure: the therapy was to be based on mercurial ointments, and a down payment was required for the purchase of the mercury. But the treatment never started, because Ratti, no longer wishing to be treated, asked the healer for his money back. When Fanti refused, arguing that he had already prepared the mercurial compound and that the patient must respect the terms of the agreement, the carpenter turned to the Protomedicato. It is quite clear what had made him change his mind: "I told a few friends that I had decided to use the mercury ointment, and they discouraged me from doing so, saying that I was crazy . . . ; and I went to Dr. Cingari and Dr. Valsalva for advice, and they both told me not to make such a mistake unless I wanted to be poisoned . . . ; and the barber next door . . . , to whom I told everything, scolded me not to do such a reckless thing."[25]

This carpenter had sought advice not only from his friends and his barber but also from some learned and prominent doctors indeed: Valsalva was a renowned physician and surgeon, and Cingari was a collegiate—actually, at that time, the dean of the college.[26] Once again, this case shows how patients had simultaneous contact with the official and the illicit medical realms. The choice between legal and illegal treatments was ever present for them. But at this point we can also see that the patients' use of licensed or illicit healers was less indiscriminate than it may appear at first sight. If we look at the medical system from the patients' viewpoint, we notice that the legal and the illegal sides of the system took on different roles and meanings for them. From the patients' perspective, there were basically two kinds of medical practitioners—a group to which access was easier and from which they expected effective medical services, and a higher, more remote group, to which they turned instead for protection and advice. In other words, for the patients, medical practitioners fell into two main categories: those with whom one could have a "horizontal," peer-to-peer relationship, as in the agreement for a cure; and the authorities of the official medical system, with whom the proper relationship was a "vertical" one of dependence. The first we could properly call *healers;* for the second, the term *protectors* is probably the most appropriate. In the eyes of the patients, then, the true stratification of the medical system was defined by the distinction between "healers" and "protectors," in spite of the official image of the three-tiered hierarchy.[27] Underlying this distinction, one can perceive the long-lived coexistence of two models of healing: a "horizontal" model, based on a contractual relationship between persons of equal status, and a "vertical" one, whereby healing was understood and acted out as dependence on a patron.[28]

The category I termed "healers" included unlicensed empirics as well as low-ranking licensed practitioners such as barbers. To these the sick turned, usually after a self-diagnosis, for services whose quality and effectiveness they felt they could control to some extent. A "healer" typically would be called in for a specific ministration, such as, for instance, bloodletting — a very common remedy that the sick often prescribed for themselves, as many individuals examined in the Protomedicato confessed.[29] When the treatment was longer and complex, patients managed to exert some control over it by binding the healer to an agreement for a cure. While barbers were usually asked for specific, one-at-a-time services, illicit healers were often engaged instead to perform a longer cure under a contractual agreement. The distinction was far from clear-cut, however, since some barbers would occasionally agree to promise a cure. For example, in 1687 a jeweler "infected with the clap" filed charges with the Protomedicato against a barber who had "boasted he would cure him, saying that he didn't want any payment until he, the plaintiff, healed, and that once he had cured him, he would be satisfied with a small gem for compensation."[30] This barber was clearly behaving like an illicit healer, as by this time only such healers would enter into an agreement for a cure. From the point of view of the medical authorities, this kind of behavior was reprehensible because it dispensed with proper medical supervision: a barber lapsed into illicit practice whenever he drew blood on a patient's request rather than by a physician's order. We could say that the official medical system discouraged all kinds of healing based on self-help. Patients were not supposed to have access to medical care independently of the paternalistic control of the medical authorities. Self-therapy was banned from the official medical system; interestingly, the statutes of some medical colleges forbade even physicians to treat themselves.[31]

The horizontal relationship between patients and "healers" (exemplified by the agreement for a cure) contrasted with the vertical dependence of the patients on those upper-rank practitioners who were perceived as "protectors." These were the medical authorities and the learned physicians in general, from whom people expected protection and advice rather than effective medical service.[32] Dispensers of directions to the sick, as well as to all lower-level practitioners, the physicians were seen as learned and powerful patrons who could steer a safe course amidst the perils and dangers of illness. As a supreme medical authority, the Protomedicato was viewed in much the same way.

A powerful patron can be used as a resource. And indeed, the protomedici's authority was, as we know, manipulated by the sick as a means of pressuring healers to keep to the terms of the agreement for a cure. It is also clear that the protomedici were sometimes seen as mediators between patients and "healers." This is shown, for instance, by Ippolita Riccioli's recantation of her charges: after denouncing Fabricio, as you may recall, Ippolita asked the protomedici to petition the healer on her behalf so that he would come back to her. Obviously, she was not thinking of the protomedici as judges in charge of punishing illegal medical practice; she saw them instead as powerful mediators — persons of authority and social clout whose support she was trying to enlist to help with the difficulties and perplexities of dealing with a healer. For sick persons, filing charges against an unlicensed practitioner could also be a way to gain access to the medical authorities and benefit from their patronage — for instance, by receiving a physician's advice free of charge. Unlike Ippolita Riccioli, some patients played their cards successfully to this end. On December 13, 1758, the protomedici met at the house of Dr. Galli. For their inspection, two pitchers — one longish and thin, containing scented water, and another of round shape with some reddish liquid in it — were displayed on a table. These had been brought to Dr. Galli, so that he would examine them, by Lucia Zaffi, a widow who owned a shop in the parish of San Leonardo. This woman's deposition is worth hearing, as she tells her story very clearly:

> I've been suffering for some time past from a pain inside my throat, and fearing it was ulcerated, I complained about it to Gioseffo the baker . . . ; and he suggested that I consult with that charlatan known as Boschetti, who is currently practicing in Bologna's public square . . . ; and on the 11th of this month of December, the day of the Vow, I went to see the charlatan at his inn, . . . and he offered to treat me with one of his medical secrets, adding that he absolutely wanted to be paid, whether I was cured or not, and gave me two pitchers . . . ; which are the same I see on this table.
>
> But after I told a friend that I had consulted with said Boschetti . . . , that person suggested that I first see Dr. Galli and ask his opinion of the charlatan's

prescription, and that I let him inspect the two liquids before using them, and so I did . . . ; and Dr. Galli having charitably examined my throat, and having told me that, as far as he could see, it was not ulcerated at all, he prescribed a different medicine, and I made up my mind not to use the drinks of the charlatan anymore.[33]

By denouncing the charlatan, this patient managed to obtain a medical resource—a learned physician's advice—that otherwise would have been utterly beyond her reach. As for Dr. Galli, a celebrated physician and the founder of the Bologna School of Obstetrics,[34] his charitable behavior indicates once more how strongly the members of the medical elite felt a personal obligation to behave as the gracious and benevolent patrons of the sick.

II. THE OBSTRUCTED BODY: POPULAR IMAGES OF SICKNESS AND HEALING

My illness is obstruction, which the doctors call ascites.
—Ippolita Riccioli to the protomedici, 1672

Healing and protection—this was the twofold demand that the people of early modern Bologna addressed to the medical system. It was to meet these two needs that, in the patients' view, the medical system branched out into two different kinds of practitioners—healers and protectors. How was this twofold demand related to healing practices? How was it linked to popular perceptions of the body and illness?

The most striking feature in the patients' description of illness is the perception of disease as something that moves inside the body. "A pain in the stomach, which kept moving around," are the words that Agata Aspertini used to characterize her disease, as we saw above. And this is how an eyewitness described the progress of illness in a pregnant woman inadequately treated by a surgeon: "She had a flow in her neck, from which the humor descended to her right breast . . . , and built a tumor that turned into incurable cancer." The movement of disease in the body was linked to the flow of humors: "I had a tumor in my right knee, caused by the flow which was discharging there." These are common people speaking; but not very different is a statement by a midwife licensed by the Protomedicato. She described the worsening condition of a woman during her lying-in as follows: "I found her in very bad shape, because the *pangs of childbirth had moved to her head,* due to the burning feeling she had at the back of her head."[35] The patient's symptom — a burning pain behind her neck — was taken as a sign that the trauma of labor had moved within the woman's body.

The movement of disease inside the body was seen as channeled by the flow of humors. Not only was blood viewed as the main seat of illness,[36] but humors, or bodily fluids, were considered to be the fountainhead of the corruption and rotten matter associated with disease. Let us examine how a Bolognese day-laborer perceived and described his illness in 1632, when the city was in the aftermath of a major plague epidemic. In mid-August, when quarantine measures were still in place, Tommaso Pascarini, "a young peasant in his thirties," came to the Ospedale della Vita, requesting treatment for a swelling on his neck. Suspecting a case of bubonic plague, the hospital officers questioned him closely about his whereabouts since the onset of his illness. Tommaso gave them a brief history: "I began feeling some pain, and a lump, looking much like a pimple, grew on the right side of my neck, with a little swelling; and I didn't much heed it because it didn't give me trouble or pain."[37]

He kept on leading his normal life: "I went to the main square and waited near the stairs of San Petronio with other harvesters, hoping to be hired." A few days later, he went to see a butcher for whom he had worked a few months earlier, and asked him for "the money that he owed me for my service; and not only did the same Rocco the butcher refuse to pay me, he even punched me on my head and neck, on the right side, where I had that lump." "And in consequence of this punching, the lump got aggravated a bit, and this caused more humor to run to it. . . . I didn't work because this lump gave me a fever . . . , and since the pain in the neck was hurting more and more, this morning I came to the hospital." A few days later, Tommaso was questioned again: "Heaven be praised, I am very well, not having any fever and feeling healthy and strong; and this lump in my neck . . . broke down and is draining a lot of water . . . ; for which reason I believe it's not a bad and contagious disease but only a swelling caused by the beating I got . . . because at first I had just a little inflammation; and I hope in two or three days to be totally recovered."[38]

In Tommaso's words, we can notice, first of all, the causal link he established between the "aggravation" of the lump and the flow of humors toward the inflamed part; and secondly, the perception of the discharge of liquid from the lump as a positive sign of recovery. Similar views of the physical process of healing were voiced in the words of many other patients. Evacuation of the corrupted humors was seen as crucial for recovery and therefore as an essential aspect of therapy. When the body was unable to expel the corrupted humor spontaneously, evacuation had to be induced by medical means. In this framework, medication's first object was to effect a discharge of humors; and in point of fact, this is how patients evaluated the success or failure of therapy. In 1687, for instance, a man "infected with the clap" filed a suit against a barber who had prescribed him a potion, alleging that this medicine "locked up the clap inside my body, so that instead of feeling better, I got worse every day."[39] A medication that trapped the disease inside the body was clearly counterproductive. Conversely, a medication capable of producing multiple evacuations was considered highly effective. For example, a decoction prescribed to an ailing actress gave good results because, a witness argued, "it made her sweat, urinate, and have a bowel movement, so that the same day she was able to leave the house, and that very same evening she went back to the theater."[40] A remedy capable of inducing a triple evacuation was very powerful indeed!

Evacuation was the main purpose of most of the remedies used by popular healers. In 1691, the cobbler Andrea Volta was prosecuted for selling a compound that he described as causing a double evacuation: "a special medication of my own, which if taken by mouth induces vomiting and belly discharge."[41] When tried in 1670 for prescribing oral medications, the surgeon Gio. Batta Terrarossa pleaded that his remedies were merely evacuative. He was perfectly aware that he had violated the Protomedicato's rule — he knew very well that "nobody should administer by mouth, under penalty of excommunication." However, the pills he had prescribed were simply intended to ease evacuation: "They helped the patient spit large quantities of matter . . . ; they made a great deal of rotten matter come out of his mouth."[42] Terrarossa explained very clearly the evacuative purpose of his methods of treatment: "The physical intent of my medications was to draw out of the patient's head that salty mucus that descended to the opening of the stomach and filled the lung with viscous matter, as one could see from the patient's spit being mixed with pus and blood, as sticky as birdlime."[43]

At the trial of another barber-surgeon, accused by an unidentified witness of having administered oil by mouth to a wounded person, the defendant testified that his prescription was meant to be merely evacuative:

> I usually give medicine by hand, but never by mouth. . . . I know very well that I cannot give anything to anyone by mouth. To relieve the wounded person, I gave him an enema and I treated him as I felt it was proper for his wounds . . . ; and I ordered the people of his household to get some almond-

oil, half of which to apply externally to his body and stomach, and half to give him by mouth to soothe the stomach . . . so that if the stomach contained any hemorrhaged blood he could vomit it out.[44]

Almond-oil, in fact, was commonly used as an emetic. This barber's therapeutic purpose was obvious: he wished to induce vomiting so as to help the patient get rid of internal bleeding. It is also clear that, unlike the protomedici, the barber did not think that prescribing an emetic was medicating "by mouth." Inducing vomiting, insofar as it had an evacuative purpose, he saw as part and parcel of his legitimate range of tasks. Furthermore, the barber's words imply that the oral prescription was just one aspect of a complex procedure aimed at "soothing the stomach" by anointing it externally and internally.

The discharge of diseased matter was also among the purposes of ointments, a remedy often used by lower-rank healers. The surgeon Terrarossa explained to the protomedici how he used to anoint "the soles of the patient's feet, his upper stomach, his loins, the nape of his neck, and his wrists," so that this "would make him spit a lot and clear out a large quantity of dirty, stinking matter from his nose."[45] By acting on the skin, the boundary between the inner and outer body, ointments partook of the beneficial purpose attributed to a large number of popular healing practices—the purpose of drawing impurities up to the surface of the body so that they could be more easily expelled. Such was the function of bloodletting, emetics, and purges, as well as steam baths and other procedures aimed at inducing profuse sweating. It was likewise the function of popular healing techniques such as the cautery, cupping, vesicatories, and scarification—all of which were based on the application of caustic or blistering agents to the skin so as to produce an open, draining sore. The corrupt matter inside the body—it was believed—would be attracted to the open sore and thus discharged.[46]

Underlying all these therapeutic procedures was the idea that disease impaired or altogether stopped the body's natural capacity to purge itself. Disease implied a disruption of the proper balance between the body's input and its output. Like the basic dichotomies of hot and cold, humid and dry,[47] the distinction between the inner and outer body had been a major symbolic opposition in western medicine ever since its earliest formulations in the Hippocratic treatises. In a study of the metaphors of the body in the Hippocratic Corpus, Mario Vegetti has pointed out that the most frequently employed image of the body was that of a container in which the humors are constantly flowing—mixing, clashing, and interreacting with each other. In this vision of the body, fluids were the primary element, much more important than the solid organs: Hippocratic medicine emphasized secretions and excretions while ignoring the notion of the body as an organism, a unified whole made up of interdependent parts. As a consequence, therapy was centered on the proper balance between what enters and what exits the body. "Anomalous discharges (of excrement, sweat, phlegm, blood) were seen as the pathologic symptoms which had to be eliminated by properly modifying intake (of food, drink, air, etc.). If we search the Hippocratic Corpus for an explicit anthropology, we can find it precisely in this metaphor of the body as a container with an input and output."[48]

Mikhail Bakhtin saw strong similarities between the Hippocratic vision and what he called "the grotesque image of the body." Grotesque bodily imagery, for Bakhtin, was a central and resilient feature of European popular culture, to be found also in learned culture in the works of the great humanist and physician François Rabelais. In fact, according to Bakhtin, the Hippocratic texts were one of the most important literary sources for Rabelais's concept of the body.[49] A main feature of grotesque body imagery is a weak barrier between the body and the surrounding environment; the body is portrayed in unrestrained openness to the world. Particularly important, in this vision, are all orifices, as channels between the body and the world. According to Bakhtin, this view was also characteristic of Hippocratic medicine. "Ancient medicine, as reflected in the Hippocratic Corpus, lent great importance to bodily evacuations. In the physician's eyes the body was first of all represented by the elimination of urine, feces, sweat, mucus, and bile."[50]

This same emphasis on bodily excretions can be found in the perception of disease and in the techniques employed by popular healers in seventeenth-century Bologna. The grotesque body was an open body, whose orifices were the site of fluid exchange, of free circulation between the self and the world. As tersely described by Bakhtin, it was a body with a gaping mouth.[51] Health consisted precisely in this complete openness to the world. From patients' descriptions of disease and their quest for medical services, we can see that illness was perceived precisely as the loss of the body's natural condition of openness. The sick body was described first of all as a closed body, one that needed to be forcibly opened for the expulsion of the disease trapped inside. Like a river or a channel, the body is at constant risk of "oppilation," or obstruction. "I suffer from oppilation, which the doctors call ascites," said Ippolita Riccioli to the protomedici in 1672.[52] *Oppilation,* a term originally indicating the obstruction of a flow of water, was often used by the people of Bologna to signify a wide array of illnesses, from dropsy to amenorrhea, all of which were thought to involve the pathologic retention of humors inside the body.[53] For the people of Bologna, a healthy body was in constant fluid motion. In sickness, by contrast, the flow of humors was interrupted, and the communication channels with the world were clogged and stopped up.[54]

This view of the body echoed religious themes. Whereas in ancient and medieval medicine the humors had been the very symbol of life (the body's "radical moisture" was seen as a fundamental vital principle),[55] in early modern religious texts they were more often considered vehicles of corruption and mortality. "Les humeurs mettent le corps en pourriture, et ce à cause de plusieurs maladies, et de là procède la mort" ("Humors pollute the body, and this because of many diseases, wherefrom comes death"), we read in an edifying text from the *Bibliothèque bleue*.[56] In Counter-Reformation Bologna, the term *oppilation* signified not only a pathologic condition of the body but also a state of spiritual disease whereby sinners closed their souls to the word of God and their mouths to confession. Saint Antoninus drew an explicit parallel between the sacrament of penance and medical evacuation: "Penance is a purging of ill humors, that is, an evacuation of vices." He further drew a correspondence between the spiritual remedy of confession and medical evacuation: "Confession is like a rhubarb decoction, which causes vomiting."[57] We find the same metaphorical use of medical terms to indicate religious concepts in *Pastarino's Preparations to Medicate Oneself in These Dangerous Times of the Plague,* a pious pamphlet written in 1577 by a Bolognese apothecary. "And what are these oppilated pores other than our ears, deaf to sermons, and our mouths, closed to confession? These need to open up because thereby illnesses are revealed, bad humors purged off."[58] We can still find the analogy between purge and confession in the Catholic culture of the eighteenth century, for instance in *Del governo della peste,* by Ludovico Antonio Muratori.[59]

In the grotesque vision of the body, obstruction epitomizes the diseased condition. The "oppilated" body is unable to rid itself of impurities; it needs external help to effect the evacuations that are necessary for well-being. Health is based on the body's capacity for cleansing. Conversely, illness consists precisely in the loss of that capacity. In view of all this, we can understand why turning to a healer was conceptually associated with self-medication. A healer was supposed to help the sick body perform, by artificial means, the self-cleaning hindered by disease.[60] From this viewpoint, therapy was seen as an artificial replica—an imitation—of the body's excretory functions. Thus, the healer's intervention was conceptualized as an extension of the body's natural self-cleaning, and in this sense it fell under the category of self-help. This also explains why inferior practitioners, those whom the people perceived as healers, did not hold a social position of authority over patients: it was not only because their services were associated with lowly bodily functions such as evacuation but also because their role was simply to assist the body's self-help. Consequently, in this case, the relationship between patient and healer had a "horizontal" configuration. Healers could intervene aggressively on the sick body, but they did not have a role of authority or supervision over the patient's life.[61]

This is the view of therapy which we find among patients and popular healers alike. In learned medicine, by contrast, the concept of therapy was remarkably different. In doctors' eyes, evacuation had a secondary role, its primary function being the elimination not of corruption but of corporeal surplus.[62] What the doctors stressed above all, with respect to the balance between bodily input and output, was a methodical control of the diet — a well-regulated regimen to which the body must submit. Seventeenth-century learned medicine, in Bologna as elsewhere, was still profoundly influenced by the Galenic paradigm. Although Galen's status as a scientific authority had long been under severe attack, especially in the field of anatomy, Galenism still reigned paramount in therapeutic practices (and it is therapy that concerns us here).[63] Mario Vegetti has pointed out that the Galenic view of the body differed significantly from the Hippocratic one. Although the Galenic doctrine was a synthesis of Hippocratic and Aristotelian themes, Galen opted for Aristotle's model of the body as a system of solid organs, rather than the Hippocratic view centered on bodily fluids. No longer seen as a hollow container wherein the humors flow unceasingly, the body was viewed by Galen, in Aristotelian fashion, as an integrated system of solid organs ranked by purpose and function. Galen's view of the body, Vegetti observes, could be compared to the political concept of *polis* — a well-ordered system of government based on the hierarchical integration of different social strata.[64] Galenic doctrine emphasized the hygienic, preventive role of medicine — the "good government of the body" — rather than therapeutics. There was no need for aggressive therapeutic procedures. As a system of organs with specific and interrelated purposes, the body could be safely left to its natural functioning as long as it was governed by a "rule of living." Hence the primacy of diet, and the secondary role attributed to evacuatory therapies.[65]

In learned medicine, therefore, therapy was associated with the exercise of authority — the governance of the body. We can better understand, at this point, why physicians saw diet — the prescription of "a rule of living" — as their primary and exclusive responsibility. Regardless of the official ideology of the three-tiered hierarchy, prescribing diets seems to have been what doctors primarily did, in actual practice. For example, here is how a doctor described his role during a surgical procedure performed in orthodox fashion — namely, with the surgeon carrying out the manual intervention and the physician supervising the patient's diet.

> I applied myself methodically to support the surgical procedure by keeping the [patient's] blood in a well-fermenting state, and in well-regulated movement, by means of altered broths; and with an appropriate diet I sought to inhibit what would, through an excess of nutrition, impress too much movement to the blood and result in the accumulation of undigested nutritive juice, apt to increase the heterogeneity of parts in the blood, lest these parts be carried to the wounded limb, weakened by the fracture and pain.[66]

The doctor's task, in this case, is described as one of supervision over the process of nutrition.[67] The passage quoted above comes from a physician's testimony in a trial concerning matters of payment. Both the physician and the surgeon testified that the patient was to blame for the length and difficulty of treatment, because he had "not kept himself to the prescribed regimen" on account of his "proclivity to disorderly conduct" and his "constitutional inclination to drink."[68] Prescribing a diet implied control over the patient's behavior, and patients generally acknowledged that the physician's "rule of life" required obedience.[69] Because of this element of dependence and authority, the relationship between physician and patient took on a "vertical" configuration.

Cultural rules regarding food, from table manners to medical and religious dietary norms, can be seen as a "relational idiom" of gestures and behaviors which ritually expresses various social relations, including trust and mistrust, inclusion and exclusion, rank differences, submission, and authority.[70] The connection between dietary rules and social authority, which may escape us today, was probably quite obvious to the people of a Counter-Reformation city such as seventeenth-century Bologna, who were accustomed to the fasting rules imposed by the church. Indeed, the people of Bologna may well have suspected that fasting during Lent was related as closely to mundane power as to divine law. This is what we glimpse from the testimony of a maidservant accused of "swearing and blasphemy against the institution of Lent" and brought to trial in the Inquisition Tribunal of Bologna in 1697. On the first Thursday of Lent in that year, a group of people had been sitting around the kitchen fire in the house of a notary in Medicina, a village in the Bolognese territory. They were Signora Maria Caterina, the notary's daughter; Domenico, a manservant; and a maid, Antonia Mingozzi. While the group was "talking together about fasting and Lent," Antonia burst out: "A curse on that damned breed of insolents that started Lent and fasting!"

> At which, the said Domenico and Signora Maria Caterina screamed: What did you say? And I answered: Nothing, what did I say; and they said: Lent was established by our Blessed Lord; and I said: Oh really? *I thought it had been established by some cardinal or some such big-wig;* and they said: This is a matter for the Inquisition. And I told them: Well, I've said it, there's nothing I can do now.[71]

In this maid's eyes, Lenten fasting was simply one of the ways in which masters cut down on their household expenses by depriving servants of food. She shrewdly perceived that, beneath a religious veneer, the rule of fasting reinforced mundane hierarchy and power. Her blasphemous words were deliberately hurled at that "breed" of "cardinals and big-wigs," whose rule benefited the masters by allowing them to legitimately starve their servants.

The trials for "blasphemy against fasting in the time of Lent" which were heard by the Bolognese Inquisition in this period show that observance of the church's dietary rules was widespread among the common people. Those who did not observe the prescribed abstinence from meat were viewed as outsiders and aroused suspicions in the community. This is shown by the trial of Rosa Paleotti, a "former Turk," as she is designated in the court records. A slave girl donated as a child by a Venetian nobleman to a Bolognese marquise, Rosa had been baptized and raised in her patroness's household.[72] When we meet her in the Inquisition records in 1699, Rosa was no longer under the marquise's protection but was living, as she herself said, as a *putta libera* ("a free maid"), earning her living as a singer. She was denounced to the Inquisition by her fellow musicians, who were shocked by her stubborn habit of eating meat during days of abstinence and by her gruff response to their reproofs: "Get off my back, because I want to eat whatever pleases me."

Summoned by the inquisitor, Rosa argued that she had been given leave to eat meat on forbidden days by her physician, Dr. Albertini. This was confirmed by the doctor, who testified that Rosa suffered from "an inflammation," or "abscess," of the liver. "That's why I recommended that she eliminate all kinds of acids, aromatics, and salts which are bad for her condition . . . , and I gave her permission to eat meat every day, regardless of whether it was Friday, Saturday, or a Vigil, as well as during Lent; and I was tolerant on this issue because she told me that she had been raised as a Turk, never eating fish or dairy products, and that she felt sick every time she ate them." The physician's argument was not challenged by the inquisitor, and Rosa was simply admonished not to eat meat on forbidden days unless she had a fever or could present a written permit from a doctor.[73]

The diffusion of *fedi quaresimali*—certificates issued by physicians exempting patients from fasting—indicates that, in the seventeenth century, medicine was extending its sway over the field of dietary controls traditionally exercised by the church.[74] During the Counter Reformation, both physicians and clergymen shared an interest in dietetics and in the curative properties of fasting for the health of both body and soul. Of Cardinal Giulio de' Medici, for example, it was said that "he fasts throughout Lent and the vigils of Our Lady, on Good Friday and Saturday, taking only bread and water; . . . and whenever he dines, he entertains two physicians at his table, with whom he talks over the quality of the food being eaten."[75] Famous Counter-Reformation physicians such as Paolo Zacchia and Alessandro Petroni, a friend of Ignatius Loyola's, wrote treatises on dietetics.[76] We have also seen how seriously the protomedici of Bologna took their role of "guardians of the mouth" and food inspectors for the city—tasks that were surrounded by an aura of almost priestly authority. To go back to Saint Antoninus's analogy between sacraments and medicines, it is significant that the saint compared the eucharist to an "electuary," the internal medicine that, in principle, only a physician could prescribe.[77] One might argue that their increased role in the control of diet was one of the ways in which early modern physicians strengthened and legitimized their social authority. It is interesting to note that, before the Counter Reformation, a physician's authority had not been recognized as legitimate by religious authorities. Medieval canonists had unanimously maintained that a patient did not commit a sin by disobeying his physician, because the latter did not hold any legitimate authority (in the sense of legal guardianship) over the patient.[78] This traditional opinion was reversed during the Counter Reformation. The Roman Catholic scholar and physician Gian Battista Codronchi, for instance, wrote in *De christiana ac tuta medendi ratione* that disobeying one's physician was sinful, because a doctor held legitimate authority over his patient.[79]

This is a culture in which the physician took upon himself the role of *custodian,* controller of the body's intake, and protector of its vulnerable interior. Behind this role laid a widespread social perception of illness as a poison that could enter the body from the outside, especially through the mouth.

This pervasive fear of poisoning is proved by the popularity of theriac, the antipoison medication par excellence. It is also indicated by patients' behavior: before taking a medicine prescribed by the surgeon Terrarossa, for instance, the archpriest Petroni had one of his servants drink some of it first, to check that it was not noxious. Well aware of such fears, the charlatans who applied for licenses to sell their remedies offered to swallow them in front of the protomedici, as proof of their safety.[80]

This pervasive fear of poisoning was probably reinforced by the Protomedicato's insistent admonition to lower-rank healers never to administer oral medications. The medical authorities' prohibition was probably perceived by the people as somewhat akin to the church's dietary rules. This is suggested by the patients' troubled reaction whenever a healer made them break a religious fast. In 1746, for instance, a patient filed charges against an apothecary who had prescribed him an oral medication. What had turned the patient against the practitioner was the fact that the latter's prescription conflicted with the church's command of abstinence from meat on certain days. According to the patient: "He gave me four doses of a tobacco-colored powder and ordered that I take one, dissolved in meat broth, every morning, regardless of whether it was an ordinary day or a fast day. But . . . I was uneasy about taking the powder with meat broth on Fridays and Saturdays."[81]

Breaking two rules at the same time (the medical prohibition against taking oral medications from anybody but a physician, plus the church's commandment of fasting) was too much for this patient. He probably felt that illness, as a state of weakness and danger, required even greater respect for the rules of established authorities.

I do not know whether the grotesque, joyously open body described by Rabelais in the most happy of utopias ever actually corresponded to the lived experience of human beings. Certainly, the concept of disease which we find in seventeenth-century Bologna seems to confirm the importance of the grotesque for understanding the popular perception of the body in early modern Europe. But it also suggests that the weak boundary between the body and the world—emphasized by Bakhtin as an aspect of joyous openness—could be felt instead as vulnerability, as fear of penetration by disease.[82] The "oppilated" body is closed in two ways: it is no longer capable of expelling the disease hidden inside; and its main orifice—the mouth—is a vulnerable area that needs to be guarded. In this vision of the body, therefore, therapy has two basic meanings: it may mean an intensification of self-cleaning efforts with the help of a *healer*, but it may also mean putting oneself under the tutelage of an authoritative *protector*.

Chapter 6

THE DISAPPEARANCE OF THE
AGREEMENT FOR A CURE

Je suis d'avis de m'en tenir, toute ma vie, à la médecine. Je trouve que
c'est le métier le meilleur de tous; car soit qu'on fasse bien ou soit
qu'on fasse mal, on est toujours payé de même sorte.
—Molière, *Le médecin malgré lui,* act 3, scene 1

I

In a culture in which illness was perceived through the image of the obstructed body, there were two main therapeutic needs: evacuation therapies, aimed at the artificial discharge of the corrupted humors that could not be expelled by natural means; and the regulation of diet, or the control of bodily input. For patients, these two basic needs corresponded to the two groups of medical practitioners I have named "healers" (called upon to perform evacuation therapies) and "protectors" (called upon to regulate and guard access to the inner body). We can now see more clearly the grounds for coexistence, but also for potential conflict, between these two groups (which roughly correspond to the official and illegal realms of medical practice, since the "healers" can be largely identified with the unlicensed practitioners).

Patients saw both groups as performing necessary therapeutic tasks, but their attitudes to them, as we know, differed greatly. From one group, the patients asked for healing; from the other, they expected protection. The relationship between patient and "healer" was horizontal and conceptually linked to self-therapy; that between patient and physician, or "protector," was vertical: it ruled out self-help and implied instead the sick person's dependence on the doctor's authority. The two were in a measure incompatible, insofar as the egalitarian relationship with the healer contradicted the hierarchical nature of the physician-patient relationship. We can expect that the more widely doctors extended their clientele networks, the more starkly the incompatibility between the two models would begin to emerge. And indeed, in the long run, the vertical model of healing won over the horizontal model. The egalitarian relationship between patient and healer, epitomized by "the agreement for a cure," steadily lost ground and finally disappeared. This, at least, is what we can glean from the history of the changing attitude to the cure agreements, as we can trace it in the documents of the Protomedicato.

As the seventeenth century progressed, two increasingly divergent concepts of medical equity confronted each other in the protomedici's courtrooms: on the one hand, the patients' customary notion, based on the agreement for a cure; on the other, the medical authorities' view of a well-regulated medical practice. We have already examined each of these views separately; it is now time to determine what happened when they interacted and finally clashed.

By the end of the sixteenth century, the Protomedicato still acknowledged, at least in part, the legal validity of a promise for a cure; whenever the parties had signed such an agreement, the medical authorities maintained that payment depended on the patient's actual recovery. But somewhere in the first half of the seventeenth century, the protomedici's attitude started to change. In 1633, for instance, the dean of the college made the following entry in his "Liber secretus," the journal in which he recorded the proceedings of the college and the Protomedicato:

> A certain butcher appealed to us, dean and protomedici, claiming to have treated another butcher's nephew, who had been suffering from the ringworm for two years. The lad was partially cured in three months thanks to some lotions and a balsam the butcher considered a medical secret of his own. However, when the butcher requested fifty silver *piastre* in payment, declaring that the patient had been healed of the ringworm, the latter refused to pay, on the ground that he was not yet totally cured. We ruled that the butcher should receive only sixteen piastre . . . , and we lowered his fee to that amount because there was no written agreement between the two; and also because, according to our statutes, the butcher was not allowed to practice medicine. Both parties left my house satisfied with the decision.[1]

Once again, we can see that the protomedici did not deem it beneath their dignity to act as mediators between sick persons and popular healers. Furthermore, the episode shows that they still believed that an agreement for a cure had some legal value, if it was recorded in written form. But, most important, we can notice in this case a clear disagreement between the view of the patient and that of the protomedici: while the patient objected to paying the agreed-upon sum because he did not feel completely recovered, the protomedici thought that the healer's right to a fee was partly invalidated for other reasons — because there was no written evidence of the cure agreement and, more important, because the healer was unlicensed. Increasingly, throughout the first half of the seventeenth century, this second point became decisive: the protomedici firmly adopted the view that a practitioner's right to a fee depended on his compliance with the rules of the medical establishment — namely, having a regular license and keeping within the boundaries specified therein. A decree issued in 1614 by the Roman Protomedicato expressly stated that illegal practitioners (including not only charlatans but also unlicensed physicians and surgeons) forfeited their right to a fee.[2] It was by taking away their right to payment that the medical authorities effectively undermined the practice of popular healers. The battle between official and popular medicine was fought less on the lofty terrain of ideas than on the more prosaic ground of economic rights.

The origins of the principle that excluded illegal healers from the right to payment can be traced back to Roman law. Although Roman law utterly ignored the very idea of medical licensing, it nevertheless provided a nascent juridical weapon for the early modern fight against illegal practice. This weapon was found in the text of the Digest, which denied "those who employ magic and exorcism" the right to be paid, "because these practices do not belong to medicine."[3] In seventeenth-century Europe, medical authorities extended this norm to all unauthorized medical practice. This proved a much more forcible way of penalizing and discouraging illegal practice than criminal prosecution, which usually, at least in the Bolognese case, as we know, simply led to the imposition of a fine. It is probably because of its practical efficacy that this norm became a staple item of European medical jurisprudence. We find it enforced not only in Bologna but also, for instance, in France, where it was a general rule that "those who are not licensed to practice in the area where they want to practice, cannot sue for payment in the courts of law."[4]

Understandably, of all the cases concerning payment which were heard by the Bolognese Protomedicato from 1605 to 1776, only three were filed by unlicensed healers (see chapter 4, table 7). The above-mentioned case involving the butcher who treated the ringworm was the last to end in a decision partly favorable to the healer. As you may recall, the butcher was granted the right to be paid (although a sum considerably smaller than the one he claimed).[5] The butcher's case actually marked the end of a trend; thereafter, the protomedici invariably denied the right to payment to all illegal healers. In 1657, when the legate referred to the college a case that an unlicensed woman healer had filed regarding a matter of payment, the woman (unnamed in the records) did not even bother to show up in the Protomedicato.[6] She probably knew that she had no chance to make good her claim in that court. Less well-versed in the ways of the Protomedicato was a certain Guarnieri, a distiller who in 1689 sued for nonpayment a patient whom he had treated for several weeks with a "purgative water" "to rid him of the pains and scabies that afflicted him."[7] With considerable professional pride, the distiller told the protomedici that "he was almost making a living" just from the sale of this purgative water. His patient, however, found it too expensive at 20 lire but was ready to settle at 10 lire. To this patient, the protomedici's ruling must have come as good news indeed: he did not have to pay anything at all for the treatment, because the distiller was not licensed to sell medicines. In addition, the healer was sentenced to a fine of 50 scudi (250 lire) for practicing illegally — a very high sum, which upon appeal, however, was reduced to 15 lire, following the usual pattern of clemency.

Deprivation of the right to payment was systematically used by the protomedici to penalize two forms of illegal practice: that of unlicensed healers, and also that of those licensed practitioners who overstepped the boundaries of their profession — for instance, barbers who prescribed oral medications or treated patients without a physician's supervision. The decree of the Roman Protomedicato, cited above,[8] specifically mentioned both cases. In fact, the same penalty was used to discourage any violation of the Protomedicato's rules by all lower-level practitioners, including apothecaries whose preparations did not comply with the pharmacopoeia.[9] The penalty was extremely effective because the Protomedicato was the only court qualified to settle disputes over payment for medicines and medical services. Barbers and apothecaries who wished to sue patients who were unwilling to pay had no choice but to appeal to the Protomedicato as the only competent judge,[10] and they knew that if they did so their practice would be under close scrutiny as to its compliance with the official medical rules.

Study of the sentences issued by the Protomedicato leaves no doubt that the threat of deprivation of the right to payment was used by the court to impose observance of the licensing system upon all lower-rank practitioners. For example, in 1678 the *procuratore dei poveri* (the "advocate of the poor," a lawyer salaried by the municipality to argue the cases of those too poor to hire an attorney) asked the protomedici to establish the "fair fee" due to the barber Carlo Marocchi, who had treated Pietro and Giovanni Mazzetti, a father and son, for "stomach pains." But upon examining the barber's professional qualifications, the protomedici found that he was not licensed at all. Accordingly, they ruled that his debtors did not have to pay him for treatment "because Marocchi was not licensed to medicate, in violation of the college's decree."[11] This barber quickly learned the Protomedicato's lesson. A few years later, when applying for a license to open a steam-bath establishment, he also requested that, in light of his newly acquired license, the protomedici allow him "to bring some patients to court, in order to collect due payment."[12]

It must be noted, however, that in imposing the loss of payment as a penalty for illegal practice, the protomedici were considerably more rigorous and heavy-handed with popular healers than with professional practitioners such as barbers. In fact, they showed some reluctance to strip a barber of his fee even when he was caught practicing without a license, as we can see in the following case. In 1618, the patient Pietro Bugognoli appealed to the Protomedicato to be exempted from paying the barber Antonio Quirini the balance of an agreed-upon fee of 25 scudi (125 lire). The patient had already given the barber two *corbe* (160 liters) of wine, valued at 6 lire and 10 soldi per corba, and believed that he did not owe him anything more because, firstly, the medications had been "unfavorable and damaging to his disease," and secondly, the barber "did not have a license or permit to medicate."[13] Thus, in this case the patient accused the healer of violating not only the cure agreement but also the licensing laws of the Protomedicato. For his part, the barber Quirini testified that he "had treated said Pietro in an orthodox manner" and had actually cured him of a serious illness. The Protomedicato's sentence was not unfavorable to the barber. Since "he had given treatment in good faith," he was entitled to a portion (albeit minimal) of the promised sum. In the future, however, he should take care not to provide treatment without first obtaining a license.[14]

In this case, the Protomedicato sided with the practitioner, granting him the right to a fee (albeit one much smaller than he had claimed) in spite of the fact that he had practiced illegally. Why so? As a matter of fact, the protomedici had to take into account the possibility that some patients might take undue advantage of the rules of the official licensing system. Patients who did not want to pay their healers could simply accuse them of not being licensed or of overstepping the limits of their profession, and thus shirk their obligation to pay what had been promised in the initial agreement. In fact, patients were quite adroit at exploiting the healers' vulnerability vis-à-vis the official medical system. In the juridical pluralism of the old regime, that labyrinthine tangle of competing jurisdictions, early modern people—even the common people—knew how to find their way to the court or magistrate presumably most favorable to their case. Obviously, it required some ability to find the charge appropriate to each of the many courts of justice. It was of no use to the patient Cristoforo Capponi, when sued for debt in 1668 before the Protomedicato by the surgeon Terrarossa, to countercharge that the surgeon "during treatment, whispered some words which I couldn't understand." The patient was clearly insinuating that the surgeon had employed magical formulas, but the prosecution of magical healing was no business of the Protomedicato's. It was a matter for the Inquisition, and the protomedici would not meddle with it. So they ignored the insinuation and sentenced the patient to pay the fee that was due.[15] Conversely, in vain did an ironsmith from Cento denounce a foreigner to the Inquisition in 1697, charging him with performing a cure on a fellow villager "with an ointment made of nettles and the fat of a male pig." The Inquisition found nothing superstitious in the treatment, and charges were dropped,[16] although the healer was obviously unlicensed. But that was the Protomedicato's affair, and no matter for the Holy Office.

Generally, however, the patients who turned to the Protomedicato knew very well which accusations would be most telling in this court and most damaging to the healer they were suing: "He made me swallow some draughts"; "he treated me with plasters, oils, and some powders and herbs, *also by mouth.*"[17] People were well aware of the rule prohibiting lower-rank practitioners from medicating by mouth, and they knew how to turn it to their personal advantage. Here also we find that "capacity to know and manipulate the system" which was displayed by accusers in early modern witchcraft trials. "The accusers were familiar not only with the ways of the Tribunal, but also with the expectations and cultural values of its officers."[18]

As justices, the protomedici were fully aware of this problem. In fact, their sentences seem to have been prompted by the effort to balance two intentions: on the one hand, they sought to use the suits brought by patients as an occasion to pressure lower-level practitioners into compliance with the licensing system; on the other, they tried to safeguard the interests of practitioners—even when the latter occasionally strayed into illegal practice—against patients' dishonesty. In 1697, the surgeon Cavazza attempted to collect payment from the shoemaker Domenico Gualandi by suing him in the Foro dei Mercanti (the Merchants' Court). Gualandi countersued Cavazza in the

Protomedicato, on the grounds that the surgeon had not medicated him according to standards (he had bled him without a doctor's prescription) and for this reason was not entitled to payment. The protomedici looked into the case by summoning as a witness a woman who had assisted the patient during his illness and who testified that the surgeon had indeed given professional care to the shoemaker ("I heard Gualandi plead with the surgeon and ask him not to leave him"). The protomedici ruled that the surgeon was entitled to payment despite his violation of the rule on bloodletting. He was simply admonished not to repeat the offense in the future.[19]

Interestingly, this case indicates a challenge to the jurisdictional prerogatives of the Protomedicato. The surgeon initially brought his suit not to the Protomedicato but to the Foro dei Mercanti — a tribunal created by the merchants to take over the ancient jurisdictions of the guilds regarding "all cases related to trading, bankruptcy, contracts, and similar issues," including litigation over payment, such as this specific case.[20] A small number of suits concerning payment which were heard by the Protomedicato between the end of the seventeenth century and the beginning of the eighteenth had originally been addressed by the plaintiff (a member of either the apothecaries' guild or the barbers' guild) to the Foro dei Mercanti, which had passed the cases on to the Protomedicato as the only competent judge over all medical matters.[21] Only a thorough study of the archives of the Foro dei Mercanti could tell us whether, and to what extent, barbers and apothecaries preferred to turn to this court rather than to the Protomedicato when trying to recover debts from their clients.[22] The reasons for such a preference would not be hard to understand. If they appealed to the Protomedicato, barbers and surgeons had to submit to the protomedici's control over their practices, a control they could avoid in the Foro dei Mercanti. It is also possible that both barbers and apothecaries perceived the protomedici as somewhat biased in favor of the sick (probably in view of the protomedici's "fair price" policy described in chapter 4). Be that as it may, in four of the seven cases sent from the Foro dei Mercanti to the Protomedicato, this change of jurisdiction had been requested by the patient, who challenged the legal competence of the Foro dei Mercanti over medical fees.[23] This seems to suggest that, unlike practitioners, patients saw the Protomedicato as disposed to favor them.

All of this points to the specific problem of balance and fairness which the protomedici had to solve in rendering justice to both patients and practitioners. On the one hand, they were expected to protect the sick by guaranteeing the proper standard of medical care; on the other, they also had to safeguard the professional interests of medical practitioners. To strip a practitioner of his fee was a serious business. Clearly, the protomedici felt that it was too harsh a punishment for those barbers or apothecaries who occasionally transgressed the licensing rules. In such cases, they often chose to close an eye, or even two.

Not so, instead, with illegal healers such as charlatans and the like: in their case, the loss of the right to payment was enforced relentlessly. Without exception, unlicensed charlatans were sentenced to return the money they had received for treatment. The same sentence was occasionally issued even against a barber, but only when his behavior appeared to be glaringly charlatan-like. For example, in 1772 the barber Carlo Gavassei was sentenced to return fifteen *paoli* to the patient Domenico Buldrini, who had brought a complaint arguing that as a result of the barber's remedy, "he felt even worse." The barber described his potion as a medical secret made of "gold, air, and silver," but when the protomedici analyzed its chemical composition, they found that it was little more than dirty water.[24] The protomedici were willing to stand by those licensed lower-level practitioners who behaved professionally, but by 1772 a barber-surgeon peddling such "secrets" was considered to be no better than a charlatan.

That the Protomedicato dealt more severely with charlatans than with barbers or apothecaries should not bring into question the protomedici's intention to act as fair judges. From their viewpoint, the false remedies of charlatans were more dangerous to the public than was an occasional brush with illegal practice on the part of licensed practitioners. The protomedici's conduct was, in fact, consistent with the ideal of medical equity that they advocated—the ideal that medical care should be canonical, that is, consistent with the doctrinal orthodoxy established by the learned authorities. They considered it their first and main duty to uphold and to further spread canonical therapies.

Patients, however, had a different notion: what they wanted was not that therapies be orthodox but that they be effective. There were, in fact, two conceptions of medical justice. For the patients, a therapeutic transaction was fair if the healer respected the terms of the cure agreement; for the protomedici, it was fair if the practitioner medicated according to the official rules. This difference between the viewpoints of patients and those of medical authorities can be seen, for example, from the fact that often a suit that was brought by a patient for breach of a cure contract (and was therefore under civil law) would be handled by the Protomedicato as a criminal case (under the rubric of illegal practice), although the plaintiff had formally brought no criminal charges against the defendant.[25]

Thus, even when patients obtained restitution of the sum paid for treatment, it was granted to them according to a principle of justice which was different from their own. The protomedici, in fact, ordered illegal healers to return their fees not because they found the healers guilty of breach of contract but because they considered non-orthodox treatments to be a form of fraud, which entitled patients to a refund as compensation for damages.

II

Patients expected treatment to be effective; the medical authorities dictated that it be orthodox. Lower-level practitioners, especially barber-surgeons, found themselves caught between these two expectations, and the pressure proved to be too much for them. Patients regarded barber-surgeons as "healers," that is, as practitioners whose work could be hired under the terms of a cure agreement and therefore was to be paid for when it produced results. The medical authorities, however, would allow barber-surgeons to claim their fees only if they complied with the official rules. Barber-surgeons were, so to speak, doubly vulnerable: they could lose their fee not only if a patient was unsatisfied with therapy but also, even in case of successful treatment, if they had not abided by the protomedici's rules. In order to be lucrative, their practice had to be both effective and orthodox. Under the compounded pressure of these two constraints—the expectations of the public and those of the medical authorities—the barber-surgeons tried to rid themselves at least of one constraint, the public's expectation that they work under the terms of the cure agreement. This was probably the main reason for the demise of the cure agreement. As shown by the Protomedicato's records, in the second half of the seventeenth century cure agreements practically disappeared from the dealings between patients and barber-surgeons. The agreements survived only among charlatans, who kept making such deals with their patients up until the second half of the eighteenth century.

The history of the cure agreement is a history of constant decline. The medieval contracts, formal documents drawn up by notaries and undersigned by physicians, were replaced by informal, often oral stipulations with lower-level practitioners—initially barbers and unlicensed healers, and subsequently only the latter. Like a splinter slowly but surely pushed out of the body, the custom of making agreements for a cure was slowly but surely driven out of professional medical practice. Dropped first by physicians and

later by barber-surgeons, it was finally altogether banished from regular practice and stigmatized as suitable only to charlatans.

As already mentioned, physicians' unwillingness to enter into cure
agreements began to be expressed in texts on medical ethics in the sixteenth
century. At the beginning of the seventeenth, in the authoritative *Quaestiones
medico-legales,* Paolo Zacchia summarized the new attitude by arguing that
such agreements were unworthy of doctors and should be left to inferior
practitioners such as barber-surgeons. According to Zacchia, a fee obtained
by bargaining lost the dignified status of an *honorarium* and took on instead
the degraded character of *merces* (wages), tainted by its association with manual work. "It goes against the dignity of the physician not only to bargain for
a fee with any patient, for whatever illness and at whatsoever moment, but to
even mention the issue of payment."[26] The prohibition on doctors making
cure agreements, underscored by the treatises on medical ethics, was also
mentioned in the statutes of some colleges, especially those newly founded
in the sixteenth century, which punished severely any violation of this rule.[27]
A significant example can be found in the statutes of the College of Physicians of Modena (1550):

> If a given fee has been agreed upon by a physician and a patient, and the pa-
> tient is slow to pay, we do not want the physician to be thus deprived of his
> due; but the dean and counsellors shall assess the fee on the basis of the days of
> treatment and the patient's social condition, and shall decide, thereupon, the
> amount due to the physician. But if a physician has been so reckless as to
> promise recovery *[salutem]* in front of witnesses and has agreed not to receive
> payment until the patient has been returned to health, in such a case we rule
> that he shall be deprived of all payment whatsoever.[28]

Here, promising a cure is considered to be an unacceptable deviation
from professional behavior. The physician who entered such an agreement
deserved to be punished and was condemned by his peers to the loss of his
fee. This severity indicates how strongly physicians felt the urgency to ban
the cure agreement from professional practice. The insertion of this norm
into the statutes shows that the college wanted to impress on every physician
the duty to support the profession's claim to payment irrespective of results.
Doctors had to present a united front in order to impose this new form of
payment on a reluctant public, which was used to the better terms of the
cure agreement. So the statutes stressed that it was downright unprofessional

for a physician to agree to pocket his fee only upon the patient's recovery. The professionally correct behavior was to request payment on each visit—namely, as the Modena statutes specified, "during the course of treatment, as everyone does, without waiting for treatment to end up with recovery."[29] We should also observe that the loss of payment which was inflicted on the disobedient physician was the same penalty imposed on charlatans; the statutes implied that by promising a cure a physician behaved like a charlatan and ought to be treated as such.

In the seventeenth century, barber-surgeons followed in physicians' footsteps by adopting the new form of professional payment. Their position was particularly difficult since they had none of the authoritative persona of "protectors" enjoyed by the physicians, and patients were accustomed to paying them upon results. Caught in the crossfire of the patients' and the medical authorities' expectations, they reacted by evading as much as possible the pressure from patients, by refusing to enter into cure agreements. By the end of the seventeenth century, barbers who would accept the traditional terms of a cure agreement had become exceedingly rare. In the few examples I found of such contracts, it is clear from the document that this was an exceptional case, one in which unusual circumstances had led the practitioner to grant the patient what was clearly regarded as almost a personal favor. Such was the case in an agreement made in 1696 between the barber-surgeon Bartolomeo Cavazza and Vicenzo, husband of the patient Diamante Lambertini:

> I hereby declare, in the presence of witnesses, that I will treat Diamante Lambertini until full recovery, for a sore that she has on her right foot, by applying remedies, which I will use always after notifying the physician; and in such a way that Vicenzo Lambertini and his family will have no ground of complaint against me, as if, for instance, I tried to prolong treatment by using caustic or bad remedies, God forbid, since it is my wish to conclude treatment as soon as possible. We agree upon seven lire to be paid once Diamante has recovered; and I'm doing this as a favor to Dr. Bonaveri, and with this agreement I rest satisfied.[30]

Although the surgeon speaks in the first person, the agreement was actually written down by Dr. Bonaveri, who was also one of the countersigning witnesses and was probably, as a family friend of the Lambertini's, the mediator of the whole transaction. Most likely, it was because of the physician's insistence ("I'm doing this as a favor to Dr. Bonaveri") that the surgeon gave the Lambertini family preferential treatment by making his fee conditional upon Diamante's recovery. A sign of the times (and of the Protomedicato's hovering presence) is the fact that the surgeon, while promising a cure, also guaranteed orthodox treatment ("always after notifying the physician") and, in doing so, ensured the lawfulness of his position. An even more telling marker of the new balance of power between patient and practitioner is the role of time in this document. The reader will probably remember that, in traditional cure contracts, the healer had to cure the patient within a specified time under penalty of losing his fee. Here, instead, the passing of time is viewed as an element potentially favorable to the surgeon, one that he could take undue advantage of. This can be explained by recalling that in the seventeenth century the way of paying for medical care had changed radically. As we saw in chapter 4, a new pattern emerged whereby patients were charged not for a whole course of treatment but instead for each single, specific service. For example, barber-surgeons' bills now listed each service rendered,[31] following the model of physicians, who indicated the number of visits. This new circumstance explains why the agreement between the surgeon Cavazza and Lambertini was such a good deal for the patient, grudgingly granted by the surgeon. Obviously, it would have been more profitable for the practitioner to be paid for each service instead of having to wait for the end of treatment and the uncertain outcome of recovery. Time was now on the practitioner's side: since patients paid for each service, the longer the treatment, the higher the payment.

Disconnecting payment from recovery also involved a fundamental change in the way in which people thought about therapy. No longer viewed as a whole, unified process oriented toward the restoration of health, therapy was now fragmented into a series of standardized procedures, each with a monetary value of its own. Therapy and the restoration of health became in this way two separate concepts. Turning to a practitioner no longer meant asking for recovery; it now meant only asking for a specific medical service, to be paid for separately, regardless of final results.

In *Le médecin malgré lui*, Molière described Sganarello's delighted discovery, when forced to don the robes of a physician, that a doctor could claim payment "whether he does well [or] whether he does damage," as quoted in the epigraph to this chapter. By the mid–seventeenth century, Molière could still hope to lampoon this claim as preposterous, but the bent of the times was inexorably against him. What Sganarello quickly found out with a rogue's enthusiasm was made possible by the disappearance of the agreement for a cure. By the eighteenth century, patients no longer linked payment for medical care to the recovery of health. When they turned to the

Protomedicato to dispute a practitioner's bill, they no longer mentioned whether they had been healed or not but merely contested the number of services performed by the practitioner. For example, when Edoardo Modona was sued for debt by the surgeon Giovanni Antonio Lodi in 1747, he requested that the court read him the surgeon's bill — since he was illiterate — and then challenged the number of services mentioned by the surgeon. He also asked the protomedici to lower the surgeon's fee in consideration of his poverty.[32] Patients no longer expected that justice be done on the basis of the agreement for a cure, but only that the protomedici establish a fair price for the medical service and, at most, that they charitably lower the fee to meet the needs of indigent patients.

III

The disappearance of the cure agreement from medical practice implied also the waning of a view of medicine which allowed for self-diagnosis and self-therapy. This change was probably due to the converging pressure that both patients and medical authorities were exerting on barber-surgeons. In order to practice legally, barber-surgeons were required to act under a physician's supervision, and not upon the patients' request. At the same time, their business depended largely on a demand for medical services which was based, more often than not, upon some kind of self-diagnosis. People who felt sick usually decided to have their blood drawn, without seeing the need to consult a physician. Their requests to barber-surgeons, therefore, were incompatible with the official rules. This was the dilemma faced by barber-surgeons in their daily practice. They had to meet the needs of clients who still viewed therapy as an aid to the self-purification of the body, with regard to which a physician's "advice" was deemed irrelevant. Many surgeons found themselves in this difficult position, caught between the incompatible demands of physicians and patients. This is just what happened in 1701 to Taddeo Azzoguidi, surgeon of Castel San Pietro. As the husband of a patient testified:

> My wife Isabella, seriously wounded, sent for Signor Taddeo to draw her blood; he . . . asked if the doctor had been consulted about this; and since the answer was no, he refused to draw blood and left. But the said Isabella, restless for the pain, again sent for Signor Taddeo and told him that she absolutely wanted a bloodletting; and Signor Taddeo answered that it was necessary first

to notify the doctor; and Isabella replied, "I do not want the doctor on my ass; if you want to draw blood, as is your bounden duty, do it, or else I'll send for some other barber."[33]

A seventy-year-old barber-surgeon, convicted in 1743 of "medicating, prescribing caustic remedies and opiates, [and] signing certificates of exemption from Lent," and charged, among other things, with having drawn blood from a girl without a physician's prescription, testified that he had repeatedly told the girl's parents to send for a physician but that they had not heeded him. His deposition confirms that, for many patients, calling a barber did not include the intervention of a supervising physician: "I visit the poor who don't have a physician, or who are not attended by the doctors. . . . I go to them when they call me . . . ; and I have drawn blood and prescribed pectoral waters *[acque pettorali]* and ointments."[34] The performance of this barber, as he himself described it, was clearly in the tradition of self-therapy; the treatment that he had prescribed for the girl was an extension of the remedies already applied by her family ("noticing she had been anointed, I told them to keep anointing her").[35]

The link between the barber's role and the tradition of self-therapy is confirmed by the fact that many patients felt confident that they could appraise the professional skills of a barber without the help of any physician. Let us hear, for example, how a stable-boy rated the skills of Alessio Porta, surgeon and apothecary in the village of Molinella, in 1745:

Feeling sick on a Sunday, just after lunch, I went to the stables and threw myself on the cot there, where I spent the night. The morning after, Signor Alessio Porta . . . happened to come by. He felt my pulse and told me it was necessary to draw blood. . . . He probably tore my vein, because he hurt me a lot. After bloodletting, he told me that I should take some medicine by mouth, and gave me I don't know what in a glass . . . ; and it was so bad that I refused to drink any more of it. He came back to visit me another time, but knowing that I could not get well in his hands, I asked him what was due for his services, and I got rid of him.[36]

But by the middle of the eighteenth century one can see in patients a new attitude toward barber-surgeons—an attitude clearly influenced by physicians and, particularly, by their disapproval of evacuatory therapies performed without a doctor's supervision. In 1759, a tailor of Castel San Pietro accused the surgeon Gordini of drawing blood from a woman who was seven months pregnant, causing her to get breast cancer: "I heard from many physicians of Bologna who visited the woman that this bloodletting gave her breast cancer."[37] The physicians' opinion now stood between patients and surgeons even in the case of bloodletting, a procedure traditionally associated with self-therapy. It is interesting to notice that patients' attitude toward this most basic among evacuative therapies (bloodletting was traditionally considered the "general evacuation") was changing radically. People began to be afraid of it and accused barber-surgeons of overusing it. (It is possible, indeed, that the new terms of payment, linked to each service rendered, might have actually led barbers to overdo this procedure.) A surgeon was criticized for drawing blood from a woman five times in six hours and for "opening three times the vein in the same place."[38] "I didn't want to allow so many bloodlettings," complained a farmer who had hired a barber to treat his wife, "ill with a fever."[39] These comments echo physicians' attitude toward bloodletting—an attitude that precisely at this time (the mid–eighteenth century) became more negative than in the past.[40]

All of this can be seen as a steady decline of traditional self-therapy and, in particular, of patients' traditional right to define recovery in lay terms. This is suggested by a cure agreement—the last one we find in the archives of the Protomedicato—signed in 1764 by a charlatan known as "Il Corso" (the Corsican), and Francesco Fossi, innkeeper in the village of Pianoro and steward in the household of Countess Zambeccari. The agreement is like all of those previously examined except for one significant detail: establishment of recovery was left to a professional surgeon rather than to the patient himself.

Il Corso promised to cure Fossi, who suffered from gallstone, by dissolving the stone "without surgery, only with his remedies and medical secrets," within a period of seven months. The patient, in turn, agreed to deposit a payment of forty-five *zecchini* in the hands of Carlo Redi, a professional surgeon ("professore chirurgo," he is called in the document) employed at the Ospedale della Vita. Redi was also entrusted with establishing whether the stone was gone or not. At the end of the seven months, the healer would receive the forty-five zecchini only "after the surgeon performed a test with a syringe and declared under oath in a written statement that the patient no longer has the stone."[41] The other terms of the agreement were unfavorable to the patient: he would lose his money if he refused to submit to the syringe test (a painful procedure) or if he decided to interrupt the treatment.

This contract shows that the traditional, horizontal relationship between patient and healer had been infiltrated by the vertical element of professionalism; certification of recovery now required a judgment based on the technical expertise of a professional.

What happened next? Il Corso began treatment in early April and by May asserted that the patient was healed. The innkeeper, however, complained of pain and felt that he was still affected by the disease. As his son related to the protomedici: "It ended up with my father being visited by Redi . . . ; and after the test with the syringe, in which my father almost died of pain, it was concluded that, unfortunately, he was still suffering from the stone and had the same ailment as before."[42] After a short absence from Bologna, Il Corso wished to resume the treatment, but the patient refused and filed a suit in the Protomedicato (the charlatan, in turn, appealed to the cardinal legate). After establishing that the remedy used was "fallacious," the protomedici sentenced Il Corso to pay trial expenses and forbade him to prescribe internal medications in the future. The text of the sentence does not mention the restitution of the deposit to the patient, but it contains an interesting comment on cure agreements in general. Such contracts, the protomedici stated, ought to be considered "iniquitous and dishonest, invalid, not to be allowed even to regularly licensed practitioners."[43]

What did the protomedici mean by saying that agreements for a cure were "iniquitous and invalid"? We know that, from the sixteenth century on, medical ethics considered such agreements as unsuitable for physicians, but that nonetheless, at the turn of that century, the protomedici still recognized the agreement as a legally valid transaction, which they were called upon to endorse in their role as magistrates. By the second half of the eighteenth century, their attitude had changed radically, as we can observe in the case of Il Corso versus Fossi. The protomedici now viewed the agreement no longer as simply unprofessional but as legally invalid. In this, they followed the jurisprudence of their own times. During the seventeenth century, in fact, some European jurists already had started to argue that agreements for a cure should not be considered a valid form of contract.

IV

This new opinion of the jurists was another crucial factor in the process leading to the disappearance of the cure agreement. Doubts as to the legal validity of cure contracts were raised first in the sixteenth century — for instance, by Gian Filippo Ingrassia, the Sicilian protomedico whose guidelines for establishing medical fees, as we saw in chapter 2, included some consideration of treatment results. Ingrassia advised that physicians relinquish once and for all the old habit of entering into cure agreements with their patients. His reasons were mainly ethical: some practitioners, he argued, might charge exorbitant fees for a cure, exploiting the fears of their patients. But he had legal objections as well, because in case of a dispute, he thought, it would be difficult to prove the validity of such agreements in a court of law.[44]

As a matter of fact, Italian court records of the sixteenth century show that the legal validity of the cure agreements was challenged in some lawsuits over medical payment. Evidence of this can be found in the *decisiones*—legal reports compiled by early modern jurists on the motivations for a court's sentences.[45] In a collection of such reports on the sentences issued by the Regio Consiglio of Naples, published in 1509 by the renowned jurist Matteo d'Afflitto, we find a discussion of the lawsuit between the surgeon Carlo Copula and the heirs of the patient Pietro de Blancha. The surgeon demanded payment of one hundred *ducati* for successfully medicating the wounded man (the patient died later of other causes). The Neapolitan court ruled in favor of the surgeon, thus acknowledging the juridical validity of the agreement for a cure. However, in reporting this decision, d'Afflitto, who had been one of the judges in charge of the case, admitted to some doubts about the sentence:

> At first I was of contrary opinion, viz. that the heirs should not be required to pay the fee promised to the surgeon, because it is not allowed to physicians to be promised payment by the patients in exchange for treatment—such promises are unlawful. On this issue, I cited the "Archiatri" law . . . as well as the "Si medicus" law. . . .
>
> But on further consideration, I saw that the "Archiatri" law refers to a physician salaried by a community, and therefore is not relevant to our case. No more is the "Si medicus" law, which concerns a physician who applies harmful remedies, in which case any promise of payment by the patient should be voided. . . . The Sacred Council unanimously ruled that in the case at hand, however, the promise was valid, and the heirs of the patient who had been cured *[convaluit]* of his wound were sentenced to pay the surgeon the sum of one hundred ducati.[46]

Similar doubts were aired in a case heard by the Rota of Florence. This time the plaintiff was a physician, Jacopo de Melioratis, of Pistoia, who sued the heirs of the patient Francesco Bottegari, whom he had treated for a fistula. The terms of the agreement specified seven months of treatment, for which the patient should pay fourteen scudi. At the time of the trial, this amount had been paid, but since the treatment had been prolonged for fourteen more months, the physician demanded an additional payment. The agreement in this case did not require a cure: the physician had simply agreed to render his services to the patient for a given period of time, in exchange for a salary, without promising recovery. In other words, the contract was similar to a hiring contract (*patto di condotta*) between a physician and a community. This explains why the physician had found the agreement acceptable; by this time, physicians were refusing to sign cure agreements, but their business was largely based on patti di condotta with groups or communities and even, as in this case, private citizens. In ruling in favor of the physician, the Florentine court explicitly considered the contract between de Melioratis and Bottegari as fundamentally equivalent to a patto di condotta. In fact, the court assumed that the contract between the physician and his patient had been tacitly renewed, just as usually happened with patti di condotta between physicians and communities (if not explicitly rescinded, the hiring contract was supposed to be implicitly renewed year after year).[47] Although upholding the validity of this specific contract, the jurists who handled this case entertained some doubts as to the validity of agreements between doctors and patients:

> Having issued the sentence, we expressed some doubts among ourselves that the salary requested should be actually paid, because a patient's promise to the physician does not seem to be legally binding according to the "Archiatri" law. . . . We found that Matteo d'Afflitto had also expressed doubts on this issue with reference to a sentence of the Neapolitan Council in favor of a physician. D'Afflitto, however, stated that the "Archiatri" law applies only to physicians whose salary is paid by the community: these indeed are not allowed to receive additional payment from patients, and any promises made to them are not binding.[48]

The jurists questioned the legitimacy of the agreement between patient and practitioner on the ground of two Roman laws: the "Archiatri" law, part of the Code of Justinian, and the "Si medicus" law, included in the Digest. We have examined these laws in chapter 2, when comparing Roman and barbaric legislation on medical matters. It may be helpful to cite again the relevant parts of these laws, so that the reader can see the textual grounds on which the jurists based their doubts. Here is the pertinent section of the "Archiatri" law:

> The town physicians should be aware that their salaries come from the public, and in consequence they should honestly treat the poor rather than shamelessly

serve the rich. They will be allowed to accept what their patients offer them once they have been cured, but not what those who are dangerously sick promise in exchange for health.[49]

First of all, we should note that this law concerned only public physicians who received a salary from a community. The law did not allow them to request additional payments from the sick (and thus serve the rich rather than the poor). In and of itself, the text of this law did not prohibit agreements between physicians and patients in general, but prohibited such agreements only for those physicians who were already salaried by the community. As to the law "Si medicus," it dealt with a particularly reprehensible case of medical sharp practice: "If a physician, whom someone entrusted with treating his eyes, uses harmful medications to the point of almost making the patient blind, in order to compel him in bad faith to sell his goods to himself, the governor of the province shall punish the physician for this illegal action and shall order that the goods sold be returned to the patient."[50]

Here, also, the law does not prohibit all agreements between patient and practitioner, but only those based on medical fraud. In the case mentioned, a physician applied harmful medications to his patient's eyes, worsening his condition and thus increasing the patient's fear of going blind, in order to press him to sell his property to the physician himself on unfair terms. In such a case, the patient's consent to the agreement was extorted through fraudulent pressure. This vitiates the contract and makes it voidable.[51] While both laws seem clearly to indicate the intention to combat abuses in medical practice, they did not deny the legality of agreements signed in good faith. This was, in fact, the traditional interpretation of these laws by medieval jurists.[52] In the cases decided by the Regio Consiglio of Naples and by the Rota of Florence, as we have seen above, the jurists, in spite of their doubts, opted for the traditional interpretation of the two laws, restricting the invalidity of the contract only to those cases in which the physician was a town doctor or acted in bad faith.[53]

Starting in the second half of the sixteenth century, in contrast, jurists increasingly adopted the view that all agreements between physician and patient were legally invalid. They read the "Archiatri" and "Si medicus" laws as prohibiting any form of agreement between physicians and patients, not only those signed in bad faith. For example, Pinhel, in an argument that many other jurists quoted as the last word on the controversy, criticized the traditional, restrictive interpretation of the two laws and maintained that both referred to all doctors.[54] Like other jurists who followed his interpretation, Pinhel based his argument on the analogy between physicians and lawyers. As a matter of fact, some texts of the Digest and of the Code of Justinian expressly prohibited lawyers from entering into agreements with their clients while the legal case was pending, and especially vetoed lawyers' practice of bargaining for a portion of the property that might be awarded to the client if he won the case. Thus, Roman law absolutely prohibited legal advisors from striking a deal for a fee with their client during legal proceedings. Here is the relevant passage from the Digest:

> If a lawyer has been promised a honorarium and if he has come to an agreement on legal services: let us see whether he can claim the agreed-upon sum. This is what our emperor and his divine father wrote about these agreements: "It is a bad custom to exact a promise of payment in exchange for legal counsel. By law, if an agreement on future payment is signed while the case is still pending, such an agreement will be null. But if the agreement is signed once the legal case is solved, the lawyer will be entitled to ask for a reasonable payment, even when payment was promised as a percentage of what the client obtains by winning the case *[nomine palmarii],* as long as the amount that the client gives the lawyer does not exceed the limits established by law to lawyers' fees."[55]

The early modern jurists argued that if a lawyer was prohibited from entering an agreement with his client while the case was still pending, the same prohibition should also apply to a physician, because client and patient were similarly vulnerable.[56] Contracts between doctor and patient, like those between lawyer and client, were always vitiated by patients' and clients' fear *(metus)* of losing, respectively, their life or their property. As argued by Vincenzo Carocci, the author of an influential treatise on leases and contracts: "One could say that the patient is necessarily forced into the agreement by the hope of regaining health, just as a client is driven by the hope of winning the case."[57] Accordingly, any agreements between a physician and a patient, including agreements for a cure, are vitiated by fear and therefore should be considered legally invalid.

This opinion prevailed among early modern jurists, although controversy on the issue persisted throughout the seventeenth century and well into the eighteenth.[58] In 1736, H. Lampe summarized the discussion in his learned legal-historical treatise on the medical profession.[59] Lampe disagreed with those who, like Paolo Zacchia in *Quaestiones medico-legales,* had argued that the agreement was unsuitable for physicians but acceptable for surgeons and other lower-level practitioners. In contrast, Lampe believed that the text of the "Si medicus" law concerned all medical practitioners. Furthermore, it did not make sense to maintain that the agreement was illegal only if the patient's fear *(metus)* could be proven, because by definition, fear was inherent in the condition of the sick, just as it was in that of litigants. For Lampe, once more, the analogy between lawyer and physician resolved the issue. Just as it was prohibited for a lawyer to bargain about a fee when the legal case was still pending, even more so should such bargaining be prohibited to physicians, since life is more important than property.[60] Thus, even bona fide agreements for a cure ought to be considered to be against the law.

The analogy between physician and lawyer which was underscored by these jurists was a time-honored commonplace,[61] as was the companion analogy between patient and client. The thirteenth-century legal scholar Odofredo used it in his *Lectura super codice,* when discussing the law that prohibited all kinds of agreements between lawyers and clients:

> Gentlemen, this is a very honest law. Keep this in mind: since the lawyer takes upon himself to help his client in good faith, he cannot buy anything from him or come to any agreement with him while the legal case is still pending.
>
> In fact, you should know that patients and clients share the same nature and the same behavior. The client is always running after his lawyer, and even on holy days leaves his village to go see his lawyer and ask him what to do; therefore, if he signs a contract with him, this will not be valid, because for fear of losing his suit, he is willing to give anything. . . .
>
> And the same can be said of the patient: the patient has no other lord and master than his physician; and if the physician buys from the patient, the transaction is not valid, because the law assumes that the only agreement the patient can make with the physician is for a cure. Therefore a sale (from the patient to the physician) is not valid because, fearing death, the patient is willing to give anything.[62]

Odofredo sees the relationship between lawyer and client, or physician and patient, as featuring the same bond of domination and dependency as that between patron and client—or even master and servant, as the above passage indicates. According to medieval jurists, any transaction between master and servant was presumably invalidated by fear *(metus)*: "Fear and a relationship of domination and servitude invalidate the transaction."[63] An unbalanced power relationship (as between master and servant, or husband and wife) cannot lead to an equitable transaction, because of the strong likelihood that the weak party would be intimidated into consent, which would invalidate the agreement. It should be noticed, however, that Odofredo refers not to a cure agreement signed in good faith, but to a sale contract between patient and physician, presumably involving conditions unfavorable to the former. Odofredo clearly distinguished between agreements signed in good faith and those signed in bad faith. It is precisely this distinction which early modern jurists wiped out, by condemning all agreements between physician and patient. Furthermore, Odofredo's lively description of the patient's subservience to his physician was only an anecdotal, incidental notation. In the seventeenth-century legal treatises on the privileges of the sick, in contrast, this same image became the basis of a new juridical theory on the social weakness of the sick, and the consequent need to afford them legal protection. The starting point of this theory was once more the commonplace analogy between patient and client. For example, in *De infirmitate eiusque privilegiis* (1603), Tommaso Azzio maintained, "The lawyer cannot come to an agreement with the client, because the latter is willing to give up everything for fear of legal action; and so does the patient with the physician, for fear of death."[64] But new consequences were drawn from the analogy, namely that even bona fide agreements for a cure were against the law, as argued by Heinrich von Bode in his *De iuribus infirmorum* (1693):

> It is concurring opinion that some people are forbidden to make contracts with the sick, in compliance with the "Si medicus" and "Archiatri" laws. A physician cannot legally make a contract with a patient during illness; and if a sale contract is signed, it must be voided. . . . In fact, a patient agreeing to sign a contract in such circumstances does so for fear of death rather than out of his own free will. What is established by the "Quisquis" law of the Codex, in the section "De postulando" (that no promises or agreements shall be made between lawyer and client when the case is pending) should also be applied to physician and patient, for reasons of analogy. . . .
>
> From the prohibition, expressed in the "Archiatri" law, against physicians' accepting what the sick offer in exchange for their health, it should be inferred that all agreements and promises made with the intention to recover health should be considered invalid.[65]

The illegality of the agreements between physician and patient was argued by these jurists on the basis of a wider conceptualization of the sick's right to protection. By prohibiting the cure agreement, they argued, the law ensured protection of the sick from medical abuses. One of the privileges of the sick was precisely the right to be legally protected from such iniquitous transactions as cure agreements.

Let us pause briefly to compare this juridical theory with the social reality we have observed in the courtrooms of the Protomedicato. The jurists presented the agreement for a cure as an inequitable transaction. But was it really so? Definitely not from the point of view of the patients. To them, the agreement was perfectly equitable as long as both parties kept their promises. Unquestionably, many of these agreements were signed by both patient and healer in good faith. Moreover, the cure agreements that we have examined so far (except perhaps for the one between innkeeper Fossi and Il Corso, whose terms were unusually unfair to the patient) do not confirm the jurists' image of a helpless patient in the clutches of an all-powerful physician. Although the patient's dread of sickness and death was undoubtedly an aspect of the agreement, the practitioner, in turn, was faced with fear of failure and loss. The cure agreement forced practitioners to face the limits of their skills and knowledge every time they undertook treatment. Treating someone on these terms made sense only if the healer, having visited the patient, felt reasonably confident of being able to cure him. Linking payment to results thus protected patients from charlatanism (which is nothing but false promise). Moreover, by binding the healer to a promise of good results and by giving the patient the right to evaluate the results, the agreement strongly limited medical dominance in the transaction. The practitioner's obligation to perform a cure was the balancing element in the agreement—the element that equalized the relationship between patient and healer, making it truly contractual.

In contrast, the jurists believed that a genuine contractual relationship between patient and healer could not exist, because any agreement between the two would be invalidated by the patient's fear. This juridical argument, which at first sight seems so sensitive to the interests of patients, can only stand if one ignores a crucial aspect of the agreement: the promise of a cure. And in fact, while the jurists insisted on the obligations that the agreement imposed on the patient, they never mentioned the obligation imposed on the healer—the obligation to effect a cure.[66] Had I researched the history of the cure agreements exclusively through the texts of early modern jurists, I would never have learned that the agreement was based on making payment conditional upon results, as this significant detail is never mentioned in early modern juridical literature.

Reading early modern jurists on this issue, I was at first extremely puzzled, because their description of the cure agreement seemed so utterly out

of touch with what happened in the courtrooms. In court, the patients described the cure agreement as a good-faith exchange of promises between
two parties who considered themselves on an equal level. The jurists, instead,
described it as a reprehensible abuse of power imposed by an all-powerful
practitioner on a helpless patient. And in a disconcerting twist, precisely
while insisting on the need to safeguard the interests of patients, they eliminated (from sight, from memory, from discussion) what truly protected patients against medical fraud — the promise of a cure.

Compared with the courtroom record, the jurists' view of the cure
agreement seems totally unsupported — a learned fiction with very little
bearing, or no bearing at all, on patients' actual experience. By suppressing
any mention of the promise of a cure, this juridical fiction presented a dis-
torted picture of the agreement as structurally skewed in favor of the healer
and, therefore, inequitable.

It is important to point out that by suppressing all mention of the
promise, the jurists not only ignored the facts but also passed over in silence
a long juridical tradition with which, undoubtedly, they were very familiar.
In order to assert the invalidity of the agreement between patient and healer,
they had to advance a rather shaky new interpretation of the "Si medicus"
law and the "Archiatri" law, one that was totally at odds with the medieval
commentaries. In fact, a gloss to the Digest (much quoted, in the Middle
Ages, as a cornerstone of all juridical doctrine on the patient-doctor relationship) clearly upheld the legal validity of the cure agreement. The gloss
examined the case of a physician who undertook by contract to cure a patient affected by gout, with payment contingent upon recovery.[67] The issue
raised in the gloss was whether or not the physician was entitled to payment
if the patient relapsed after a temporary recovery. Obviously, in the glossator's
mind, the promise of a cure was a legally binding aspect of the doctor-patient agreement. If the patient had been promised recovery, was the physician
entitled to payment if the recovery had been short-lived? Beyond all doubt,
the gloss assumed that a cure agreement signed in good faith was fully valid
from a legal point of view — or else the issue it raised would not make any
sense.

This gloss was cited and discussed for centuries by commentators on
the civil law.[68] It was, beyond all doubt, a very well known juridical text. Yet
it was never mentioned by those early modern jurists who argued that the
cure agreement was unlawful. (A few admitted incidentally that their views
were at odds with the gloss, but did not seem to think much of it.)[69]

Early modern jurists might have had more reasons than one for ignoring this gloss. One of those reasons might have been that it concerned a section of the Digest that dealt with leases and contracts. The context of the gloss is, in fact, significant and deserves some attention. The law that was commented on dealt with the case of a contract to build a house: during construction, the building was ruined by an earthquake. Since the damage resulted from natural causes, the law established that the builder was liable for damages (in this case, for the cost of rebuilding).[70] Obviously, the glossator saw an analogy between these circumstances and those of a physician whose patient relapsed owing to natural causes — in both cases, he argued, the party performing the work was liable for damages resulting from the workings of nature. The gloss, therefore, implied a classification of labor which included physicians and craftsmen in the same class: both were to be paid at the completion of their work, on the basis of results, and both could be hired by contract.

In the early modern age, in contrast, jurists employed a completely different classification of labor: their professional opinion was that the physician's work ought to be considered a liberal art, intrinsically different from the labor of craftsmen. As a liberal art, the jurists argued, the doctor's work could not be hired by contract (here, also, they seem to have willingly shut their eyes to the overwhelming evidence of the *patti di condotta*). They conceded that medical work could be hired by contract only if the practitioner was a slave, as had occurred in Roman antiquity.[71] Similarly, in *Tractatus locati et conducti* Carocci argued that the issue of relapse mentioned in the gloss concerned only lower-level practitioners such as surgeons and farriers, whose services were of a servile nature and could, therefore, be hired by contract.[72]

Thus, the jurists' disregard of this gloss to the Digest may have been due to their assumption that it no longer applied to physicians, whose work, as a liberal art, did not fall under the rules of contracts. There is no doubt, however, that the very existence of the gloss was an embarrassment for the jurists, because it contradicted what they were keen on arguing, viz., that medicine had always been considered a liberal art. The gloss proved instead, with incontrovertible evidence, that in a not too distant past, the physician's work had been considered to be on a par with the manual work of the craftsman. But above all, the gloss embarrassed the jurists because it contradicted the general principle that they were trying to establish — namely, the invalidity of all agreements between physicians and patients. Giving recognition to the traditional doctrine embodied in the gloss would have meant recognizing the fact that, historically, the agreement between healer and patient was based on the promise of a cure. This was precisely what the jurists had to ignore if they wished to argue the invalidity of the cure agreement.

Why were the jurists so determined to condemn the cure agreement? After all, physicians — who had higher stakes in the issue — denounced the agreement not as illegal but only as unsuitable for upper-rank practitioners. The jurists were especially responsible for surrounding the agreement with an aura of reprobation, for presenting it as morally objectionable and against the law. There is evidence that their interest in the issue was intense: the debate over the cure agreement involved the most famous legal scholars in Europe and was the topic of several seventeenth-century legal dissertations.[73] Why all this interest?

I mentioned earlier that the analogy between physician and lawyer played a fundamental role in the jurists' argument regarding the invalidity of the cure agreement. The fact is that when dealing with the agreement between doctor and patient, early modern jurists were also dealing with an issue that concerned them very closely — the issue of payment for legal services. An important element of similarity in the histories of the legal and the medical professions is the issue of remuneration. Lawyers' fees, like physicians', seem originally to have been dependent on results. There are clear traces of an ancient tradition (probably as ancient as the agreement for a cure) whereby a lawyer would receive his fee *(palmarium)* only when he won a case (in fact, the palmarium was a percentage of the property won by the litigant).[74] A lawyer's honorarium, like a physician's, was promised by the client and was paid only when the work had been successfully completed.[75] A long-standing debate addressed the issue of when a lawyer should be paid — at the beginning of, during, or at the end of a legal case — just as a similar debate concerned the appropriate timing of payments to physicians. Medieval jurists maintained that lawyers, like physicians, should be paid at the completion of their services.[76] Analogously, just as the jurists discussed whether a physician should treat his patient without charge in case of relapse, they also discussed whether a lawyer who promised to plead a case for a given fee ought to offer his legal services for free when the case was appealed.[77]

The professionalization of both medicine and law required the suppression of the traditional view that regarded legal and medical services as similar to a craftsman's labor and thus compensable upon successful completion. This is why the jurists were so keen on attacking the cure agreement. They also were trying to get rid of a traditional principle that stood in the way of their claim to be paid regardless of results. By condemning cure agreements, they were attacking something that hindered not only the development of the medical profession but also that of the legal profession. In fact, the same professional strategy allowed both lawyers and physicians to overcome these traditional impediments to the development of their professions. Significantly, just as the statutes of some medical colleges prohibited physicians from signing agreements for a cure, so also the professional associations of lawyers forbade their members to sign contracts in which they agreed to receive payment only if they won the case.[78] The same professional ethics upheld the principle that a lawyer should receive his salary even if he lost the case, as long as his conduct complied with professional standards, just as a physician should be paid even if the patient died, as long as the prescribed therapy had been canonical.[79] In his treatise on the privileges of the sick, the jurist Azzio used once again the analogy between lawyer and physician to refute the traditional opinion that doctors should treat their patients without charge in case of relapse. "Just as a lawyer who has represented a client in a legal case is not required to represent him again without charge when the case goes on appeal . . . so, too, physicians are not required to treat a second time without charge those they have already treated once."[80]

Clearly, in presenting the cure agreement as legally invalid, the jurists were directly prompted by their professional self-interest, which made it crucial for them to establish that remuneration of the liberal professions should be unhinged from traditional shackles. Thanks to their control over the interpretation of the law, the jurists were able to present as a rule of general interest what was in truth the special interest of the liberal professions.

V

Early modern jurists wove the legal fiction of the invalidity of cure agreements very skillfully. They did it by presenting themselves as champions of the sick and of justice, rather than advocates of their own professional interest. Their rejection of the agreement for a cure was offered to the public as being entirely justified by ethical reasons. To this purpose, the jurists used the moral principles of Christian paternalism: the strong have the duty to protect the weak and should not take advantage of them. Counter-Reformation precepts for physicians taught that it was a mortal sin for a doctor to demand high fees from patients, exploiting their fear of dying.[81] Christian and professional ethics agreed in viewing the physician as the dominant party in the therapeutic relationship. From a professional, as well as Christian, viewpoint, the strong should not profit from the frailties of the weak. The cure agreement was immoral precisely because it was seen as the instrument by which the physician could prey upon the patient's vulnerability. With the same judicious mixture of professional and Christian precepts, the jurists condemned the promise of a cure. It was not only unprofessional behavior ("the vice of those less worthy in the profession," as Paolo Zacchia wrote)[82] but also a sin of arrogance, because recovery could come only from God.

This complex of ethical and juridical arguments underlay the new attitude of the Bolognese protomedici toward the agreement for a cure. The new professional ethics smoothly merged with the traditional "estate-ethos" of the medical elite. In the medical elite's self-image, as we saw earlier, the therapeutic role was marginal; the elite physician saw himself, first of all, as a gracious patron who offered protection rather than recovery. The task that these physicians attributed to themselves in medical practice was first of all a protective role: a general supervision over the regimen of the body. Professional ethics supported this image of the physician as a custodian and patron, morally obliged to protect the patient.

Relatively detached from the tensions of day-to-day involvement in practice, the medical elite envisioned the doctor-patient relationship as vertical and hierarchical, centered on sick persons' dependency on the physician's authority. In their view, justice meant protection. Even their supervision of lower-rank practitioners and popular healers was linked to this principle. By ensuring the compliance of all medical procedures, even the most menial ones, with the rules issued from above, the protomedici tried to bring all healing acts under their own control.

Their vision excluded any possibility of a horizontal therapeutic relationship. The medical authorities were unable to see that the agreement for a cure implied an attempt by the sick to establish a more balanced relationship between themselves and their healers. The agreement for a cure was based not only on a principle of equity (represented by the mutual exchange of promises in good faith) but also on a principle of equality. In the cure agreement, healer and patient stood on equal ground: the healer's expertise was measured against the exacting yardstick of efficacy by the sturdy common sense of the patients. Such a state of things was inadmissible to the medical authorities, just as it was inadmissible to the jurists, who, in fact, passed it over in silence.

There is a hidden irony in the justice that the Protomedicato rendered to the sick. They were often granted what they asked for, but for reasons dif-

ferent from those which had prompted their pleas. They asked the protomedici to implement the cure agreement; ironically, it was precisely the
protomedici's intervention in the relationship between healers and patients,
with the pressure it put on lower-rank practitioners, that forced the agreement out of medical practice.

The history of the cure agreement has shown us that the vertical
model of healing was destined to prevail over the horizontal model. In the
eighteenth century, more clearly than in the past, the therapeutic relationship
had become a relationship of dependency. The social authority of the physician over the patient therefore predates the great transformation of medicine
in the second half of the nineteenth century, which enormously reinforced
the prestige and social clout of physicians. What the sociologists today call
the doctors' "professional dominance"[83] is not simply a consequence of new
medical technologies but is rooted in the early modern codification of the
doctor-patient relationship in accord with the vertical model of patronage.
Modern medical dominance is certainly based on the erasure — from history
as well as from memory — of the ancient horizontal model of healing which
I have called the agreement for a cure.

It took many centuries to eradicate this model and replace it with the
vertical doctor-patient relationship envisioned by the jurists in the ancien
régime. This vertical relationship not only survived but thrived in the society
of the nineteenth century. Indeed, it still thrives today; it is a piece of ancien
régime that we still carry with us.

There is one last paradox related to this issue which deserves mentioning. I showed how the majority of jurists in the seventeenth and eighteenth
centuries argued against all contractual agreements between physician and
patient. But the traditional opinion advocating the legality of such agreements (as long as they were signed in good faith) did not completely disappear,[84] and in the early nineteenth century, paradoxically, it was resurrected as
the new common opinion. Early-nineteenth-century jurists argued that contracts between doctor and patient were legally valid because one ought to re-
ject the assumption that physicians intend to exploit the patient's condition
of fear. They argued that such a generalized suspicion had been justified in
ancient times, when physician were often slaves or belonged to the lower
classes, but seemed nonsensical in modern times, when medical men were
gentlemen with a professional moral code.[85] By the early nineteenth century,
jurists could acknowledge the validity of contracts between doctors and patients without any qualms of conscience. Why so? Probably because by that
time the agreement for a cure had completely disappeared, even from the

dealings of lower-rank practitioners (in fact, the three-tiered hierarchy no longer existed, since by then physicians and surgeons were professional peers).[86] Once the promise of a cure had been expunged from medical practice, and the balance of power between patient and doctor had been irrevocably altered in favor of the latter, jurists were free to redefine the doctor-patient relationship as a contract.[87] But the nineteenth-century relationship between doctor and patient was no longer a contract in the ancient egalitarian sense. Like many other contracts on which nineteenth-century society was based, the contract between doctor and patient hid a heavy imbalance of power behind the appearance of consensual agreement.

In the same way, the contractual form of the modern patient-doctor relationship is simply a thin veneer disguising the overwhelming dominance of the medical profession. Nothing could be more different from the ancient, egalitarian balance between patient and healer than the modern relationship between doctor and patient. To appreciate the difference, we only have to think, just for a second, how much our medical system would have to change if we could ask our physicians to deliver recovery in exchange for payment. What was once a social reality is now the wildest of all medical utopias.

VI

Finally, let us return to the patients' viewpoint. We have seen how, by the end of the eighteenth century, they no longer received a promise of a cure but were given a promise of protection and orthodox treatment instead. Recovery was no longer something that the patients had a right to ask for, even in dealing with unlicensed practitioners. Even quacks demanded payment regardless of the outcome of treatment, as the charlatan Boschetti told Lucia Zaffi in 1758 ("He wanted to be paid even if I had not been cured," lamented the woman).[88]

Of course, the disappearance of the promise of a cure did not mean that patients stopped asking for recovery. After all, they had other resources beside the earthly medical system. The therapeutic horizon of the people of a Catholic, early modern city was much broader than our modern, limited perspective. When seeking help during illness, these patients often looked upward to heaven—to the invisible presence of the saints, with their supernatural thaumaturgic powers. It is within the history of healing miracles that we should follow the historical development of the patients' obstinate search for a cure.

I am not suggesting that we view miraculous healings as an alternative to the limitations that the professionalization of medicine imposed on the patients' quest for health. Actually, turning to a saint made perfect sense in a society that viewed the therapeutic transaction as a vertical relationship of dependence on authority. In a very insightful book, Peter Brown has shown that the relationship with a saint was essentially a vertical relationship of dependence on the thaumaturgic power of a heavenly patron.[89] Healing miracles were perfectly consistent with the vertical model of healing imposed by the medical elite—a model in which the legitimate therapeutic power came from above. The official reports of miraculous healings in eighteenth-century Bologna typically include a chain of patrons and mediators on the way to recovery (physician, confessor, patron saint). The saint is at the top of the hierarchy.[90]

In early modern Bologna, saints were actually the supreme embodiment of the ideal of the doctor as patron. Patients sought from them what real-life physicians would no longer promise—recovery. And at the same time, with the saints one could come to a bargain, as testified by votive offerings. According to Peter Brown, the relationship with the saint is a paradoxical mixture of vertical and horizontal elements: a powerful patron, the saint is also a friend and a fellow-being, a companion in our human condition. In early modern Bologna, the saint was indeed the ideal medical practitioner—a "patron" and a "healer" at the same time. Turning to a saint, patients could ask simultaneously for recovery and protection.

The history of the agreements for a cure should probably include the vows addressed to the saints in exchange for healing. Significantly, one of the very few seventeenth-century jurists who defended the validity of the cure agreement likened it to a vow to the divinity: "Just as the vow binds the person who . . . made a promise to God in exchange for health, so the patient is bound to pay what has been promised to the healer in exchange for recovery."[91]

Although this view was exceptional among the jurists, it was probably shared by some of the common people. There is, for instance, an impressive painting by Goya, a self-portrait of the artist as an old man, together with the physician who cured him of a dangerous illness. The painting is formally conceived as a votive offering, though addressed to a doctor instead of a saint. In an inscription under the painting, Goya wrote that he made it for the doctor Arrieta out of gratitude for his restored health.[92] The picture is a secular *ex-voto;* as such, it suggests that, even by the early nineteenth century, the relationship between patient and doctor could be consecrated by gratitude. It poignantly conveys what I have tried to trace in this book — the depth and complexity of feeling that could bind patient and healer.

My readers have likely noticed that this book was not chiefly meant as a contribution to the history of the medical profession. The disappearance of the cure agreement is undoubtedly an aspect of the process we call the professionalization of medicine. But what I have attempted to describe here was not so much the rising power of a profession, as the vanished world of meanings that patients and healers gave to their encounter in the past. What I found fascinating in researching the history of the cure agreement was the discovery, through scattered and long-forgotten sources, of a notion of justice profoundly different from the one that regulates medical practice today. The history of the cure agreement is but a fragment in a wider history of the notions of justice we have lost.

Appendix
EXAMPLES OF CURE AGREEMENTS,
1244–1764

DOCUMENT 1: GENOA, 1244

In nomine Domini amen. Ego Rogerius de Bruch de Bergamo promito et convenio tibi Bosso lanerio sanare et meliorare te de infirmitate quam habes in persona tua, silicet in manu et pede et in bucha bona fide omni adiutorio Dei hinc isque ad mensem unum et dimidium proxime venturum tali modo quod de manu poderis te inbochare et incidere panem et calciare et melius ire et parlare quam modo non facis et ego met facere debeo omnes expensas que et quas in hoc necessaria erunt et tu debes mihi dare et solvere ea occasione lib. septem ianuinorum et non debes comedere de aliquo frutame neque de carne bovina nec de sicca neque de pasta lissa nec de caulis et si predicta tibi non observabo nichil mihi dare debes. Et ego Bossus predictus promito tibi dicto Rogerio dare et solvere tibi infra diem tercium postquam predicta mihi observabis et sannatus ero et melioratus lib. septem ianuinorum. Alioquim penam dupli tibi stipulanti spondeo et inde omnia bona mea habita et habenda tibi pignori obligo. Insuper nos Alchisius de Bergamo et Johannes de Papia lanerii promittimus tibi dicto Rogerio quod si dictus Bossus non observabit ut supra tibi promisit. quod non tibi observabimus sub dicta pena et obligatione bonorum nostrorum. Actum eodem loco. Testes Daniellus Bullus et Opico Bonus Viccinus lanerius. Die eadem. circa vesperas.

[C. Mancini, "Un singolare contratto del 1200," *Atti e memorie dell'Accademia di Storia dell'Arte Sanitaria,* ser. 2, 36, no. 2 (1965)]

DOCUMENT 2: BOLOGNA, 1316

Universis hoc presens instrumentum publicum inspecturis pateat evidenter, quod sapiens sir dominus magister Johannes de Anglio medicus asumpsit et suscepit curam et medicamen nobilis viri domini Bertholucii nati quondam domini Guidonis de Samaritanis civis Bononiensis fiendam per magistrum Johannem pro quinquaginta florensis boni et puri auri et recti ac justi ponderis ad pondus Bononiense pactis et conventionibus infrascriptis. Videlicet quod idem magister Johannes promisit eidem domino Bartholucio curacionem et medicacionem . . . de infirmitate, qua patitur, omnibus suis medicinis aquis et confectionibus, emendis suis magistri Johannis sumptibus et expensis ita et taliter, quod idem dominus Bartolucius usque ad quatraginta dies proxime secuturos sentiet convalesentiam et melioramentum tali modo, quod poterit aliqualiter ducere manum, brachium pedem, cossam cum tibia ac se fibullare et se calciare cum manu predicta et se lavare manum sanam cum manu nunc patiente. quibus omnibus sic peractis et ante dictum tempus quadraginta dierum, idem dominus Bertholucius promisit et convenit eidem magistro dare et solvere in continenti viginti quinque florenos auri ex predicta summa quinquaginta florenorum pro medicinis factis et fiendis in posterum pro deliberatione totaliter facienda. Deinde predictus magister promisit et convenit curare, medicare et liberare in totum predictum dominum Bertholucium, ita quod ipse sentiat liberaliter sanitatem de predicto lactere patiente, quam sentit de alio lactere nunc sano, qua sanitate sic habita et percepta idem dominus Bertholucius promisit et convenit eidem magistro in continenti ad suam requisitionem dare et solvere superfluum dicte summe, sive alios vigintiquinque florenos auri boni legalis et puri, ut superius est expressum. Insuper dominus Raynerius, quondam domini Jacobini de Arzellata capellanus Sancte Marie Maioris, per stipulationem solempniter fuit confessus, eidem magistro Johanni se habere in deposito de petitione dicti domini Bertholucii quinquaginta florenos predictos, promittens eidem magistro eosdem florenos eidem solvere in omnibus et per omnia sicut superius est expressum, qua solutione facta ab altero predictorum, alter intelligatur a dicto magistro in omnibus liberatus. Cum praedictis praedictis promissionibus, obligationibus, renuntiationibus et aliis in dicto instrumento insertis; ex instrumento Jacobi dominici de Mascheronis notarii hodie facto Bononie in domo dicti domini Bertholucii presentibus dominis Alberto de Panzonili iuris perito, Antonio quondam Ungarelli, qui asseruerunt predictos cognosse contrahentes, Jacobo Rambaldi de Tarvisio quem ipse dominus Bertholucius constituit procuratorem ad denuntiandam predictam memoram Bertholomeo domini Raynerii de Arzellata testibus et domino Bertholucio domini Cathelani de Malavoltis. Et sic dicti magister Johannes testis et procurator dicti Bertholucii, ut patet instrumento procuratorio scripto manu dicti notarii facto dicta die, loco et presentibus dictis testibus una cum dicto notario venerunt dixerunt et predicta scripbi fecerunt.

[A.S.B., Comune, Ufficio dei memoriali, 1316, fol. 131v]

Document 3: Candia, 1348

Manifestum facio ego Theodoro Temisto medicus physicus atque cerurgicus habitator burgi Candide et promitto cum meis heredibus tibi Nicolao Lulino habitatori Candide et tuis heredibus quia teneor et debeo medicare et sanare te de malo sive passione tui dexteri pedis, continuando revisitare et videndo te omni die, in eo quod michi pertinet in cura atque arte et scientia physica videlicet cirurgica nec recedere de civitate sine tuo consensu, tenear itaque te perfecte curavisse et sanavisse dicto malo, hinc per totum mensem aprilis proxime venturum vel antea Deo concedente, tu vero pro solucione autem mea debes dare et solvere yperpera cretensia centum cum ad dictum terminum vel antea te sanavero perfecte et pro maiori mea securitate et cautela dicte peccunie ad requisitionem meam dedisti et presentavisti Nicolao Mairangelo habitatori Candide presenti et confesso et contento, par unum dresatoriorum perlarum pro tuo signo et pignore quod tibi convento esse sufficiens pignus et ipsum, postquam te sanavero, si me non appacaveris, teneatur illud par dresatoriorum presentare in quoqumque loco fuerit opus, quandocumque voluero ut inde possim habere solucionem predictorum centum yperperorum. . . .

Manifestum facio ego Nicolaus Lulino suprascriptus et promitto cum meis heredibus tibi Theodoro Temisto medico suprascripto et tuis heredibus quia si per totum mensem aprilis proxime venturum vel antea Deo concedente me curaveris et perfecte sanaveris de malo sive passione mei dexteri pedis secundum ordinem carte quam hodie michi fieri fecisti . . . sum contentus dare et deliberare tibi yperpera cretensia centum cum ad dictum terminum vel antea me sanaveris perfecte et pro maiori tua securitate et cautela dicte peccunie, ad requisitionem tuam, dedi et presentavi Nicolao Mairangelo par unum dresatoriorum perlarum pro tuo signo et pignore quod tibi convento esse sufficiens pignus et ipse postquam me sanaveris, si te non appacavero teneatur illud par dresatorium presentare in quoqumque loco fuerit opus quocumque volueris ut inde possis habere solutionem predictorum centum yperperorum.

[G. Rizzi, "Contratti medioevali fra medico e malato," *Minerva medica* 38, 1, no. 22 (June 1947): 521–24]

Document 4: Bologna, 1476

Sia noto e manifesto a ciaschuna persona che vedera o liegera la prexente scritta come io M. Zohane da Ragusa prometto liberamente guarire Antonio nipote di Maestro Hannibale q. Michaelis de Malpighi da Bologna della tigna e senza dolo e fraude infra il tempo e termine de' uno mexe proximo che verrà e più li prometto che ditto male non li tornerà più. Anchora li prometto fare tornare li capilli sopra la sua testa belli e in quantità come suole havere. E il ditto Maestro Hannibale mi promette dare tri ducati: li quali lui li dipone in mano di Maestro Domenico Daloro cittadino di Bologna; i quali tri ducati mi promette dare o fare dare al preditto maestro Domenico. Et io lo debbo fare cauto e sicuro che ditto male più non li tornerà e come l'avo fatto cauto e sicuro, come è detto, lui mi debbe fare dare li preditti tri ducati al preditto maestro Domenico.

[U. Stefanutti, "Sulla liceità giuridica e deontologica dei patti conclusi 'prima della cura' fra medici e pazienti (secoli XIV, XV e XVI)," *Giustizia e Società,* no. 4 (1965): 370.]

Document 5: Avignon, 1477

Pactum pro Magistro Petro de Narbona, sirurgico, et honesta muliere Guilemeta Julliane, uxore Paquerii Auvray, servientis Regii, habitatoris avenionensis.

Anno Domini Millesimo CCCCLXVII, et die decima tercia mensis Junii, in mei notarie &, personaliter constitus discretus vir Magister Petrus de Narbona, civis et habitator avenionensis, gratis & promisit et convenit honeste mulieri Guillemine Juliane, uxori Pasquerii Auvray, servientis Regii, habitatoris avenionensis, presente &, ipsam sanare et curare, et sanatam sive curatam reddere infra sex menses proxime futuros de quadam fistula sive morbo fistule, appelata fistula lacrimosa, quam ipsa habet in facie, subtus et juxta ocolum sinistrum. Et hoc mediante summa trium scutorum, quos ipsa Guillemina eidem magistro Petro dare et solvere promisit et convenit pro cura predicta per ipsum de ipsa fienda et laboribus suis impendendis circa ipsam curam; et hoc quamprimum ipsam Guilleminam de dicta fistula sanata et curata fuerit. Cum pactis sequentibus fuitque de pacto inter ipsos quod idem Magister Petrus de Narbone teneatur et debeat ipsam Guilleminam plenarie et omnino sanare et sanatam reddere infra dictos sex menses. Et in casum in quem ipsam non curaret sive sanaret et sanatam et curatam non redderet, quod ipse Magister Petrus de Narbona de hiis que fecerit nihil habere debeat.

Item ulterius est de pacto, quod si in futurum dicta fistula revertatur, seu iterum reveniat eidem Guillemine, quod ipse Magister Petrus teneatur et debeat ipsam sanare, sive curare et curatam reddere suis sumptibus et expensis et absque eo quod ipsa teneatur aliquid eidem solvere.

Pro quibus tenendis & . . . Actum in domo habitationis ipsius Guillemine, presentibus ibidem Poneto Lonzerii, textorio de Avenione, Lardinio de Terramondo, argentario, et Johaneto Reginati, habitore avenionensi, testibus & et me Silvestre.

[P. Pansier, "La pratique de l'ophtalmologie dans le moyen-âge latin," *Janus* 9 (1904): 25–26.]

DOCUMENT 6: MESSINA, 1484

Magister Franciscus de johanne medicus de trivisu prout ipse discit se nominarj sponte se obligavit curare et deo duce sanare et ad convalentiam reducere magistrum Paulum Palumbum civem messanensem ibidem presentem etc. de infirmitate sua qua habet de catarru pectustrictu sine asma pro ducatis aurejs quatuor venetis quos presentialiter ut constitit ipse magister Paulus traddidit in deposito penes magistrum Petrum de la ferra civem messanensem ibidem presentem et ipsos ducatos iiijor. recipientem ut constitit itaquod sanato ipso Paulo et convalente de ipsa infirmitate inde ad mensem j ipse magister Franciscus valeat consequi et habere dictos ducatos iiijor et eo non convalente ipsi quatuor ducati restituantur dicto Paulo hoc tamen declarato quod omnes medelas et medicamina dictus magister Franciscus debeat facere sumptibus proprijs.

Presentibus Antonello Spagnolo, Angelo Calapay et Angelo Groppulo.

[G. Pitré, *Medici, chirurgi, barbieri e spziali antichi in Sicilia* (Florence, 1942), 148 n. 1]

DOCUMENT 7: POITIERS, 1620

Personellement establys Me Alexandre Desloriers M^e opérateur et distillateur estant de présent aud. Poictiers, d'une part et François Riffault escuier Sr du Bouschault et de Condat demeurant en ceste ville d'aultre. Entre lesquelles partyes ont esté faicts les marchés et obligations qui s'ensuivent: sçavoir que led. Desloriers a promis et sera tenu de traicter et médicamenter led. Riffaut d'une hernie venteuse du costé droict jusque à parfaite guérison, moyennant la gràce de Dieu et, luy fournira de tous médicamens à ce requis et nécessaire, moyennant que led. Riffault a promis et sera tenu bailler aud. Desloriers, la somme de soixante et quinze livres tr. De laquelle somme, led. en a présentement baillé et payé aud Desloriers la somme de dix livres tr. qu'il a eue, prinse et reçue a la vue de nousd. no.^{res} en pièces de sept sols et autres bonnes monnoies de poix et prix de l'ordonnance, s'en est contenté et quitte led. Riffault, et le parsus montant à la somme de soixante cinq livres, led. Riffault sera tenu de payer aud. Desloriers, lorsqu'il sera parfaitement guéri de lad. hernie, au dire de deux médecins de cettes ville. Ce que dessus a esté stippullé et accepté par les partyes lesquelles a l'accomplissement et entretenement ont promis leur foy et serment, obligé et engagé tous et chascun leurs biens présens et futurs, dont et jugé et condempné et soubmis. Faict et passé aud. Poictiers en l'estude des no.^{res} soulsignés après midy le 1er jour de juillet mil six cens vingt.

[*Bulletin de la société française d'histoire de la médecine* 9 (1912): 451]

DOCUMENT 8: BOLOGNA, 1696

Adì 16 Aprile 1696.

Io sottoscritto alla presenza degli inc.ti testimoni servirò a medicare a tutta cura la Diamante Lambertini per la piaga che essa tiene nel piede destro, mettendovi li rimedi, che continuamente mi servirò, comunicandoli però sempre al Sig. Medico acciò Vicenzo Lambertini e sua famiglia non havessero occasione di lamentarsi di me ponendovi diversi rimedi caustici o longhi per portar avanti la cura che Iddio mi guardi, havendo premura conchiudere il più presto sia possibile per il concordato di lire sette qual se tutta volta essa Diamante sia guarita, e lo faccio per amor del Sig. Dottor Bonaveri, che così mi chiamo contento. In fede io Bartolomeo Cavazza afermo quanto di sopra, croce di Vicenzo Lambertini quale afferma e promette quanto di sopra, Io Giacomo Bonaveri fui parte a quanto di sopra e scrissi di comissione delle parti, io Gio.Batista Volta fui presente a quanto di sopra e udii il concordato.

[A.S.B., Coll. Med., b. 342.]

DOCUMENT 9: BOLOGNA, 1698

Io infrascritto havendo osservato l'infermità di Giuseppe Pecoroni che ha dalla parte destra della sua vita principiando nella faccia mi dichiaro e m'obbligo di guarirlo della sud. infermità per questo Natale prossimo a venire senza alcuna pretensione d'alcun danaro con patto però che (se) havrò guarito detto male o infermità il d. Pecoroni sia obligato a farmi un regalo di lire centro di quattrini. In fede di ciò mi sottoscrivo

Antonio Maria Mondini

afermo quanto sopra ma non nel tempo che dice (in venti giorni in più).

[A.S.B., Coll. Med., b. 342.]

DOCUMENT 10: BOLOGNA, 1764

Con la presente il S. Francesco Fossi abitante all'osteria nuova, si obbliga a far pagare e consegnare solennemente al Sig. Giuseppe Maria Pietri di nazione corsa dimorante a Bologna la somma di 45 zecchini stati depositati in mano del Sig. Carlo Redi ogni qualunque volta per ciò e non altrimenti che il sud. Sig. Giuseppe Maria Pietri senza taglio, coi suoi rimedi e segreti disciolga perfettamente la pietra nella vescica dentro il termine di sette mesi al sud. Sig. Francesco Fossi, che sta da molto tempo indisposto per il detto male, e d. somma si abbia come sopra a pagare doppo che il professore chirurgico avrà fatto l'espremento con la siringa e asserirà con fede giurata che più non abbia l'ammalato la detta Pietra, né in tutto né in parte e che sia perfettamente disciolta e la vescica sia libera dalla sud. Pietra. Si dichiara inoltre che quando dal sud. Sig. Giuseppe Maria Pietri si ordinerà al professore di siringare l'ammalato a suo piacere e quanto conviene per vedere se sia perfettamente guarito e che dall'ammalato non si volesse ciò fare debba il deposito della somma concedersi senza alcun contrasto o dilazione del più avendo l'ammalato cominciato a prendere i medicamenti che dal sud. Sig. Giuseppe Maria Pietri gli si daranno per sciogliere la suddetta pietra e questo non volendo continuare la suddetta cura del termine predetto si intende sempre che la somma concordata debba essere consegnata senza alcuna eccezione al sud. Sig. Pietri dichiarandosi inoltre che il contratto vaglia tanto in Bologna che fuori che rinunciando ad ogni legge e statuto che potesse ciò intervenire e contradire facendo che in simil modo da me sottoscritto abbia tutto il valore esso a forza e favore del Sig. Giusseppe Maria Pietri et in fede di ciò mi obbligo in forma. . . .

Se squingi in caso non si terminasse la sud. cura per difetto di non ritrovarsi medicine il sud. Professore non possa mai contare il tempo vacante nel numero delli sette mesi sopradetti, come anco si obbliga il sud. Professore per essere per tutto il mese d'Ottobre nella città di Bologna con le medicine per terminare la sud. cura, ed il deposito in questa vacanza di tempo resti in mano del depositario si e no fatta la guarigione come sopra; e non essendoci il sud. Professore nella città per tutto il mese d'ottobre possa il sud. infermo prendere il suo denaro dal d. depositario o se mai venisse la febre all'infermo, e che per tal difetto non prenda il rimedio suddetto, non possa mai contare in conto di cura quelli giorni nel numero delli sette mesi prescritto ma doppo passata la febre debba prendere il rimedio come sopra e questo a di' 7 Aprile 1764.

Io Giuseppe Maria Petri mano mia propria, et in fede di ciò Io Francesco Fossi mano mia propria.

Carlo Redi ha ricevuto il sud. deposito di quarantacinque zechini rimessi.

[A.S.B., Coll. Med., b. 349, *contra Josephum Pietri de Corsica.*]

NOTES

ABBREVIATIONS

A.C.A.B.—Archivio della Curia Arcivescovile di Bologna

A.S.B.—Archivio di Stato di Bologna

A.S.B., Coll. Med.—Archivio di Stato di Bologna, Archivio dello Studio, Collegio di medicina ed arti

A.S.B., Sanità—A.S.B., Reggimento, Assunteria di Sanità

A.S.C.—Archivio di Stato di Cagliari

A.S.M.—Archivio di Stato di Milano

B.A.R.—Biblioteca Angelica, Roma

B.C.A.B.—Biblioteca Comunale dell'Archiginnasio, Bologna

B.L.R.—Biblioteca Lancisiana, Roma

B.U.B.—Biblioteca Universitaria, Bologna

C.G.J.C.—Corpus glossatorum juris civilis

H.A.B.W.—Herzog-August Bibliothek, Wolfenbüttel

INTRODUCTION: THE VOICES OF THE SICK

1. H. Cohen, "The Evolution of the Concept of Disease," in *Concepts of Medicine,* ed. B. Lush (Oxford, 1961).

2. Pedro Laín Entralgo, *Doctor and Patient* (London, 1969), 107–8. Significantly, this shift in the doctor-patient relationship was pointed out by a historian whose main concern was not the progress of medical sciences but the cultural world of ancient medicine. See Laín Entralgo's important works: *La curación por la palabra en la Antigüedad clásica* (Madrid, 1958); and *Enfermedad y pecado* (Barcelona, 1961). On the relationship between doctor and patient in ancient times, see also C. A. Behr, *Aelius Aristeides and the Sacred Tales* (Amsterdam, 1968); and, more recently, D. Gourevitch, *Le triangle hippocratique dans le monde gréco-romain: Le malade, sa maladie et son médecin* (Rome, 1984).

3. N. D. Jewson, "The Disappearance of the Sick Man from Medical Cosmology," *Sociology* 10 (1976): 225–44.

4. D. Guthrie, "The Patient: A Neglected Factor in the History of Medicine," *Proceedings of the Royal Society of Medicine* 37 (1945): 490–94.

5. D. Porter and R. Porter, *In Sickness and in Health: The British Experience,*

1650–1850 (London, 1988); idem, *Patient's Progress: Doctors and Doctoring in Eighteenth-Century England* (Stanford, Calif., 1989). See also R. Porter, ed., *Patients and Practitioners: Lay Perceptions of Medicine in Pre-Industrial Society* (Cambridge, England, 1985); idem, "The Patient's View: Doing Medical History from Below," *Theory and Society* 14 (1985): 175–98; and L. McCray Beier, *Sufferers and Healers: The Experience of Illness in Seventeenth-Century England* (London, 1987). E. Shorter, *Bedside Manners: The Troubled History of Doctors and Patients* (New York, 1985), is a rather controversial work and, in my opinion, a very superficial one, especially in its account of pre-nineteenth-century medicine.

6. Virginia Woolf, "On Being Ill," in *Collected Essays* (London, 1967), 4:194–95.

7. Ivan Waddington, *Power and Control in the Doctor-Patient Relationship: A Developmental Approach* (Leicester, 1978); idem, "The Development of Medical Ethics," *Medical History* 19 (1975): 36–51; idem, *The Medical Profession in the Industrial Revolution* (Dublin, 1984). For a comment on Waddington's thesis, see D. Rüschemeyer, "Professionalisierung: Theoretische Probleme für die vergleichende Geschichtsforschung," *Geschichte und Gesellschaft* 6, no. 3 (1980): 320–21.

8. This assumption is seen, for example, in G. Panseri's study on the origin of "medical police" in the eighteenth century. Panseri asks, "How could it happen that, suddenly, the doctor's attention turned to the world of the poor, peasants and artisans, which up to that point had been so despised as to be ignored?" ("La nascita della polizia medica: L'organizzazione sanitaria nei vari stati italiani," in *Scienza e tecnica nella cultura e nella società dal Rinascimento a oggi,* Storia d'Italia, Annali, vol. 3 [Turin, 1980]), 157.

9. D. Jacquart, *Le milieu médicale en France du XIIe au XVe siècle* (Geneva, 1981); F. Lehoux, *Le cadre de vie de médecins parisiens au XVI et XVII siècles* (Paris, 1976); K. Park, *Doctors and Medicine in Early Renaissance Florence* (Princeton, N.J., 1985); R. Palmer, "Physicians and Surgeons in Sixteenth-Century Venice," *Medical History* 23 (1979): 451–60; idem, "Physicians and the State in Post-Medieval Italy," in *The Town and State Physician in Europe from the Middle Ages to the Enlightenment,* ed. A. W. Russell (Wolfenbüttel, Germany, 1981), 47–61; M. Pelling and C. Webster, "Medical Practitioners," in *Health, Medicine, and Mortality in the Sixteenth Century,* ed. C. Webster (Cambridge, England, 1979), 165–235.

10. Park, *Doctors and Medicine,* 113.

11. See chap. 5, below, pp. 128–29.

12. A.S.B., Coll. Med., b. 345, trial of Antonio Arconati, 1723.

13. See chap. 2, n. 70.

CHAPTER 1: A DOCTORS' TRIBUNAL

1. "The College of Arts is divided into the two Colleges of Philosophy and Medicine, with different statutes . . . and officers, although in most things they work

as a joint body, since the majority of doctors belong to both colleges" (A.S.B., Coll. Med., b. 208). The two colleges were distinct, just as the doctoral degrees in medicine and in philosophy were distinct. However, just as it was possible to receive a degree *in utraque censura* (both medicine and philosophy), many doctors in fact belonged to both colleges. From the end of the sixteenth century to the end of the eighteenth century, the lists of members of the College of Philosophy and the College of Medicine were partly overlapping: see B.C.A.B., MS. B 683, "Cattalogo de Collegiati nel Collegio de Signori Dottori di Filosofia estratto dall'insigne Sig. Dott. Gaetano Monti dai libri originali di d. Collegio," and "Cattalogo de Collegiati nel Collegio de' Signori Dottori di Medicina dall'anno 1485 all'anno 1782." This latter list shows gaps and inaccuracies; I was able to complete it and revise it for the years 1593–1793 thanks to the information provided by the official records of the college. Throughout this book, translations from non-English sources are mine unless otherwise noted.

2. The colleges were abolished by a decree of the Amministrazione Dipartimentale del Reno dated November 13, 1797. See L. Simeoni, *Storia dell'Università di Bologna* (Bologna, 1940), 2:145. The College of Medicine, however, managed to prolong its existence, if not its authority, for a few more years—until 1799. See A.S.B., Coll. Med.—b. 295, Acta Collegii, 1788–99; b. 306, "Diario Rusconi," 1790–1800.

3. The College of Arts adopted new statutes in 1507 (A.S.B., Coll. Med., b. 216, "Statuta Collegii Medicinae et Philosophiae," and "Statutum philosophorum"). The oldest statutes (dated 1378, 1395, and 1410) were published by Carlo Malagola in *Statuti delle Università e dei Collegi dello Studio bolognese* (Bologna, 1888), 425–522. The College of Medicine was founded on the model of the College of Jurists. See Albano Sorbelli, *Il Liber secretus iuris caesarei* (Bologna, 1938), 1:lxvi ff.

The statutory number of fifteen members (twelve numerary and three supernumerary) had already been established in the oldest statutes of the college, dating from 1378, 1395, and 1410, and is underscored again in the revised statutes of 1507 (rubr. 1). The College of Philosophy was also limited by statute to a fixed number of fifteen members (ten numerary and five supernumerary), with analogous requirements for admission (A.S.B., Coll. Med., b. 216, "Statutum Philosophorum," rubr. 1).

Other rules introduced after the statutes of 1507 regulated the requirement of a one-year appointment as lecturer at the Studio as a criterion for admission. In 1609, the so-called "Constitutio Justiniana" (issued by Cardinal Legate Giustiniani) established that the one-year teaching appointment as a precondition for entering the college was to be only in the topics of physic and surgery, either theoretical or applied. The text of the "Constitutio Justiniana" was attached to a seventeenth-century manuscript copy of the statutes of 1507 (A.S.B., Coll. Med., b. 216).

4. The nature of the college has often been misunderstood. For example, G. Minelli anachronistically mistakes the college for a professional association in the modern sense; see Minelli, *All'origine della biologia moderna: La vita di un testimone e protagonista. Marcello Malpighi nell'Università di Bologna* (Milan, 1987), 40. The elitist nature of the college was clearly among the reasons that led to its abolition during the French occupation. "The colleges belonged to those who became members,"

complained a document issued on Messidor 6, in the ninth year of the Napoleonic era (Simeoni, *Storia dell'Università di Bologna*, 2:152).

5. The statutes and lists of members of the Società dei Barbieri (the barbers' guild) of 1320 are still extant (A.S.B., Capitano del popolo, Società d'Arti, b. IV). We also have the barbers' statutes of 1376 and the list of members of the Società degli Speziali (the apothecaries' guild) of 1318. These two documents can be found in A.S.B., Codici Miniati.

On the apothecaries, see G. Baldi, "Gli Statuti dell'Arte degli speziali di Bologna," in *Atti del III Convegno di studi dell'Associazione Italiana di Storia della Farmacia* (Pisa, 1958); and idem, "Matricole ed elenchi di speziali bolognesi dal 1318 al 1866," in *Atti del Congresso internazionale di storia della farmacia* (Aosta, 1969).

6. The medical students were associated as members of the Universitas of Medicine and Arts. "Universitas" was the name of the students' fraternity (see Malagola, "Statuti dell'Università di Medicina ed Arti," in *Statuti*, 213–307).

7. For example, the Medical College of Florence seems to have been of the first kind, as it originally developed out of the guild of physicians and apothecaries; see Raffaele Ciasca, *L'Arte dei medici e degli speziali nella storia e nel commercio fiorentino dal XII al XV secolo* (Florence, 1927), 78, 142. And so was the Medical College of Mantua, in which all doctors wishing to practice in the city had to enroll; see G. Carra and A. Zanca, "Gli Statuti del Collegio dei medici di Mantova del 1559," in *Atti e memorie dell'Accademia Virgiliana di Mantova* (Mantua, 1977), 17, 29. The medical college of Milan, originally open to all practitioners according to the medieval statutes, became exclusive with the new statutes of 1517, which tightened admission requirements (one of the conditions was that the applicant's family have belonged to the nobility for at least 120 years); see A. Bottero, "I più antichi statuti del Collegio dei medici di Milano," *Archivio storico lombardo*, n.s., 7 fasc. 1–4 (1942): 30. The medical college of Parma was also limited to twelve numerary members, according to the statutes of 1440; see M. Varanini, "Gli statuti dell'almo collegio medico parmense," *Salsomaggiore illustrata*, no. 3 (1942): 52.

For a general overview of medical colleges in north-central Italy in the late Middle Ages, see Irma Naso, *Medici e strutture sanitarie nella società tardo-medievale* (Milan, 1982), 85–97; and idem, "Il Collegio dei medici di Novara negli ultimi anni del Quattrocento," *Studi di storia medievale e diplomatica* (Milan, 1979), 265–361. For bibliographical information on medical colleges and their statutes, see G. Gonetta, *Bibliografia statutaria delle corporazioni d'arti e mestieri d'Italia* (Rome, 1881).

8. For example, in the statutes of 1395 it is established that the ordinary and extraordinary lectureships in medicine "de mane et in nonis" salaried by the city of Bologna could be assigned only to members of the college (rubr. 26). See Malagola, *Statuti*. Again, in the statutes of 1507 (A.S.B., Coll. Med., b. 216) it is confirmed that the ordinary morning lecture on medicine should be reserved for a college member (rubr. 15; see also rubr. 16–18 for other rules on lectureships).

9. A.S.B., Coll. Med., b. 208, "Atti, Partiti, Statuti et Altro per le Aggregazioni

dal 1606 a tutto 1651." In a discussion of the statutes in 1622, some college members argued that the number of supernumeraries could be changed at the discretion of the college.

10. Ibid. The supernumeraries were divided into three groups: the first group (from the thirteenth to the fifteenth position) shared the privileges and duties of the college, from which the second group (from the sixteenth to the nineteenth position) and the third group (from the twentieth to the twenty-third position) were excluded. The doctors assigned to the twentieth to the twenty-third positions were admitted "in potentia" and could not sit in the college, even though they immediately had to pay the fee required for admission.

In 1729 it was established that supernumeraries could serve as protomedici only temporarily to replace absent numeraries (A.S.B., Coll. Med., b. 216, "Declarationes, Ordinationes, et Provisiones de novo habitae in Collegio Med.").

11. By the end of the eighteenth century, the fee for admission to the College of Medicine was 591 *lire* and 10 *soldi* (A.S.B., Coll. Med., b. 246, "Direttorio per l'Economato delli Almi Collegi di Medicina e Filosofia," 1799).

12. In the council of the barbers' guild (limited to twelve members), priority status for admission was reserved for the sons or brothers of a deceased member (A.S.B., Codici Miniati, "Statuti della Società dei Barbieri," 1556–1715).

13. A.S.B., Assunteria di Studio, Diversorum, b. 93.

14. A.S.B., Coll. Med., b. 296. The decision was issued by the cardinal legate. The college confirmed it with a resolution dated 1622: "collegium semper intelligatur apertum . . . dummodo non sint plures quam duo de una et ead. familia et agnatione actu aggregati" (b. 208, doc. 6).

15. The college doctors Ippolito Poggioli and Luigi Magni both had paternal uncles who were collegiates. Poggioli and Magni were admitted to the college in 1663; for their *civilitatis probationes*—i.e., testimonies on their citizenship and family— see A.S.B., Coll. Med., b. 353. Likewise, Tarsizio Riviera (admitted in 1790) had a paternal uncle, Bartolomeo Riviera, who had been admitted as an honorary member in 1781; see G. Gandolfi, *Elogio di Tarsizio Riviera* (Bologna, 1807), v; M. Medici, *Compendio storico della scuola anatomica di Bologna dal Rinascimento delle Scienze e delle Lettere a tutto il secolo XVIII* (Bologna, 1857), 405. Paolo Salani, admitted in 1677, was the stepson of Gio.Carlo Mattesilani, a member of the college from 1651 to 1707 (b. 341). Carlo Antonio Sivieri, who was admitted in 1663 and died in 1664 (b. 353), and Giacinto Maria Sivieri, who was admitted in 1691 (b. 342), were the sons of two brothers.

16. The importance of agnatic kinship was also stated in the general rules on Bolognese citizenship, as defined in the city's statutes; see *Statuta civilia et criminalia civitatis Bononiae . . . illustrata a P. C. Sacco* (Bologna, 1735–37), 2:183–84.

17. G. Fantuzzi, *Notizie degli scrittori bolognesi* (Bologna, 1786–90), 5:57.

18. A.S.B., Coll. Med., b. 340, "Civilitatis Probationes" of Bartolomeo Ferrari.

19. A.S.B., Coll. Med., b. 341, "Civilitatis Probationes" of Antonio Gioseffo Magnani. I have not systematically researched each collegiate's family connections on

the maternal side, and I report here only those mentioned by contemporary witnesses in the candidates' civilitatis probationes.

On the importance of maternal kin in the selection of functionaries recruited to high magistracies in eighteenth-century Rome, see the research results and interesting observations of Renata Ago, "Burocrazia, 'nazioni' e parentele nella Roma del Settecento," *Quaderni storici* 13, 1, n. 67 (1988): esp. 86 ff.

20. A.S.B., Coll. Med.—"Civilitatis Probationes" of Gioseffo Cucchi (b. 332), Giovanni Antonio Cucchi (bb. 247 and 353), and Antonio Magnani Cartari (b. 341). For the admission of Gio. Agostino Cucchi, see b. 250, "Sententiae et decisiones tam in prima, quam in secunda instantia, in causa Excell. D. Io. Augustini Chucchij Philosophi, et Medici Bon. ad favorem ejusdem contra Collegia Bonon. Phil. & Medicinae."

In 1626, when Giacomo Cucchi was admitted to the College of Philosophy, it was established that he could not attend the sessions of this college when his father Antonio and his brother Gioseffo (members of the Colleges of Medicine and Philosophy) were present, because of the rule that prohibited simultaneous membership in the college by three members of the same family or "agnatic line" (A.S.B., Coll. Med., b. 208).

On the Cucchi Cartari family, see G. B. Guidicini, *Cose notabili della città di Bologna* (Bologna, 1870), 3:178, 4:299.

21. A.S.B., Coll. Med., b. 196, "Civilitatis Probationes" of Melchiorre Zoppio. On Zoppio, see S. Mazzetti, *Repertorio di tutti i professori antichi e moderni, della famosa Università e del celebre Istituto delle Scienze di Bologna* (Bologna, 1848), 331.

22. A.S.B., Coll. Med., bb. 341, 238, 349, "Civilitatis Probationes" of the three members of the Donelli family.

23. A.S.B., Coll. Med., b. 234, text of the *Privilegium palatinatus.*

24. That is, they could create "knights of the golden spur" *(equites aurati).* The college did occasionally bestow these privileges: for example, the title of "public notary" was granted by the college to Lelio Mariani, of Lucca, on January 5, 1663 (A.S.B., Coll. Med., b. 207, doc. 33). On March 31, 1637, the college legitimized two boys and a girl (b. 219, "Liber secretus, 1626–1630").

25. They granted it, for instance, to Durando Pelocio, a French student who received his medical doctorate at Bologna in 1548 (A.S.B., Coll. Med., b. 207, doc. 29). The college first appointed a knight in 1545 (b. 217, "Liber secretus, 1504–1575," c. 60).

26. A.S.B., Coll. Med., b. 246, "Direttorio per l'economato delli Almi Collegi di Medicina e Filosofia," 1779. On the fees required for a degree, see n. 93, below.

27. On this project and its failure, see Charles Webster, *The Great Instauration: Science, Medicine, and Reform, 1626–1660* (New York, 1976), 300–308; and Harold J. Cook, *The Decline of the Old Medical Regime in Stuart London* (Ithaca, N.Y., 1986), 105. On the Royal College of Physicians, founded in 1518 on the Italian model, see Charles Webster, "Thomas Linacre and the Foundation of the College of Physi-

cians," in *Linacre Studies,* ed. R. Maddison, M. Pelling, and C. Webster (Oxford, England, 1976).

28. In Bologna, critical opinions about the oligarchic character of the college seem to have been present within the college itself. In 1663, an anonymously printed broadsheet circulated in the city, denouncing "errors and abuses introduced in the colleges of medicine and philosophy" (A.S.B., Coll. Med., b. 338, *Errori e Abusi introdotti nelli Collegi di Medicina, e Filosofia*). Among other things, the broadsheet argued that, according to the statutes, "one cannot be admitted to the college unless he is a Bolognese doctor and citizen, which disposition gives ipso facto a right to admission to all those who are such." The anonymous author of the broadsheet seems to suggest that all Bolognese doctors had the right to become members of the college.

The broadsheet was probably written by Ippolito Poggioli, who had become a supernumerary member of the college that same year. On August 21, 1663, the dean of the college, Montalbani, confiscated the broadsheet from a copyist who stated that he had received it from Poggioli's father. On January 15, 1664, Poggioli was suspended from the college (A.S.B., Coll. Med., b. 338).

29. Manfred Stürzbecher, *Beiträge zur Berliner Medizingeschichte* (Berlin, 1966), 34, 65. See also R. A. Dorwart, "The Royal College of Medicine and Public Health in Brandeburg Prussia, 1685–1740," *Medical History* 2 (1958): 13–23.

30. A.S.B., Coll. Med., b. 217, "Liber secretus, 1504–1575." On the evolution of the Protomedicato in the sixteenth century, see L. Ricci, "Il Protomedicato e i controlli sanitari in Bologna dal XVI al XVIII secolo" (*tesi di laurea,* Facoltà di Magistero, University of Bologna, 1969–70).

31. "Ordinationes Fori Protomedicatus," in *Liber pro recta administratione Protomedicatus* (Bologna, 1666), 3.

32. These two powers of the dean are described in articles 4 and 34 of the statutes of 1507 (A.S.B., Coll. Med., b. 216).

In the statutes of 1378 and 1395, the dean's jurisdiction was limited to the disputes among the members of the college. In the statutes of 1410 (rubr. 3), instead, we find his powers defined according to the following formula: "Cognoscere summarie, et de plano, sine strepitu, et figura iuditii, de omnibus, et singulis litibus, quaestionibus et differentiis, quae verterentur, vel verti possent inter praefactos Doctores . . . aut cum quibuscumque aliis singularibus personis litigare volentibus cum Doctoribus." This formula is also found in the statutes of 1507 (art. 4). As regards the rules on unlicensed practice, a list of practitioners licensed in medicine or surgery was established with the statutes of 1410 (rubr. 21; see Malagola, *Statuti,* 515–16).

33. On the jurisdictional powers of the guilds, see A. Pertile, *Storia del diritto italiano* (Turin, 1892–1903), vol. 6.1, pp. 111 ff.

34. "Sommario del breve di Nostro Signore Papa Gregorio XV, concesso al Collegio di Medicina, & suoi Protomedici" (1621), in *Liber pro recta,* 23.

35. B.U.B., MS. 1052, "Informatione in materia del Protomedicato"; A.S.B., Reggimento, Assunteria di Studio, b. 149.

36. Pertile, *Storia del diritto,* vol. 2.2, pp. 212 ff.

37. See, for instance, S. Mazzetti, *Memorie storiche sopra l'Università e l'Instituto delle Scienze di Bologna* (Bologna, 1840), 56–57: "The popes entrusted the public health policies to the Medical College, under the name of the Protomedicato, concerning the licensing in the different branches of medicine, the control over practitioners, the punishment of offenders, the judgment on the qualifications of doctors, surgeons, etc., the inspection of apothecaries' and grocers' shops—all powers that were taken away from the college after the French invasion of 1796 and entrusted to special commissions instituted by the government."

38. G. Olmi, "Farmacopea antica e medicina moderna: La disputa sulla Teriaca nel Cinquecento bolognese," *Physis* 19 (1977): 234–37.

39. A.S.B., Coll. Med., b. 217, "Liber secretus, 1504–1575," c. 140.

40. I examined the complete series of the minutes of the college's sessions (Acta Collegii) from 1576 to 1799 (A.S.B., Coll. Med., bb. 265–95) and that of the Acta Prothomedicatus (bb. 318–29). The latter series is incomplete; the records for the years 1570–1604 and 1702–44 are missing.

41. For a case in which the college overrode a decision of the Protomedicato, see, for instance, A.S.B., Coll. Med., b. 318, Acta Protomedicatus, 1605–17, minutes for June 10, 1605.

42. A.S.B., Coll. Med., b. 319, *"Nomine totius Collegii iudicent, cognoscant, provident, iustitiam faciant et exequant,"* decree issued on August 14, 1628.

43. A.S.B., Coll. Med., b. 319, decree issued on January 5, 1629.

44. *Liber pro recta,* 10.

45. A.S.B., Coll. Med., b. 258, "Ristretto degli atti e decreti più notabili fatti nel Collegio e Protomedicato di Medicina dell'anno 1562 all'anno 1792," decree issued January 14, 1671, reissued April 9, 1672.

46. A.S.B., Coll. Med., b. 261, "Responsio petitionis factae ab Academia parisiensi Collegio medicorum Bononiae circa usum approbationis chirurgorum." This correspondence with Paris is dated 1749.

47. *Liber pro recta,* 8. On the ceremony for the preparation of theriac, see F. Cavazza, *Le scuole dell'antico Studio bolognese* (Milan, 1896), 262 ff.

48. A.S.B., Coll. Med., b. 213; *Liber pro recta,* 5.

49. On the Neapolitan Protomedicato, see L. De Rosa, "The *Protomedicato* in Southern Italy, XVI–XIX Centuries," *Annales Cisalpines d'histoire sociale,* ser. 1, no. 4 (1973): 103–17; P. Franco, "Il Protomedicato napoletano," *Pagine di storia della medicina* 9, no. 2 (1965). On the conflicts with the Medical College of Salerno, see Salvatore De Renzi, *Storia documentata della scuola medica di Salerno* (Naples, 1857), 587–88. In Piedmont, the Protomedicato was formed by royal appointment; see Pertile, *Storia del diritto,* vol. 2.2, p. 212. On Protomedicati in early modern Italy in general, see D. Gentilcore, "All That Pertains to Medicine: Protomedici and Protomedicati in Early Modern Italy," *Medical History* 38 (1994): 121–42.

The Spanish Protomedicato was named directly by the Crown, as well; see P.

Iborra, *Historia del Protomedicato en Espana (1477–1822)* (Madrid, 1885–86); this work was reissued by J. Riera and J. Granda-Juesas in *Acta Historico-Medica Vallisoletana* 24 (1987). The most detailed work on this institution is the important volume by J. Tate Lanning, who extensively studied the history of the Protomedicato in Spain and in the colonies; see Lanning's *The Royal Protomedicato: The Regulation of the Medical Profession in the Spanish Empire* (Durham, N.C., 1985). I thank Stuart Schwarzt for kindly pointing out this book to me. See also the essays in the special issue of *Dynamis,* vol. 16 (1996), on the Spanish Protomedicato from 1593 to 1808.

50. This conflict over the university lectures led to a lawsuit between the college and the Senate (1678–90), which originated from the fact that the Senate had refused to pay the lecturers' salaries, asserting that the number of lecturers exceeded the needs of the students (for documentation on this lawsuit, see A.S.B., Coll. Med., b. 210).

51. M. Fanti, "Le classi sociali e il governo di Bologna all'inizio del secolo XVII in un'opera inedita di Camillo Baldi," *Strenna storica bolognese* (1961): 157 ff.

52. B.C.A.B., MS. B 4184, "Titoli dei due Collegi di legge Canonica e Civile e del Collegio di Medicina nel governo e nell'amministrazione della Dogana, detta fra noi Gabella Grossa."

The Congregazione della Gabella Grossa, of which the syndics elected by the colleges were members, imposed tariffs on foreign goods imported into Bologna as well as on merchandise exported from the city. It was also responsible for the maintenance of the navigable canals that connected Bologna to the river Po (the levies from the goods transported by water were supposed to be used for this purpose). Many documents on the Canal Navile, Bologna's main navigable canal, are to be found among the records of the College of Medicine (A.S.B., Coll. Med., b. 201). The administration of the Customs House was certainly an important aspect of the college's public responsibility.

53. A.S.B., Coll. Med., b. 208, "Atti Spettanti al Coll. di Filosofia e Medicina nella causa d'Aggregazione del Dott. B. Bonaccorsi, 1622–1646." For Bonaccorsi's civilitatis probationes, see b. 196; more information on him is in b. 259. On Bonaccorsi, see also G. N. Alidosi, *Li dottori bolognesi di teologia, filosofia, medicina e d'arti liberali dall'anno 1000 per tutto marzo del 1623* (Bologna, 1623; reprint, Bologna, 1980), 39. See also Fantuzzi, *Notizie* 2:285.

The guild of the Bombasari included "sellers of cotton cloth and dealers in cotton wadding"; see Luigi Dal Pane, *Economia e società a Bologna nell'età del Risorgimento* (Bologna, 1969), 192.

54. *Liber pro recta,* 23.

55. Naso, *Medici e strutture sanitarie,* 94, 154.

56. A.S.B., Coll. Med., b. 214. Against this healer the Protomedicato released a warning, prohibiting him from practicing (b. 197).

57. For example, on May 23, 1712: A.S.B., Coll. Med., b. 258, "Ristretto degli atti e decreti." For similar disputes between the Protomedicato of Castile and the po-

litical authorities over licensing or permits for the sale of medicines, see J. L. Valverde, F. Sanchez, and L. Vinuesa, "Controversias jurisdiccionales del Protomedicato castellano," *Asclepio* 30–31 (1978–79): 410. On the Protomedicato of Castile, see R. Roldan y Guerrero, "Los origines del Tribunal del Real Protomedicato de Castilla," *Archivio Iberoamericano de historia de la medicina y antropologia medica* 12 (1960).

58. A.S.B., Coll. Med., b. 213. The Protomedicato of Bologna managed to maintain exclusive authority over medical licensing in Bolognese territory, despite attempts at interference by the Roman Protomedicato. On this issue, see F. Garofalo, "Il collegio dei medici di Bologna e di Roma circa l'esercizio della professione," *Atti e memorie dell'Accademia di Storia dell'Arte Sanitaria,* no. 3 (1965). Bologna successfully resisted this interference in spite of the fact that, at least formally, the Roman Protomedicato held jurisdictional authority over all of the Papal States. See F. M. Ponzetti, "L'archivio antico dell'Università di Roma," *Archivio della R. Deputazione romana di Storia patria* 59, no. 2 (1936): 259.

59. See, for example, J. P. Frank, *Sistema compiuto di Polizia medica* (Milan, 1786).

60. A.S.B., Sanità, "Elenco di recapiti esistenti nell'Archivio di Sanità," 1579–1793. These archival records have been cursorily examined in a brief study by E. Rosa, *Medicina e salute pubblica a Bologna nel Sei e Settecento* (Bologna, 1978), 35–36. For general information on the development of similar institutions in the late Middle Ages and the early modern period, see C. M. Cipolla, "Origine e sviluppo degli Uffici di Sanità in Italia," *Annales Cisalpines d'histoire sociale,* ser. 1, no. 4 (1973): 83–101.

61. As late as 1662, a decree of the college required that all candidates for the doctoral degree in medicine should take a loyalty oath to the Galenic and Aristotelian doctrines (A.S.B., Coll. Med., b. 296). In the broadsheet *Errori e abusi* (see n. 28, above), this oath requirement was severely criticized: "They require new doctors to swear under oath that they will teach the doctrines of the Ancients in philosophy and medicine, as if philosophy and medicine were, like theology, based on principles of faith" (b. 338). On the persistence of Galenism in the Italian universities, see Nancy Siraisi, *Avicenna in Renaissance Italy: The Canon and Medical Teaching in Italian Universities after 1500* (Princeton, N.J., 1987).

62. A.S.B., Coll. Med., b. 218, "Liber secretus, 1575–1594." At times, the protomedici received requests for advice from outside Bologna. See, for example, b. 207, no. 44, "Voto dell'Almo Collegio di Medicina ricercato dalla sacra Consulta di Roma in causa vertente fra li terracinesi e l'Ecc.ma Casa Gabrielli per una nova risiera nell'anno 1776," for a case concerning the effects of a rice field on the salubrity of the air.

63. A.S.B., Coll. Med.—b. 258, "Ristretto degli atti e decreti," September 24, 1729; b. 323.

64. A.S.B., Coll. Med., b. 258, "Ristretto degli atti e decreti," July 18, 1743.

65. A.S.B., Coll. Med., b. 340.

66. The different roles of these two institutions within the political systems of the old Italian states were pointed out by Pertile (*Storia del diritto,* vol. 2.2, pp. 212–14): "Originally, the Magistrato di Sanità had the task of preserving the state from contagious diseases by inspecting and approving ships coming from abroad. Later on, the Magistrato di Sanità extended its authority over all matters concerning public health, holding jurisdiction over all related civil and criminal cases. Also, the protomedico had civil and penal jurisdiction over matters within its competence. Furthermore, it cooperated with the Health Magistrate in an advisory role, besides examining and approving physicians, surgeons, apothecaries, and midwives, and visiting apothecaries' shops at least once a year" (212).

67. On London, see Webster, *Great Instauration,* 288; on the Prussian case, see Stürzbecher, *Beiträge,* 40, 64.

68. The citizenship requirement was waived only for honorary members. The first to be admitted to the college as an honorary member was Marcello Malpighi in 1691; see H. Adelmann, *Marcello Malpighi and the Evolution of Embryology* (New York, 1966), 617–18. Other honorary members of the college were Antonio Leprotti and Pier Paolo Molinelli (1742), Domenico Maria Gusmano Galeazzi (1743), Giacomo Pistorini (1768), Bartolomeo Riviera (1781), and Gaetano Uttini (1789).

69. The records of the civilitatis probationes, kept in chronological order, are in A.S.B., Coll. Med.—b. 196 (1530–1606) (incomplete; actually contains materials up to 1612); and b. 238 (1709–41). Other records of the proceedings are scattered in the files of the college's notaries: b. 332 (1612–22); bb. 338, 353 (1657–63); b. 340 (1677–81); b. 341 (1677–91); and b. 342 (1698). Biographical information about the college doctors can also be found in bb. 208, 234, 247, 250, 259, 348.

I was not able to locate the civilitatis probationes for the years 1622–62 and 1742–93 (they were probably included in bb. 333–37, missing from the archives of the medical college since World War II). I have filled this gap with the biographical information on the collegiates contained in other sources, primarily a list of the doctors of medicine and philosophy compiled by Bartolomeo Albertini, notary of the college, and published by his successor Gio. Battista Cavazza: *Catalogus omnium doctorum collegiatorum in artibus liberalibus et in facultate medica incip. ab A.D. 1156* (Bologna, 1664). This source systematically points out which collegiates were the sons or grandsons of other college members. Other sources include Alidosi, *Li dottori;* P. S. Dolfi, *Cronologia delle famiglie nobili di Bologna* (Bologna, 1670; reprint, Bologna, 1973); Fantuzzi, *Notizie;* B.C.A.B., MS. Montefani, "Bibliografia bolognese," b. 24; and P. Ascanelli, *I fascicoli personali dei Lettori Artisti dell'Assunteria di Studio dell'Archivio di Stato di Bologna* (Forlì, 1968).

In the list of 130 collegiates for the years 1593–1793 I did not include the honorary members, listed in n. 68, above, because they did not participate actively in the public functions of the college and the Protomedicato.

70. For instance, the well-known Bolognese surgeon Gaspare Tagliacozzi, the son of a silk weaver and the grandson of a *gargiolaro* (hemp worker), is called a "no-

bleman" in several notarial records written after his admission to the college in 1576 (M. T. Gnudi and J. P. Webster, *The Life and Times of Gaspare Tagliacozzi, Surgeon of Bologna, 1545–1599* [Milan, 1950], 226); for Tagliacozzi's civilitatis probationes (A.S.B., Coll. Med., b. 196), see 393–97.

71. The following members of the college were the sons of silk merchants: Bartolomeo Bonaccorsi (whose controversial admission to the college is mentioned above), Alessandro Guicciardini and Angelo Antonio Livizzani, admitted in 1663 (A.S.B., Coll. Med., b. 353); Leone Cattellani, admitted in 1681 (b. 341), whose father was described as a "public banker and silk merchant"; Gioseffo Maria Garani, admitted in 1691 (b. 341); Gerolamo Giglioli, admitted in 1691 (b. 341), whose father is said to have "managed a veil-gathering business." On Bologna's silk industry, see Carlo Poni, "Per la storia del distretto industriale serico di Bologna, Secc. XVI–XVII," *Quaderni storici* 25, 1, n. 73 (1990): 93–167.

72. For instance, the father of Gio. Antonio Roffeni, who became a member in 1622 (A.S.B., Coll. Med., b. 332), was a "grain merchant and the owner of several bakeries." The college members Giuseppe Antonio Pozzi and Gioseffo Pozzi, who were both admitted in 1725 (b. 238), and who, as far as I know, were unrelated to each other in spite of having the same family name, were also the sons of two "wholesale grain merchants."

73. A.S.B., Coll. Med., b. 196, "Civilitatis Probationes" of Giovanni Fantuzzi and Vincenzo Montecalvi. On Fantuzzi, see also Dolfi, *Cronologia*, 307; and Fantuzzi, *Notizie* 3:296–97. On Montecalvi, the author of commentaries on Aristotle, see G. Ghilini, *Teatro de' Uomini letterati* (Venice, 1647), 2:241; and Fantuzzi, *Notizie* 4:72–74. On the Montecalvi family, see Dolfi, *Cronologia*, 601–2.

74. A.S.B., Coll. Med.—b. 353, "Civilitatis Probationes" of Sicinio Oretti; b. 342, "Civilitatis Probationes" of Francesco Oretti. "A rather decayed family, although today it counts Sicinio, doctor of philosophy and medicine" (Dolfi, *Cronologia*, 155).

75. Antonio Gandolfi was admitted in 1593 (A.S.B., Coll. Med., b. 196; about his family, see Dolfi, *Cronologia*, 123). Lanspergio Belvisi the son and grandson of notaries, was admitted in 1593; his family is described as "noble and ancient" in his civilitatis probationes (b. 196; see also Dolfi, *Cronologia*, 319). Agostino Odofredi was admitted in 1612 (see Alidosi, *Li dottori*, 21; Mazzetti, *Repertorio*, 225; and Dolfi, *Cronologia*, 124). Pompeo Bolognetti was admitted in 1651 (see Alidosi, *Li dottori*, 164–65; Fantuzzi, *Notizie* 2:253–54; and Dolfi, *Cronologia*, 179–86). Count Gio. Carlo Mattesilani, admitted in 1651, was made a marquis by the king of Poland in 1685 (Dolfi, *Cronologia*, 714; Fantuzzi, *Notizie* 5:363–64). On the Cucchi Cartari and Magnani families, see Dolfi, *Cronologia*, 211, 475–84.

76. Domenico Maria Borghi, admitted to the college in 1663 (A.S.B., Coll. Med., b. 353), was the son of a goldsmith and the grandson of a *varottaro* (furrier), massaro of the furriers' guild. Gaspare Ferri, admitted in 1603 (b. 196), was the son of a massaro of the Bisilieri. Angelo Michele Sacchi, admitted in 1612 (b. 196), and Virgilio Bianchi, admitted in 1622 (b. 332), were the sons of two massari of the Lana (woolworkers' guild). Orazio Dolci, admitted in 1622 (b. 332), was the son and

grandson of massari of the butchers' company. Ippolito Poggioli the younger, admitted in 1663, was the son of a massaro of the drapiers' guild (his paternal uncle, also named Ippolito, had been a member of the College of Philosophy [b. 353]; on Ippolito Poggioli the elder, see Fantuzzi, *Notizie* 7:79).

77. A.S.B., Coll. Med., b. 341, "Civilitatis Probationes" of G. M. Garani.

78. A.S.B., Coll. Med., b. 196; Alidosi, *Li dottori,* 116–17; Fantuzzi, *Notizie* 3:209–14. Domenico Sebastiano Bonomi, admitted in 1691 (b. 341), was also the son of a tailor. Gerolamo Ermani, admitted in 1612 (b. 332), was the son of a carpenter.

79. A.S.B., Coll. Med.— b. 341, "Civilitatis Probationes" of Giacinto Maria Sivieri; b. 353, "Civilitatis Probationes" of Carlo Antonio Sivieri.

80. A.S.B., Coll. Med., b. 238, "Civilitatis Probationes" of Carlo Filippo Brusa.

81. The following members of the college were the sons of apothecaries: Pier Giacomo Aldrovandi, admitted in 1663 (A.S.B., Coll. Med., b. 353); Francesco Cavallina, admitted in 1713, the son and grandson of officers of the apothecaries' guild (b. 238); Gerolamo Donduzzi, admitted in 1713, also the son and grandson of apothecaries (see Fantuzzi, *Notizie* 3:262); Gottardo Bonzi, admitted in 1735, whose father owned two apothecary shops and whose grandfather had been a merchant of ironware (b. 238); and Giacomo Bartolomeo Beccari, admitted in 1735, the son of a "grocer-apothecary" (b. 238).

82. A.S.B., Coll. Med., b. 196, "Civilitatis Probationes" of Alessandro Recordati.

83. A.S.B., Coll. Med., b. 238, "Civilitatis Probationes" of Gaetano Monti. On Giuseppe Antonio Monti, see Fantuzzi, *Notizie* 6:91–94.

84. See Fanti, "Le classi sociali," 150 ff. On Baldi and his description of the social classes in Bologna, see also Dal Pane, *Economia e società,* 391 ff, 416.

85. P. A. Orlandi, *Notizie degli scrittori bolognesi e dell'opere loro stampate e manoscritte* (Bologna, 1714), 92; G. B. Rossi, *L'attioni memorabili fatte da . . . Confalonieri del popolo et Massari delle Arti già dominanti la città di Bologna raccolte da diversi manoscritti et autori* (Bologna, 1681).

86. The term *noble merchants* is used in describing the tribunes' social composition in an account of "the state, the government, and the magistrates of Bologna," written at the end of the sixteenth century; see S. Verardi Ventura, ed., "L'ordinamento bolognese dei secc. XVI–XVII: Edizione del ms. B 1114 della Biblioteca dell'Archiginnasio: *Lo stato, il governo et i magistrati di Bologna,* del Cavaliere Ciro Spontone," *L'Archiginnasio* 76 (1981): 319. See also idem, ed., "L'ordinamento bolognese dei secc. XVI–XVII: Introduzione all'edizione del ms. B 1114 della Biblioteca dell'Archiginnasio: *Lo stato, il governo et i magistrati di Bologna,* del Cavaliere Ciro Spontone," *L'Archiginnasio* 74 (1979).

87. *I Gonfalonieri del Popolo o Tribuni della Plebe dall'anno 1500 a tutto il 1769* (Bologna, 1769).

88. On the Anziani and their role, see Verardi Ventura, ed., "L'ordinamento bolognese dei secc. XVI–XVII: Introduzione," 354 ff; and "L'ordinamento bolognese

dei secc. XVI–XVII: Edizione," 313–19. The members of the medical college who also served as Anziani include Giovanni Fantuzzi; Gio. Antonio Roffeni (Dolfi, *Cronologia, 657); Ovidio Montalbani (Dolfi, *Cronologia*, 74); and Cesare Zoppio. For Fantuzzi and Zoppio, see G. N. Alidosi, *I Signori Antiani, Consoli e Gonfalonieri di Giustitia della città di Bologna dall'anno 1456 accresciuti sino al 1670* (Bologna, 1670); and B.C.A.B., MS. Gozzadini 396, "Registro de signori Antiani . . . 1670–1770."

89. A.S.B., Coll. Med., b. 259. Some of Montalbani's writings are directly concerned with his role as a magistrate. See especially his *L'honore de i Collegi dell'Arti della città di Bologna* (Bologna, 1670), a description of the Bolognese guilds which was clearly related to his experience as a Tribune of the Plebs. Fantuzzi (*Notizie* 5:57–64) mentions among Montalbani's works a collection of legal opinions, *Legalia Responsa in Causis Varis,* which, however, I was not able to locate in the Bologna libraries or archives.

90. As shown, for instance, by the encyclopedic work on medical and legal matters published by Paulus Zacchius [Paolo Zacchia], the pope's physician-in-chief, at the beginning of the seventeenth century (1612–30): *Quaestiones medico-legales* (Lyons, 1662). Some of the Bolognese protomedici also wrote on legal medicine. See G. Pozzi and M. Bazzani, *De ambigue prolatis in judicium criminationibus, consultationes physico-medicae nonnullae* (Bologna, 1742).

91. A.S.B., Coll. Med., b. 259. On Cesare Zoppio, see also Mazzetti, *Repertorio,* 331; and Dolfi, *Cronologia,* 290.

92. A.S.B., Assunteria di Studio, Requisiti dei Lettori, b. 55 (Lettera S, vol. 126).

93. The following fees are listed in the "Direttorio per l'Economato delli Almi Collegi di Medicina e Filosofia" of 1779 (A.S.B., Coll. Med., b. 246):

—the fee for the doctoral degree in medicine and philosophy, "as citizens" *(alla cittadina):* 657 lire and 10 soldi;
—the fee for the doctoral degree in medicine and philosophy, "as foreigners" *(alla forestiera):* 218 lire and 10 soldi;
—the fee for the doctoral degree with knighthood: 86 lire and 10 soldi (in addition to the regular fee);
—the fee for the doctoral degree in surgery: 96 lire and 10 soldi;
—the fee for the license to practice as an apothecary: 20 lire;
—the fee for the license to practice as a second-level surgeon: 30 lire;
—the fee for the license to practice as a first-level surgeon: 5 lire;
—the fee for licenses to practice as "bath attendants *[stufaroli],* dentists, charlatans": 5 lire.

Licenses for midwives and for apprentices to apothecaries were free. The logs of the college *(libri delle distribuzioni)* show how fees were divided among the collegiates (for example, A.S.B., Coll. Med., b. 308, "Libro delle distribuzioni,

1666–1747"). The logs with the college's income for 1666–1700 and 1721–65 are included in b. 307.

94. Beginning in 1593, the Senate reserved one thousand lire per year as payment to the protomedici for this task (A.S.B., Coll. Med.—b. 296; b. 307, "Libro del Economo, 1697–1700").

95. *Liber pro recta,* 52.

96. Ibid., 23–24.

97. Article 34 of the statutes of 1507 (which repeated article 21 of the statutes of 1410) stated: "Prior nostri Collegii, . . . teneatur et debeat . . . delinquentes punire, mulctare et condemnare . . . et per notarium dicti Collegii dictam mulctam, vel condemnationem ad discum Ursi et ufficialibus eiusdem in publica forma assignari facere." The judge at the Disco dell'Orso was in charge of collecting public money. On this office, see Archivio di Stato di Bologna, *Inventario generale dei fondi* (Bologna, 1977), 25.

According to the statutes of 1395 (rubr. 19), the task of prosecuting and punishing those found guilty of unlicensed medical practice belonged to the *podestà* and not to the dean of the college.

98. In 1582, two *esploratori* (constables)—one for the city and one for the countryside—were hired to "watch over those who dare to draw blood, medicate, and administer all kinds of oral medications without license" (A.S.B., Coll. Med., b. 214). Beginning in 1614, the Protomedicato also employed on a regular basis a courier, or messenger *(nunzio esecutore)* in charge of dispatching executive writs (*Liber pro recta,* 10–11).

99. See *Liber pro recta,* 14, for prohibitions concerning apothecaries, and 17, for those concerning barbers. The ban on barbers' drawing blood from women, especially from the foot, was also included in the statutes of the medical college of the city of Modena (1550): "nec audeat alicui mulieri aegrae aut sanae sanguinem mittere maxime e vena tali inscio medico." See V. Casoli, "Gli Statuti del Collegio dei Medici della città di Modena riformati da Giovanni Grillenzoni medico modenese, 1501–1551," *Rivista di storia critica delle scienze mediche e naturali* 1 (1910–12): 103.

On the Hippocratic aphorism concerning abortion as a consequence of bloodletting from the foot, see Hippocrates, *Aphorisms* (Cambridge, Mass., 1979), 4:166–67 (aph. V, xxxi). For the different interpretations of this aphorism in the European medical tradition, see J. Bauer, *Geschichte der Aderlässe* (Munich, 1870). The belief that drawing blood from the saphenous vein would cause an abortion is reported as common knowledge in a manual written by a barber-surgeon: P. P. Magni, *Discorsi sopra il modo di sanguinare* (Rome, 1586), 19–20. On Magni's text, see G. Pomata, "Barbieri e comari," in *Medicina, erbe e magia* (Milan, 1981), 168.

100. *Liber pro recta,* 18–19.

101. A.S.B., Coll. Med., b. 195.

102. *Liber pro recta,* 16.

103. A.S.B., Coll. Med., b. 197.

104. *Liber pro recta,* 12. See also F. Garofalo, *La giurisdizione civile e criminale del Protomedico e del collegio dei medici di Roma* (Rome, 1950). The Neapolitan Protomedicato also had jurisdiction over civil matters. In 1752, however, Charles III rescinded its power to settle litigation, limiting its authority to the supervision of medical practices (D. Gatta, *Regali dispacci, nelli quali si contengono le sovrane determinazioni . . . nel Regno di Napoli* [Naples, 1773–77], 4:561).

Also, in Vienna in the eighteenth century the Medical Faculty had civil and criminal jurisdiction; see Erna Lesky, *Österreichisches Gesundheitswesen im Zeitalter des aufgeklärten Absolutismus* (Vienna, 1959); C. Steiner, *Die Bader und Barbiere (Wundärzte) in Wein sur Zeit Maria Theresias, 1740–1780* (Vienna, 1975), 87–91.

105. "Secundum usum mercantiae" (in the manner of merchants); "sine strepitu et figura iuditii" (without the clamor and ceremony of a formal court). See rubr. 4 of 1507 statutes (A.S.B., Coll. Med., b. 216; see above, n. 32). As stated in a public notice issued by the Roman Protomedicato in 1614 (which appears as an epigraph to this chapter): "Those who feel aggravated in any way by physicians, surgeons, barbers, and others, because of medications, and bleeding, malpractice, or an unreasonable cost of medicines . . . by appealing to us, will receive swift justice, be they foreigners or . . . Roman citizens" (A.S.B., Coll. Med., b. 233).

On the "summary procedure" adopted in mercantile courts, see M. Taruffo, *La giustizia civile in Italia dal '700 ad oggi* (Bologna, 1980), 11. On the *ius mercatorum* binding anybody having business with merchants, see Francesco Galgano, *Storia del diritto commerciale* (Bologna, 1976), 38.

106. A.S.B., Reggimento, Assunteria d'Arti, Miscellanea, b. 1.

107. In the archives of the College of Medicine I found records for more than 300 trials between 1570 and 1776. Of these, 195 are criminal cases and 131 are civil cases. It should be mentioned that the distinction between civil and criminal cases is not clearcut. For instance, a civil suit filed by a healer against a nonpaying customer could become a criminal trial of the healer, if it could be proved that he had practiced without a license (see chap. 6, pp. 142–43).

There are some gaps in the documentation, as the Protomedicato's proceedings for 1570–1604 and 1702–44 are missing. But some information about these periods can be gleaned from the "libri secreti" (secret books) of the college—the diaries written by the dean, who was ipso facto a protomedico—which provide some account, albeit brief and incomplete, of the activities of the Protomedicato. Very rich sources for these periods, including transcripts of interrogations and other trial materials, are contained in the files *(filze)* of the notaries of the college. Unfortunately, the records for the period 1615–63 are missing from the filze. Some of these lacunae in the college's archive have been mentioned by G. Cencetti, *Gli archivi dello Studio bolognese* (Bologna, 1938), 48–56. In spite of these gaps, the richness of the extant documentation allowed me to make an in-depth study of the history of the college over an extended period of time.

108. The analogy between the infirm and the poor was pointed out, for in-

stance, by C. Benincasa (*De paupertate ac eius privilegiis,* in *Tractatus . . . de variis verbis Juris* [Venice, 1584], 18:154r). A juridical literature specifically concerned with the "privileges" of the sick developed in the first years of the seventeenth century; see Th. Actius [T. Azzio], *De infirmitate eiusque privilegiis et affectibus* (Venice, 1603); and chap. 4, below, pp. 117–18.

109. P. Sella, *Il procedimento civile nella legislazione statutaria italiana* (Milan, 1927), 228–33. See also F. Menestrina, *Il processo civile nello stato pontificio* (Turin, 1908).

110. E. Grendi, "Ideologia della carità e società indisciplinata: La costruzione del sistema assistenziale genovese," in *Timore e carità: I poveri nell'Italia moderna,* proceedings of the conference "Pauperismo e assistenza negli antichi stati italiani," March 28–30, 1980 (Cremona, 1982), 61–62.

CHAPTER 2: PROMISING A CURE

1. In the archives of the Protomedicato I found records for 195 criminal cases against healers, for most of which only a brief summary of the proceedings is given in the records. Detailed documentation of the court's proceedings (including denunciation, examination of witnesses, etc.) is extant for only 74 trials; significantly, 55 of these were initiated by a charge or complaint filed by a patient.

2. A.S.B., Coll. Med., b. 195.

3. A.S.B., Coll. Med., b. 236.

4. G. Rizzi, "Chirurghi e pazienti davanti al notaio," *Humana Studia,* 2d ser., 2, no. 4 (1950): 1–7; idem, "Contratti medievali tra medico e malato," *Minerva medica* 38, 1, n. 22 (June 1947): 521–24; idem, "Un contratto notarile quattrocentesco per operazione di cataratta," *Atti del II Convegno della Marca* (Fermo, 1957); C. Mancini, "Un singolare contratto del 1200," *Atti e Memorie dell'Accademia di Storia dell'Arte Sanitaria* 2d ser., 31, no. 2 (1965): 47–48; U. Stefanutti, "Sulla liceità giuridica e deontologica dei patti conclusi 'prima della cura' fra medici e pazienti (secoli XIV, XV e XVI)," *Giustizia e società,* no. 4 (1965). The text of a contract for a cure is quoted and discussed in E. Dall'Osso, "Un oculista medico-condotto del Trecento," *Giornale Italiano di Oftalmologia* (October 1956). These essays do not analyze the documents historically; they just present them as odd anecdotes.

For a brief description of the cure contract from the perspective of a social history of medicine, see I. Fischer, *Ärztliche Standepflichten und Standesfragen: Eine historische Studie* (Vienna, 1912), 105–8. This work is still very useful on the history of payments for medical services; see 98–153. Cure contracts are also briefly discussed by M. S. Mazzi, *Salute e società nel Medioevo* (Florence, 1978), 92–94; I. Naso, *Medici e strutture sanitarie nella società tardo-medievale* (Milan, 1982), 199; M. R. McVaugh, *Medicine before the Plague: Practitioners and Their Patients in the Crown of Aragon, 1285–1345* (Cambridge, England, 1993), 174–81; J. Shatzmiller, *Jews, Medicine, and Medieval Society* (Berkeley, Calif., 1994), 125–27, 131; and L. García-Ballester, "Medical Ethics in

Transition in the Latin Medicine of the Thirteenth and Fourteenth Centuries: New Perspectives on the Physician-Patient Relationship and the Doctor's Fee," in *Doctors and Ethics: The Earlier Historical Setting of Professional Ethics,* ed. A. Wear, J. Geyer-Kordesch, and R. French (Amsterdam, 1993), 54, 67 n. 88.

5. A.S.B., Comune, Ufficio dei Memoriali, year 1316, fol. 131v (notary Antonio di Alberto Gota, May 5, 1316). The original text of this document appears as document 2 in the Appendix, below. A transcription of the document was also published without commentary by Karl Sudhoff, "Ein Arztvertrag aus dem Jahre 1316 im Staatsarchiv zu Bologna," *Archiv für Geschichte der Medizin* 5 (1912): 399–400.

6. "Sic quod pars illa non erat in potestate mei; ymo videbatur mihi quod esset tamquam res mortua vel aliena" (quoted by P. Capparoni, "Un'auto-osservazione clinica inedita del secolo XV," *Rivista di storia critica delle scienze mediche e naturali* 1 [1910–12]: 74).

7. The document, which appears in its entirety as document 1 in the Appendix, below, is also published in Mancini, "Un singolare contratto del 1200," 47; and Rizzi, "Contratti medievali," 522, col. 1.

Mancini published two other contracts from Genoa. In the first (1226), a Master Giovanni promised to cure a patient, Guglielmo, at his own expense, "of the spot which you have in the head and in the brain," so as to restore sight "to your left eye, after removing all the spots and blindness." For his part, Guglielmo promised to pay the healer five Genoese lire "as soon as I begin to see from my aforementioned left eye, well enough to be able to return to my own business and errands." He would pay five more lire upon completion of the cure (Mancini, "Singolare contratto," 48).

The second agreement was between the same Master Giovanni and a shield-maker, Enrico da Vedano. The patient promised to pay the healer forty Genoese soldi if he recovered from gallstones *(de male lapidis):* "stones, which I have in my bladder or body" (Mancini, "Singolare contratto," 48).

Rizzi, "Contratti medioevali," reports two other agreements signed in Crete and now kept in the Venice State Archive. One of them appears as document 3 in the Appendix, below.

8. On Crete, see Rizzi, "Contratti medievali"; on Zara, see idem, "Chirurghi e pazienti"; on Ferrara and Dubrovnik, Stefanutti, "Sulla liceità giuridica"; on Avignon, P. Pansier, "La pratique de l'ophtalmologie dans le moyen-âge latin," *Janus* 9 (1904): 25–26; on Messina, G. Pitré, *Medici, chirurghi, barbieri e speziali antichi in Sicilia* (Florence, 1942), 148; on Hildesheim, J. Machner, *Das Krankenwesen der Stadt Hildesheim bis zum 17. Jahrhundert* (Hildesheim, 1907), 19; on Poitiers, *Bulletin de la société française d'histoire de la médecine* 11 (1912): 451. Other French agreements for a cure from the sixteenth century are published in *La France médicale* (1907): 384. Some French documents are included in the Appendix, below. See also the examples of cure contracts published in A. Toaff, *The Jews in Medieval Assisi, 1305–1478: A Social and Economic History of a Small Jewish Community in Italy* (Florence, 1979), 174–85; M. Luzzati, "Il medico ebreo e il contadino: Un documento pisano del 1462," in *La casa*

dell'ebreo: Saggi sugli Ebrei a Pisa e in Toscana nel Medioevo e nel Rinascimento (Pisa, 1985), 51–57, document on 56–57. Other examples of such contracts, found in Provençal archives, are described in J. de Duranti La Calade, "Notes sur les rues d'Aix au XIVe et au XVe siècle," Annales de Provence 9 (1912): 122–25; N. Coulet, "Documents aixois (première moitié du XVe siècle)," Razo: Cahiers du centre d'études médiévales de Nice 4 (1984): 115–25; L. Stouff, "Documents arlésiens," ibid., 4 (1984): 126; J. Schatzmiller, Médecine et justice en Provence médiévale: Documents de Manosque, 1262–1348 (Aix-en-Provence, 1989), 193 (doc. no. 62), 194 (doc. no. 63), 235 (doc. no. 82). More documents are published in Le corps souffrant: Maladie et médications, vol. 4 of Razo: Cahiers du centre d'études médiévales de Nice (1984). For Sicilian examples, see H. Bresc, Un monde méditerranéen: Economie et société en Sicile, 1300–1450 (Rome, 1986), 2:478. For Catalan examples from 1307–8, see M. McVaugh, "Bernat de Berriacho (fl. 1301–43) and the Ordinacio of Bishop Poná de Gualba," Arxiu de Textos Catalans Antics 9 (1990): 253–54.

9. For Spain, see M. E. Muñoz, ed., Recopilación de las leyes, pragmáticas, reales decretos, y acuerdos del Real Proto-Medicato (Valencia, 1751), chap. 13, art. 9, p. 168; for France, J. Verdier, Essai sur la jurisprudence de la médecine en France (Alençon, 1762), 2:497–521; and for Germany, J. Schultz, Dissertatio Juridica de contractu medici cum aegroto (Danzig, 1679), 7–8. I examine the jurists' debate on the validity of the contracts for a cure in chap. 6, below.

10. M. Pelling and C. Webster, "Medical Practitioners," in Health, Medicine, and Mortality in the Sixteenth Century, ed. C. Webster (Cambridge, England, 1979), 208, 214, 218. Evidence of suits filed by patients or healers for breach of contract in the Court of Chancery and the Court of Common Pleas is examined by C. Rawcliffe, "The Profits of Practice: The Wealth and Status of Medical Men in Later Medieval England," Social History of Medicine 1, no. 1 (April 1988): 673–77. (This study, however, does not analyze the content of the agreements.) The custom of making cure agreements in late medieval England is also documented by the legal cases reported by M. P. Cosman, "Medieval Medical Malpractice: The Dicta and the Dockets," Bulletin of the New York Academy of Medicine 40, no. 1 (January 1973): 22–47. Some of the cases mentioned by Cosman involved charges of broken promise of a cure, for which patients were requesting the return of advance payment (see 25, 29, and 32). Anne Digby (Making a Medical Living [Cambridge, England, 1994], 17) argues that the custom of making contracts for a cure, once mainstream practice, had declined in England by the eighteenth century, although surviving on the fringe of the medical profession. She gives one example of such an agreement, with the clause specifying payment by results, from Gissing, Norfolk, in 1740 (228–90).

11. Pitré, Medici, chirurghi, 148; the document appears as document 6 in the Appendix, below.

12. "De instructione Medici secundum Archimathaeum," in Collectio salernitana, ed. S. De Renzi (Naples, 1852), 5:333; S. Bongi, ed., Bandi lucchesi del secolo XIV, tratti dai registri del R. Archivio di Stato di Lucca (Bologna, 1863), 145. The surgeons

from Lucca promised to cure their patients "for an appropriate and reasonable fee, to be collected only after restoring health." Similar promises can be found in the advertising notices used by German practitioners of the fourteenth and fifteenth centuries, published in K. Sudhoff, "Vier Niederlassungsankündigungen von Ärzten aus dem 15. Jahrhundert," *Archiv für Geschichte der Medizin* 6 (1913): 309–11.

13. It was the general opinion among medical authors that patients' confidence in their healers had therapeutic effects. "Hope and trust benefit the patient during healing" ("Prodest denique aegro in medendo spes fidesque"), as stated in a text on medical deontology of the fifteenth century: A. Benedetti, "De medici atque aegri officio," in *De re medica* (Basel, 1549), 546. See also L. Botallo, "Tractatus de medici et aegri munere," in *Opera Omnia* (1512; Lyons, 1660), 16: "As Galen said, and experience itself confirms, the patient's confidence in the physician in no small way helps defeat illness, soothe pain, and hasten the healing process."

14. G. Monticolo, *I Capitolari delle arti veneziane* (Rome, 1896), 1:341: "eo quod contra ordinem sui officii certam partem solucionis a quadam persona, quam habebat in cura, antequam curaverit ipsam infirmitatem." Beatrice was tried and sentenced by the Giustizia Vecchia, the court that held jurisdiction over the guilds. Later, she was pardoned by the Maggior Consiglio, which cancelled her fine.

15. Monticolo, *Capitolari,* 1:348. Naso (*Medici e strutture sanitarie,* 198) reports the case of a patient from Asti who, in 1480, filed charges against his physician for "having requested four ducats even before prescribing the medication."

16. The original text of the document is printed in A. Gloria, *Monumenti della Università di Padova, 1318–1405* (Padua, 1888), 2:183. Domenico da Bologna is called *medicus* in the document; Novello da Marano is not. On Novello's qualification as a *medicus ciroicus,* despite his lack of academic credentials, see T. Pesenti Marangon, "*Professores chirurgie, medici ciroici e barbitonsores* a Padova nell'età di Leonardo Buffi da Bertipaglia," *Quaderni per la storia dell'Università di Padova* (1978): 14. Commenting on this document, Pesenti Marangon observes, "On such a delicate point, the two physicians' verdict is very odd: since the prescribed medicines gave no results, their colleague should return all of the money he received for treatment" (14). I believe, however, that this kind of ruling, far from being odd, was mainstream practice in the medieval courts.

17. "Die 22 octobris dijudicatum est de condemnando magistrum Johannem Andream chirurgum ad restituendum ser Nicola Bazano de Antibaros ducatos auri octo sibi numeratos pro parte solutionis pro cura ser Georgii filii sui, qui patiebatur morbum lapidis et hoc quia ex inquisitione lecta in presenti Consilio clare apparet ipsum non prestasse in cura infirmi illam diligentiam, quam prestare tenebatur. Item quod tenebatur restituere prefato ser Nicolao Bazano lapidem quem extraxit e corpore infirmi in variis petiis et quod non debeat dimitti a pallatio donec restituerit dictos ducatos et lapidem predictam supranominato ser Nicola Bazano et post hac quod dictus magister Jo. Andreas non possit amplius exercere tam in civitate quam territorio nostro artem chirurgicam sub pena ducatorum centum. . . . Die dicta ser Nico-

laus Bazano recepit a magistro Jo. Andrea ducatos auri octo et lapidem supranominatum" (Stefanutti, "Sulla liceità giuridica," doc. 2, p. 369). The request that the healer deliver the stone, which was extracted in pieces from the body of the sick man, probably reflected the healers' custom of advertising their services by showing the stones removed from their patients' bodies.

18. Rizzi, "Chirurghi e pazienti," 6–7.

19. Stefanutti, "Sulla liceità giuridica," 369, doc. 3 (A.S.B., Carte di corredo del Tribunale Civile del Podestà, year 1414, first semester).

20. See chap. 5, below, pp. 130–32.

21. Pansier, "La pratique de l'ophtalmologie," 25–26; the text appears as document 5 in the Appendix, below. Here is another clause on relapses included in a deed under seal signed in Zara in 1377—also involving the treatment of a fistula:

> Master Pietro, of the late Master Ricobaldo of Valle Sudana, town surgeon of the municipality of Zara, declares to have received from Damiano . . . , son of the late Zannino di Calcina of Zara, on behalf of [Cipri]ano of the late Donaldo de Zernoto of Arbo, twenty-one florins . . . for the treatment and cure provided by Master Pietro to Colano, son of the above-mentioned Cipriano, affected by a tear fistula that Colano had in his right eye; and in reimbursement of the expenses incurred by Master Pietro for Colano's food and drink over a period of seven months. [Master Pietro] acknowledges that, should said fistula form again in Colano's eye, Master Pietro will be responsible for medicating and curing it entirely at his own expense until Colano will completely recover. (Rizzi, "Chirurghi e pazienti," 3)

A similar clause was included in a Bolognese contract of 1476 (document 4 in the Appendix, below) and in an agreement signed in 1269 by Guglielmo da Saliceto, author of a celebrated *Chirurgia*: "Master Guglielmo da Piacenza, physician, promised Guido di Rossiglione, a German student, to cure him at his own expense from the disease of *fleume sarse* should [Guido] relapse in the next two years, for the amount of twenty-six Bolognese lire": see M. Sarti and T. Fattorini, *De Claris Archigymnasii Bononiensis Professoribus* (Bologna, 1769–72), 1:554 n. 1. *Fleume sarse* was probably a disease with a cough and discharge (*fleume* = phlegm; C. Du Cange, *Glossarium mediae et infimae latinitatis* [Niort, 1883–87], vol. 10, s.v. "fleuma": "Ita Picardi nostri Fleume dicunt pro pituita").

22. Pilius medicinensis, *Quaestiones Sabbatinae* (reprint; Turin, 1967), C.G.J.C., no. 4, quaestio 12, pp. 20–21: "Solutio. In hac quaestione posset distingui utrum ex eisdem humoribus instaurata esset infirmitas, an ex alijs. Si ex eisdem teneatur medicus, alias nequaquam, arg. ff. de solut. l. qui res ¶ aream vel aliter, utrum culpa infirmi forsan, quia non abstinuit a conviviis, an non, si culpa infirmi non teneatur, alias obligetur, arg. ff. de reg. iur. l. quod qui ex culpa."

Similarly, Bartolo di Sassoferrato [Bartolus de Saxo Ferrato] argued that the doctor should be paid again if the causes of the disease were new. If the causes were the same, the patient should not be considered healed and should be treated without charge. Bartolo specified that a relapse soon after healing would probably indicate the same cause, while a relapse after a long time would indicate new causes, in which case the doctor would be allowed to ask for extra payment. See his *In secundam Digesti veteris partem* (Venice, 1570), 2:136v; from a commentary to Digest 19, 2, 59, law "Marcius."

The *quaestiones* were controversial legal issues, which medieval glossators discussed in the presence of students on specific days of the week (for instance, Pilius's *sabbatinae* were discussed on Saturdays). On the *quaestiones* as a juridical genre, see H. Kantorowicz, "The Quaestiones Disputatae of the Glossators," *Tijdschrift voor rechtsgeschiedenis* 16 (1938): 1–67; on Pilius, see 14.

23. Among the canonists, G. Durandus [G. Durante] (*Speculum Judiciale* [1271; Bologna, 1477], rubr. "de salariis," 201 r) restated and summarized the opinion of the glossators on the issue of the physicians' fee in case of relapse. Angelus de Clavasio (*Summa Angelica de casibus conscientiae* [Venice, 1487], s.v. "medicus," no. 14, 235 v) made a slightly different case, although reaching basically the same conclusions: "Utrum medicus qui convenit pro X ducatis cum ticio liberare eum de aliqua infirmitate, puta quartana et huiusmodi: et liberat eum: scilicet in modicum tempus ticius reincidit in eadem infirmitatem teneatur iterum pro illis X eum liberare. Respondeo vi quod sic quia non extinxit infirmitatem: sed cessare fecit angustiam ipsius. Item quia non videtur curasse: cum vitiose curavit. Item quia . . . cum effectis sunt accipienda quod ideo debet intelligi cum curaret perfecte. In contrarium videtur quod non teneatur, quia de praesenti infirmitate tantum videtur cogitatum, et ideo soluto eo quod debetur sublata est obligatio in perpetuum, quia in infinitum non debet obligari. Nam infirmitas evitatur. ff. loca. l. martinus in glo. Sed tu dic quod aut rediit ex culpa infirmi, et sic non tenetur. l. quod quis ex culpa. ff. de re iur. Si non ex culpa infirmi: tunc aut statim redit, et sic tenetur quod non videtur eum liberasse, aut ex intervallo: et sic non tenetur, ut ff. de re. iur. l. quamquid."

In the late sixteenth century, Gian Battista Codronchi (*De christiana ac tuta medendi ratione* [Ferrara, 1591], 95–97) still accepted the glossators' view. This traditional opinion was shared as well by L. Ferraris (*Prompta Bibliotheca canonica juridicomoralis theologica* [Rome, 1766], s.v. "medicus"). Among jurists expert in civil law, A. Tiraquellus [A. Tiraqueau] (*Commentaria in l. Si unquam. C. de revoc. don.,* t. 6 [1535; Frankfurt, 1574], 237 n. 180) listed opinions by a number of authoritative scholars such as Bartolo and Pilius, with whom he agreed: "If the relapse occurs immediately after treatment, the physician should not be paid, because obviously the patient was not healed; on the contrary, the doctor should be paid if the illness returns after a long period of time."

Bartolo's opinion is adopted also by G. Papa [Guy de la Pape] (*Singularia* [Lyons, 1533], 76v). D. I. Bertachini (*Repertorium iuris utriusque Doctoris praestantissimi* [Venice, 1570], s.v. "medicus," 332r–334r) describes Bartolo's view as "common opinion": "Medicus, qui convenit cum infirmo de eo sanando pro certo pretio, si sanatus illico reincidit in infirmitatem, tenetur iterum eum curare" (332r). E. Speckham (*Questionum juris caesarei, pontificii et saxonici Centuria Prima* [Wittenberg, 1611], quaestio 31, fols. 78v–82r) also adopts this view of the question.

24. Rizzi, "Chirurghi e pazienti," 5–6.

25. Monticolo, *Capitolari* 1:277–78.

26. G. F. Ingrassia, *Constitutiones et Capitula, necnon Regii Protomedicatus officii* (Palermo, 1564). (I used the edition edited by Paolo Pizzutto [Palermo, 1657].) The office of the protomedico of Sicily was created in 1397; the protomedico was appointed by the king: see *Regia Imperatoriaque protomedicatus officii diplomata seu privilegia* (Palermo, 1564). On Ingrassia, see F. Orlando-Salinas, "Le tariffe per i medici nelle 'Constitutiones protomedicales' di Gian Filippo Ingrassia (1563)," *La cultura medica moderna* 9, no. 5 (1930).

On the issue of fixed fees for physicians in Italy in the early modern age, some information (mostly anecdotal) is offered in G. Del Guerra, "Gli onorari dei medici attraverso i tempi," *Economia e storia* 3 (1962): 384–89. The fixing of medical fees by state authorities was a widespread practice in the sixteenth and seventeenth centuries. For example, in Nuremberg in the early 1600s, the fees for medical services were established by the Senate. See *Leges ac Statuta Ampliss. Senatus Norimbergensis ad Medicos, Pharmacopoeos & alios pertinentia* (Nuremberg, 1612). For the same practice in other German towns, see Fischer, *Ärztliche Standespflichten,* 114–18.

27. This opinion was shared by Henry de Mondeville, a famous surgeon of the fourteenth century: "Not too long ago, people used to pay surgeons according to the amount of work performed, rather than to the gravity of the disease. In this way, ignorant and dishonest surgeons made incredible amounts of money by prolonging treatment, while the honest ones, who healed their patients as fast as they could, lived in poverty like beggars" (de Mondeville, *Chirurgia,* translated in Italian in M. Tabanelli, *Un secolo d'oro della Chirurgia francese: Henry de Mondeville* [Forlì, 1969], 1:215).

28. Ingrassia, *Constitutiones et Capitula:* "for perfectly curing a dislocation [*pro collocando aliquo luxato articulo, perfecteque sanando*] of the femur, the practitioner shall receive thirty-six *tarì;* of the tibia, thirty; of the shoulder, radius, or ulna, twenty-four; of the other bones, eighteen. . . . If these operations are not successful, [a patient] should pay as for a simple visit." Healing a hernia, extracting a gallstone, and curing scrofula "without leaving any traces of the disease" would each cost two *once.* On the value of one tarì, of one oncia (equal to thirty tarì), and of a *grano* (one-twentieth of a tarì), see D. Schiavo, *Spiegazione del tarì d'oro, moneta di Sicilia* (Palermo, 1777). Machner (*Das Krankenwesen,* 22) quotes numerous ordinances by several guilds of barber-surgeons in German towns establishing that payment could be requested by barbers only when patients were healed.

29. Ingrassia, *Constitutiones et Capitula.*

30. Pitré, *Medici, chirurghi,* 153.

31. The charge of simony against physicians treating patients for profit was commonplace in the Middle Ages; see E. S. Karnofski, "The Vision of Tainard:

Miraculum de quodam canonico guatenensi per Sanctum Donatianum curatum," in *The Church and Healing,* ed. W. J. Sheils (Oxford, 1982), 20. The charge was still mentioned in M. Navarro's sixteenth-century confession manual, *Manuale de' confessori e penitenti . . . composto dal dottor Martino Azpliqueta Navarro* (Venice, 1659), c. 23, tit. "de simonia"; and in C. Benincasa, "De paupertate ac eius privilegiis," in *Tractatus . . . de variis verbis Juris* (Venice, 1584), 18:148r: "A physician should not receive salary for having restored or for restoring health to the sick, because this is a gift which should not be sold . . . ; and if physicians receive fees in that spirit, they will commit the sin of simony, like Gehazi, who sold the blessing of health to Naaman the Syrian, and for that was struck with leprosy."

On the idea that knowledge may not be sold, see G. Post, K. Giocarinis, and R. Kay, "The Medieval Heritage of a Humanistic Ideal: *Scientia donum Dei est unde vendi non potest," Traditio* 11 (1955).

32. Antoninus, *Summa theologica* (Verona, 1740), pars 3, "De statu medicorum," p. 277.

33. P. Zacchia, *Quaestiones medico-legales* (1612–1630; Lyons, 1662), lib. 6, tit. 1, quaest. 1, p. 465. On Zacchia, see L. Allacci, *Apes Urbanae, sive de viribus illustribus qui ab anno MDCXXX per totum MDCXXXII Romae adfuerunt* (Rome, 1663), 213; P. Capparoni, *Profili biobibliografici di medici e naturalisti celebri italiani dal secolo XV al XVIII* (Rome, 1925), 134–36; A. Pazzini, *Storia della medicina* (Milan, 1951), 2:93–96.

34. *Preparamento del Pastarino, per medicarsi in questi sospettosi tempi di peste* (Bologna, 1577).

35. Such a clause was imposed even on the famous physician Taddeo Alderotti, hired as town doctor by the Venetians in 1293: "for treating diseases he shall not request more than 10 *soldi di grossi,* except for the treatment of apostemes of the liver, arthritis, leprosy, and dropsy; and if the noblemen of Venice wish to go to his house for advice, they should not pay for it" (Monticolo, *Capitolari* 1:283). Master Anselmo, hired by the municipality of Venice that same year, had also to agree by contract "to be content with the payment that the sick will give him, and to give advice at no charge to those who go and ask for it at his house" (Monticolo, *Capitolari* 1:285).

36. An example of this sales technique is described in a play by L. Ariosto, *Erbolato,* in *Opere minori,* ed. A. Vallone (Milan, 1964). On the survival of the notion that medical advice should be free and that patients should pay only for medicines, see G. Thuillier, "Pour une histoire du médicament en Nivernais au XIXe siècle," *Revue d'Histoire et d'Economie Sociale* 53 (1975): 92; and Digby, *Making a Medical Living,* 150 ff, which refers to "the earlier custom of charging mainly for medicine." Digby estimates that in England in the early years of the nineteenth century, "up to four-fifths of the cost of medical attendance had been charged up to medicines supplied." I was not able to consult on this issue L. Sasvàri, "Unpaid Healers among Greek Orthodox and Uniats in Hungary," *Orvöstort-Közl* (1979): 13–63.

37. On Cosmas and Damian as *anargiri* (healers who did not take payment for their labor), see A. Wittmann, *Kosmas und Damian: Kultausbreitung und Volksdevotion*

(Berlin, 1967), 12 ff. The ideal of the physician who cured without charge was pre-Christian. Examples of this ideal can be found in the funeral inscriptions of Greek physicians: for example, Menocritus, who lived in poverty and treated many patients without accepting compensation (*Revue Archéologique* 1 [1880]: 344), and Evenor, who did the same, although bound by contract only to treat the poor without charge (R. Bozzoni, *I medici e il diritto romano* [Naples, 1904], 136).

The idea that public physicians in ancient Greece were requested to treat the poor without charge has been criticized by L. Cohn-Haft, *The Public Physicians of Ancient Greece* (Northampton, Mass., 1956), 199–205.

38. A.S.B., Coll. Med., b. 353 *bis*. For examples of physicians who treated the poor without charge in Renaissance Florence, see K. Park, *Doctors and Medicine in Early Renaissance Florence* (Princeton, N.J., 1985), 93. The doctor's obligation to treat the poor for free is also stressed in a 1631 hiring contract between the Jewish community of Frankfurt and the physician Joseph Solomon Del Medigo; on this document, see J. S. Leibowitz, "Town Physicians in Jewish Social History," in *International Symposium on Society, Medicine, and Law,* ed. H. Karplus (Amsterdam, 1973), 121. J. Tate Lanning (*The Royal Protomedicato: The Regulation of the Medical Profession in the Spanish Empire* [Durham, 1985], 201–6) extensively documents the legal obligation of physicians and other medical practitioners (including midwives) to treat the poor without charge, in Spain and in the American colonies in the early modern period.

39. A.S.B., Coll. Med., b. 214, trial of Antonio il Romano.

40. A.S.B., Coll. Med., b. 350, trial of Andrea and Lorenzo Adriani, 1666. On the *norcini* (so called from their area of origin around the town of Norcia, in central Italy) see below, chap. 3, n. 63.

41. This was the case in Norwich, for instance, where the statutes of the guild of barber-surgeons established that unlicensed healers treating the sick without charge could not be prosecuted for illegal practice (Pelling and Webster, "Medical Practitioners," 213).

42. *Leges Visigothorum Antiquiores,* ed. K. Zeumer (Hannover, 1894), lib. 11, tit. 1, p. 292. Also in *Monumenta Germaniae Historica, Legum Sectio* 1: *Leges Nationum Germanicarum* (Hannover, 1902), 1:401–2. This is the original text:

Lex III. Antiqua:
Si medicus pro egritudine ad placitum expetatur.
Si quis medicum ad placitum pro infirmo visitando aut vulnere curando poposcerit, cum viderit vulnus medicus aut dolores agnoverit, statim sub certo placito cautione emissa infirmum accipiat.
Lex III. Antiqua:
Si ad placitum susceptus moriatur infirmus.
Si quis medicus infirmum ad placitum susceperit, cautionis emisso vinculo, infirmum restituat sanitati; certe si periculum contigerit mortis, mercedem placiti penitus non requirat; nec ulla exinde utrique parti calumnia moveatur.

The exact interpretation of these laws is controversial. Who should advance the security—the patient or the physician? I believe that it was the patient, on the basis of what we gather from the documentation on the contracts for a cure and the text of the law as translated in the *Fuero Juzgo* (see below, n. 46). This is also the opinion of A. Niederhellmann, *Arzt und Heilkunde in den Frümittelarterlichen Leges* (Berlin, 1983), 68, who follows the translation in E. Wohlhaupter, ed., *Gesetze der Westgoten* (Weimar, 1936), 291. On the other hand, both P. Diepgen (*Geschichte der Medizin* [Berlin, 1949], 1:198–99) and G. Baader ("Gesellschaft, Wirtschaft und ärztlicher Stand im frühen und hohen Mittelalter," *Medizinhistorisches Journal* 14 [1979]: 180) are of a different opinion. They believe that the physician should advance the security; in this they are probably following Fischer's lead (*Ärztliche Standespflichten,* 125).

43. On the meaning of *placitum* as contract or covenant, see Du Cange, *Glossarium mediae et infimae latinitatis* 6:346, col. 3.

44. *Leges Visigothorum Antiquiores,* 292; *Monumenta Germaniae Historica,* 402:

Lex V. Antiqua:
Si de oculis medicus ipocemata tollat.
   Si quis medicus hipocisim de oculis abstulerit et ad pristinam sanitatem infirmum revocaverit, V solidos pro suo beneficio consequatur.

P. D. King (*Law and Society in the Visigothic Kingdom* [Cambridge, England, 1972], 203) remarks that the medical profession must have been lucrative if physicians could charge a fee as much as five "solidi" to remove a cataract—even considering that payment depended on the success of treatment.

45. The law "On Physicians and Patients" belongs in the Codex Reccensvindianus of the mid–seventh century, but the designation *antiqua* indicates that it came from an earlier law code: either Leogivild's Codex Revisus (A.D. 568/69–586) or possibly even the Codex Euricianus (the earliest text of the Visigothic laws, circa A.D. 476).

The suggestion that the term *antiquae* referred to laws already included in earlier codes was advanced by Zeumer in 1894 in his edition of the Leges Visigothorum Antiquiores. See also K. Zeumer, "Über zwei neuentdeckte westgothische Gesetze," *Neues Archiv der Gesellschaft für ältere deutsche Geschichtskunde* 23 (1898): 75–112. Zeumer's suggestion is still accepted by present-day scholars: see King, *Law and Society,* 6–13.

46. *Fuero Juzgo, o Libro de los Jueces* (Madrid, 1815), libro 11, "I. Titol de los fisicos é de los enfermos," pp. 171–72:

III. Antigua. *Que el físico deve pleytear con el enfermo.*
   Si algun fisico pleytea con el enfermo, por le visitar, é por le sanar de las plagas, deve veer la plaga, é la dolor: é pues que la conosciere, pleyteye con él, é que tome recabdo por su aver.

IV. Antigua. *Si el enfermo muere pues que ha pleyteado con el físico.*

Si algun omne, é algun físico pleytea con el enfermo de le sanar sobre recabdo, sánelo quanto meior pudiere. E si por ventura murier el enfermo, nol dé nada al físico de quanto con él pleytear, nin nenguna de las partes non deven mover contra la otra.

On the relationship between Leges Visigothorum and Fuero Juzco see *Nuovissimo Digesto* (Turin, 1957–80), s.v. "Lex Visigothorum" and "Fuero."

47. For example, D. W. Amundsen, "Visigothic Medical Legislation," *Bulletin of the History of Medicine* 45, no. 6 (1971): 558; F. H. Garrison, *An Introduction to the History of Medicine* (Philadelphia, 1929), 146; M. Neuburger, *History of Medicine* (Oxford, 1925), 2:10–11; P. Laín Entralgo, *Doctor and Patient* (London, 1969), 61, 77 ff.

48. Among barbaric peoples, the Visigoths had lived the longest with the Romans. The most ancient code of Visigothic laws, the Codex Euricianus, to which the law "De medicis et egrotis" might belong, clearly shows the influence of Roman law. On this issue see King, *Law and Society,* 8–9.

49. *Codex Theodosianus,* 13, 3, 8: "Impp. Valentinianus & Valens A.A. ad Praetextatum P.V.

"Exceptis portus Syxti virginumque vestalium, quot regiones urbi sunt, totidem constituantur archiatri, qui scientes annonaria sibi commoda a populi commodis honeste obsequi tenuioribus malint, quam turpiter servire divitibus. Quos etiam ea patimur accipere, quae sani offerunt pro obsequiis, non ea quae periclitantes pro salute promittunt . . . Dat. III. Kalend. Feb. Triu. Valentiniano & Valente III A.A. Conss." (*Codex Theodosianus* [Lyons, 1566], 415). See also the text edited by T. Mommsen and P. M. Meyer: *Theodosiani libri XVI cum constitutionibus Sirmondianis et leges novellae ad Theodosianum pertinentes,* 2d ed. (Berlin, 1954).

The other laws in "De professoribus et medicis" basically list privileges granted to physicians and "professors of letters" by several emperors, starting with Constantine. Privileges included exemptions from taxes and military service, from the duty to quarter troops, and so on.

50. The meaning of the word *archiater* has been debated since the eighteenth century. Vivian Nutton ("Archiatri and the Medical Profession in Antiquity," *Papers of the British School in Rome* 45 [1977]: 191–215) summarizes the view of modern scholars: originally, the Greek word *archiatros* indicated the personal physician of a ruler. The Roman word *archiater* indicated both a court physician and a public or town physician: both were called *archiatri* in Roman juridical texts. K. H. Below, *Der Arzt im römischen Recht* (Munich, 1953), identifies archiatri with the limited number of physicians who were granted special legal privileges and exemptions.

51. This is the interpretation of the law by Nutton ("Archiatri," 209–10) and Bozzoni (*I medici e il diritto romano,* 112–13). The latter interprets *commoda annonaria* as yearly salaries. According to Nutton ("Archiatri," 209–10), the reasons for creating a number of public physicians were political rather than philanthropic. He argues that

the law should be placed in the context of the competition between Christian and pagan elites for the patronage of the urban populace.

52. *Codex Iustinianus,* 50, 10: "De professoribus et medicis," 9.

53. The intention of preventing abuses by physicians' in their dealings with the sick is clearly expressed in the law "Si medicus," also included in the Digest (50, 13): "If a physician that someone entrusted with treating his eyes used harmful medications to the point of almost making the patient blind, in order to compel him in bad faith to sell his goods to himself, the governor of the province shall punish [the physician] for this illegal action and shall order that the goods sold be returned to the patient." ("Si medicus, cui curandos suos oculos, qui eis laborabat, commiserat, periculum amittendorum eorum per adversa medicamenta inferendo, compulit, ut ei possessiones suas contra fidem bonam aeger venderet: incivile factum praeses provinciae coercet, remque restitui jubeat.")

This law described a complex case combining malpractice with the doctor's abuse of a cure agreement. The doctor applied the wrong medications to worsen the patient's condition in order to force him to sell his property at loss to pay for the treatment. In the case of such patent abuse, the sale contract was legally invalid, and the physician had to return the extorted goods. The issue in this case was not the legal validity of cure agreements in general, but rather the physician's abuse of such an agreement. The law derives from Ulpian, *Libro octavo de omnibus tribunalibus* (third century).

54. Digest 50, 13: "De variis et extraordinariis cognitionibus" (Ulpian, *Libro octavo de omnibus tribunalibus*), which also includes the law "Si medicus," cited in the previous note. This law gave the governor of the province the power to judge *extra ordinem* (with extraordinary procedure) any disputes over the payment of fees to physicians, midwives, lawyers, liberal arts teachers, and wet-nurses. In Roman civil law, the power of settling litigation originally belonged to a *judex privatus* (private judge). The extra ordinem procedure (also called *extraordinaria cognitio*) empowered public officers to settle particular disputes. Gradually the extraordinaria cognitio became the mainstream procedure in civil cases; during the Roman Empire, it was the only civil procedure. On this issue, see Bozzoni, *I medici e il diritto romano,* 200 ff.

55. Digest 50, 13: "Medicos fortassis quis accipiet etiam eos, qui alicuius partis corporis vel certi dolori sanitatem pollicentur: ut puta si auricularius, si fistulae vel dentium. Non tamen si incantavit, si imprecatus est, si, ut volgari verbo impostorum utar, si exorcizavit: non sunt ista medicinae genera, tametsi sint, qui hos sibi profuisse cum praedicatione adfirment."

56. A thorough examination of Roman sources in this respect is beyond the scope of the present study. As far as I know, the documentation on physicians in the papyri from Roman Egypt does not refer to agreements between patients and healers; see O. Nanetti, "Ricerche sui medici e la medicina nei papiri," pt. 1, *Aegyptus* 21 (1941): 301–14; O. Montevecchi, *I contratti di lavoro e di servizio nell'Egitto greco-romano e bizantino* (Milan, 1950); and I. Andorlini Marcone, "L'apporto dei papiri alla

conoscenza della scienza medica antica," in *Aufstieg und Niedergang der Römischen Welt,* ed. W. Haase (Berlin, 1993). However, ancient literary sources clearly present doctors and patients bargaining before treatment. Aelian mentions the case of a young girl named Aspasia, who had a tumor on her face: "Her father showed her to a physician, who declared he would undertake to cure her upon receiving three coins *[stateres].* The man said he did not have money; at which the doctor replied he also did not have a lot of medications" ("Pater igitur eam medico ostendit; qui se curaturum recepit, si tres acciperet stateres. At ille non habere se dixit: tum vero medicus, neque sibi medicamenti copiam esse, aiebat") (*Variae Historiae,* lib. 12, 1, ed. R. Herchner [Paris, 1858], 383). In another example, Plautus (*Menaechmi,* act 5, scene 4) makes fun of a physician who promised to cure a patient without having examined him:

> Physician: What did you say was the nature of the illness? Tell, old man . . .
> Old man: That's why I have brought you here: so that you can tell me and cure him.
> Physician: It is not difficult. I will cure him, I promise you.

57. F. Kudlien, "Die Unschätzbarkeit ärztlicher Leistung und das Honorarproblem," *Medizinhistorisches Journal* 14, nos. 1–2 (1979): 7 ff. Kudlien ("Die Unschätzbarkeit," 10) shows that the relationship between healer and patient, in the *Parangeliai* as well as in other ancient sources, was often described with the legal terms usually applied to contracts.

The way in which Galen presents his own handling of fees seems clearly to be influenced by the medical ethics that disapproved of bargaining before treatment. Consider, for instance, the case of Boëthius's wife, told by Galen in *De praenotione ad Posthumum.* Instead of negotiating his fee with the patient's husband before undertaking the cure, Galen asked his permission to administer the medications he believed necessary, for a period of ten days, and for ten more days should she show improvement. "By the fifteenth day of treatment, when every symptom of illness seemed to have disappeared thanks to the medications, Boëthius saw that he had received from me more than I had promised and asked me to complete the cure. . . . And once the woman recovered her health he sent me four hundred gold coins" (*Opera,* ed. C. G. Kühn [Leipzig, 1823], 14:646–47). The conscientious, well-educated physician, in whose image Galen wanted to portray himself, gives more than he has promised and does not request any payment other than what the patient gives him at the end of treatment out of gratitude.

58. See also Niederhellmann (*Arzt und Heilkunde,* 68): "The custom of the agreement between patient and healer probably goes back to Roman law, which allowed the physician to request payment for services rendered, only when a contract had been signed beforehand."

59. See Bozzoni, *I medici e il diritto romano,* 210; Amundsen, "Visigothic Medical Legislation," 557; and, for a more general approach, F. Kudlien, *Die Stellung des Arztes in der Römischen Gesellschaft* (Stuttgart, 1986).

As for the attitude toward women practicing medicine in ancient Rome, it is interesting to note that the law "De variis et extraordinariis cognitionibus" explicitly placed midwives on the same footing as physicians. In the early modern age, this offended many learned men, both physicians and jurists. See, for instance, the argument of a jurist, Francesco Ripa (*De peste* [Lyons, 1564], 28r): "Durantis says that a physician does not have more authority than a midwife, according to the law 'De variis et extraordinariis congnitionibus.' . . . But I could never believe this; and I think that the law can be sensibly interpreted as referring not to physicians but to slave healers who know how to treat only one type of disease, such as those of the ear, the teeth and such like. . . . God forbid that physicians, who know the causes of all illnesses and how to treat them, be put on the same footing as midwives" ("Dicit Speculator medicum non esse maioris authoritatis, quam sit obstetrix, per textum in lege 'De variis et extraordinariis cognitionibus.' . . . Sed nunquam istud crederem, unde puto quod textus ille sane sit intelligendus, videlicet quod loquatur de medico servo, qui unam morbi speciem tantum novit curare, ut sunt auricularii, dentarii et similes . . . sed physici, qui novunt omnium egritudinum causas et remedia: absit, quod eos pares esse obstetricibus dicamus"). "Speculator" was the renowned jurist Gulielmus Durantis (d. 1295), who had in fact argued for the equal status of physicians and midwives, on the basis of the text of the law "De variis et extraordinariis cognitionibus." See Durandus, *Speculum Judiciale*, 201v.

60. Nutton, "Archiatri," 213.

61. Digest, 50, 9: "De decretis ab ordine faciendis" (*Ulpianus libro tertio opinionum* [3d century A.D.]).

62. Garrison, *Introduction to the History of Medicine,* 146; Neuburger, *History of Medicine* 2:10–11; Laín Entralgo, *Doctor and Patient,* 61, 77 ff.

For a more balanced view see Amundsen, "Visigothic Medical Legislation," 553–69. I was not able to read J. L. Cassani, "La medicina romana en España y su enseñanza," *Cuadernos de Historia de España* 12 (1949): 51–69; or A. Ruiz Moreno, *La medicina en la legislación medioeval española* (Buenos Aires, 1946).

63. For instance, Bartolo (*In secundam Digesti novi partem* [Venice, 1570], 239r), when glossing the law "De decretis ab ordine faciendis" (Digest, 50, 9, 1) noted the discrepancy between ancient and modern customs in this respect. Bartolo observed that in Alessandria, for instance, the bishop had the right to license physicians ("est speciale in civitate Alexandrina, in qua electio medicorum permittitur episcopo").

64. M. A. Jaspan, "The Social Organization of Indigenous and Modern Medical Practices in Southwest Sumatra," in *Asian Medical Systems,* ed. C. Leslie (Berkeley, 1967), 233. Early modern European travelers in foreign countries noticed the practice of paying only upon recovery. See, for instance, P. Belon, *Les Observations des plusieurs singularitez et choses memorables trouveés en Grece, Asie, Indée, Egypte, Arabie, et autres pays estranges* (Anvers, 1555), 265a: "Les medecins, lors q'ils sont appelez à voir un malade en ce pays là, eux mesmes font diligence de faire recouvrer les drogues: car ils marchandent aux malades, et selon la maladie ils entreprennent de les guerir; et ne

leur sera livré tout l'argent que premierement ils ne soyent gueriz." See also the travel notes of Leonard Rauwolf, a physician from Augsburg whose "Itinerary into the Eastern Countries" was published in English in *A Collection of Curious Travels and Voyages,* ed. N. Staphorst and J. Ray (London, 1963), 218: "The physicians generally in those parts agree before hand for the cure with their patients, for a certainty, according to the condition of the patient, and his distemper, and leave security for their money, but yet it is not paid to them before the patient is cured."

65. A.S.B., Coll. Med., b. 342, *contra Antonium Mondini.*

66. Ibid. Later, Pecoroni withdrew the charge, but Mondini was fined fifty lire (the fine was reduced to twenty after a plea from his wife) and had to swear upon oath that he would never practice medicine again. For the sentence, see A.S.B., Coll. Med., b. 321, April 23, 1699.

67. See the sources cited in n. 23, above.

68. According to the statutes of Venetian physicians (1258), new members joining the guild had to take the oath that they would never intentionally prolong any infirmity (the same was requested from apothecaries). See Monticolo, *Capitolari* 1:147, 161.

69. This hiring contract is extensively quoted in L. Guerra-Coppioli, "Capitolati medici dei tempi andati," *Rivista di storia critica delle scienze mediche e naturali* 1 (1910–12): 133–34.

70. The medieval glossators and postglossators based their opinions on the law "Archiatri," which allowed public physicians to accept only gifts from their patients. For example, Bartolo da Sassoferrato, *In tres codicis libros* (Venice, 1570), ad X lib. Cod., r. "De professoribus et medicis," lex 9 (*Opera* vol. 8–9, 24r): "Medici qui salarium consequuntur ex publico . . . salarium ab infirmis non debent recipere nisi cum sanati fuerint." The topic was also discussed by J. Maynus [G. del Maino], *In primam Digesti veteris partem commentarii* (Lyons, 1569), 56r: "Physicians should not receive payment except when the infirm is healed" ("Medici non debent habere salarium nisi quando est sanatus infirmus").

This opinion was shared by canon law experts such as Durandus, *Speculum Judiciale,* rubr. "de salariis medicorum," 201v; I. Andreae, *In primum Decretalium librum Novella Commentaria* (Venice, 1581), chap. "Ad aures," p. 165a: "The physician may licitly receive a salary from a healthy man, but not from a sick one" ("Medicus a sano salarium recipit, ubi non liceret ab infirmo"). See also F. Ripa, *Tractatus de peste* (Lyons, 1564), 28v; H. Praevidellius, "De peste eiusque privilegiis," in *Tractatus . . . de variis verbis juris* (Venice, 1584), 18:171v; and Benincasa, "De paupertate ac eius privilegiis," 160v: "Physicians should not exact a salary from the sick unless their work is finished" ("Medici non debent ab infirmis salarium exigere nisi in fine operis").

In the sixteenth century this was again presented as *communis opinio* by many jurists: F. Vivius [F. Vivio], *Communes opiniones doctorum utriusque censurae* (Venice, 1566), lib. 2, opinio 176; E. Soarez, *Thesaurus receptarum sententiarum, quas vulgus interpretum communes opiniones vocat* (Venice, 1569), 164v: "The physician . . . should not demand any reward before health is restored to the sick" ("Medicus . . . nec ante praemium ullum exigeat quam sanitas infirmo restituatur"); Bertachini, *Repertorium iuris,* 333v: "A salary is not owed to the doctor except when the sick [person] is healed" ("Medico non debetur salarium nisi demum sanato aegroto"); H. Cagnolus [G. Cagnolo], *In Constitutiones et Leges Primi, Secundi, Quinti ac Duodecimi Pandectarum . . . aureae enarrationes* (Venice, 1586), lib. 1, p. 148: "It is certain that doctors' fees ought to be paid at the end, and not at the beginning of treatment, according to the text of the *jus commune* in the law 'Archiatri'" ("In medicis certum est solutio salari fieri debet in fine non in primis secundum dispositionem iuris communis L. Archiatri").

71. Speckham, *Questionum,* quaestio 26, fols. 71v–72v.

72. Ripa, *De peste,* 28v.

73. Mondeville, *Chirurgie,* in Tabanelli, *Un secolo d'oro* 1:219. In his *Chirurgie,* Mondeville vividly described the difficulties encountered by surgeons in trying to make a living from their trade (see 111 ff, 214–15, 196–201). The fourteenth-century English surgeon John Arderne also noted, "If the leech will favour to any man's asking, make he covenant with him for his travail and take it before hand" (J. Arderne, *Treatises of fistula in ano, haemorrhoids, and clysters,* ed. D'Arcy Power [London, 1910], 6).

Master Francesco da Parma, *medico delle teste* (doctor of heads) hired by the municipality of Bologna in 1465, experienced similar problems. In 1470, he wrote to the papal legate, complaining that "in his trade, it was common — after healing wounds and restoring the sick to health — to be cheated out of the fee deserved for one's hard labor, services, and industry, and even for the cost of medicines used." He requested that a way be found to make patients pay the sums agreed upon before the cure ("pro quod ei conceditur modus quidam, quo quotare possit mercedem conventam inter ipsum, et illos quibus medetur"). The cardinal legate responded by charging two civic magistrates, the Anziani and the Vessillifero di giustizia, with the authority to settle the disputes between Master Francesco and his defaulting clients (L. Muenster, "Maestro Francesco da Parma, *medico delle teste* nel servizio del Comune di Bologna [1465–1485]," *Lo Smeraldo,* no. 4 [1950]). The cardinal's response to Master Francesco's plea is reported by Stefanutti, "Sulla liceità giuridica," 369–70.

74. On doctors requesting a lien *(pignus)* before undertaking a cure, see Naso, *Medici e strutture sanitarie,* 199 ff. Roffredus Beneventanus (*Libelli Juris Civilis,* C.G.J.C., no. 2 [reprint, Turin, 1968], p. 236, col. 1) advised physicians and lawyers to request payment at the beginning of treatment, or alternatively, "to ask at least for a lien or deposit, since it is better to keep the deposit than to sue somebody." He also mentioned the medical aphorism *Dum dolet accipe* (Take while the patient is in pain). On the same topic, Durandus (*Speculum Judiciale,* 201v) had also remarked that it was safer "pignori incumbere quam personam agere" (to hold on to the lien rather than to file a suit).

75. "Dum dolet infirmus medicus sit pignore firmus." On this aphorism, see Durandus, *Speculum Judiciale,* 201v; Speckham, *Quaestionum,* 72v.

76. C. Malagola, *Statuti delle Università e dei Collegi dello Studio bolognese* (Bologna, 1888), 485–86. This norm (the only one concerning professional medical practice) returns in abbreviated form also in the statutes of 1507, rubr. 8 (A.S.B., Coll. Med., b. 216).

77. For instance, the statutes of the College of Physicians of Mantua (1559) established that one gold *scudo* per week was due to the physician who visited his patient twice a day; one gold scudo per day (computing also travel time) was due to the physician who visited a patient outside the city, at a distance of more than three thousand feet from the city walls. The text of the statutes is published with an Italian translation — often faulty, unfortunately — in G. Carra and A. Zanca, "Gli statuti del Collegio dei medici di Mantova del 1559," in *Atti e memorie dell'Accademia Virgiliana di Mantova* (Mantua, 1977), 13–31; the text cited here can be found on 30–31.

In 1600, the Medical Faculty in Vienna protested against the imposition of medical fees by the city authorities but was willing to accept fee regulation to solve disputes related to agreements for a cure. In such cases, the faculty argued, the fee should be due even when the patient died, "because health is in the hands of God" (Fischer, *Ärztliche Standespflichten*, 118).

78. Benedetti, "De medici atque aegri officio," 546.

79. L. Settala, *Animadversionum et Cautionum Medicarum libri septem* (Padua, 1628), lib. 1, chap. 21, pp. 7–8. Cf. also Ripa, *De peste*, 27v: "the doctor is not permitted to bargain over payment with the sick while the illness looms" ("non licet medico pendente infirmitate pacisci cum infirmo super salario"); and Rodericus à Castro [E. Rodrigues de Castro], *Medicus-Politicus, sive de officiis medico-politicis Tractatus* (Hamburg, 1614), 131–35.

80. Zacchia, *Quaestiones medico-legales*, 465–66: "relinquendum ergo mechanicis est, ut de mercede paciscantur"; "eorum enim opera sunt servilia."

81. Among those who argued that the agreement for a cure was incompatible with the Hippocratic oath are, for instance, Vincenzo Carrari [V. Carrarius], the author of a sixteenth-century treatise on medical ethics, and the great French jurist Jacques Cujas. See V. Carrarius, *De medico et illius erga aegros officio* (Ravenna, 1581), 33; and Jacques Cujas, *Ad tres postremos Codicis Iustiniani libros commentarii*, in *Opera omnia* (Paris, 1658), t. 2, col. 126 ("quae pactio nec iure valet nec iuriiiurando Hippocratis congruit"). However, the incompatibility is not supported by any Hippocratic texts, as Zacchia pointed out (*Quaestiones medico-legales*, 465). On the Hippocratic oath, see L. Edelstein, *The Hippocratic Oath* (Baltimore, 1944).

82. See, for example, the 1559 statutes of the Medical College of Mantua, rubr. 22 (Carra and Zanca, "Gli Statuti del Collegio dei Medici di Mantova," 30). This prohibition was also widespread outside of Italy. For instance, in Cambrai "surgeons were not permitted to make contracts for a cure with the sick" (H. Coulon, *La communauté des chirurgiens-barbiers de Cambrai, 1366–1795* [Cambrai, 1908], 194). Also, the statutes of the Medical College of Bordeaux (1542) forbade members to sign agreements for a cure (Verdier, *Jurisprudence*, 504). A Prussian ordinance of 1693 that es-

tablished fees for various medical and surgical procedures condemned the behavior of physicians who negotiated with the sick; it said that they were "lowering themselves to the level of quacks" ("einige Medici unanständlich derer Marckschreyer und anderer Empyricorum Weise gebrauchen mit den Patienten marchandiren"; quoted in M. Stürzbecher, *Beiträge zur Berliner Medizingeschichte* [Berlin, 1966], 46).

83. See Sarti and Fattorini, *De claris Archigymnasii Professoribus* 1:553, for an agreement signed by Guglielmo da Saliceto, and 569 n. 4, for one signed by Bartolomeo da Varignana (on October 11, 1283, the physician received from Aldovrandino, the marquis d'Este, 390 bolognese lire "that the said Aldovrandino owed Master Bartolomeo as fee for medical services, as per the legal instrument drawn by notary Zani Grassi"). As for Taddeo Alderotti, we are told that "he did not undertake to treat anyone except after negotiating a very high fee, which was not matching the great distance or the difficulty of the cure, but his own dignity and the wealth of those whom he was called to cure. And it was not enough to promise payment; for he wanted security for himself when going and returning, taking a large sum of money as insurance against the dangers of the journey" ("non sivisse alio se abduci ad curandum quemquam nisi pacta ingenti mercede, quae non tam esset pro loci distantia aut difficultate curationis, quam pro sui dignitate et facultatibus eorum, ad quos curandos vocaretur. Neque sat erat de mercede pacisci; nam sibi quoque cautum volebat de itu et reditu, accepta ingentis pecuniae sponsione pro securitate itineris") (Sarti and Fattorini, *De claris Archigymnasii Professoribus* 1:556); for the text of some agreements in which Taddeo requested exorbitant fees, see 2:221–22). On Taddeo Alderotti, see Nancy Siraisi, *Taddeo Alderotti and His Pupils: Two Generations of Italian Medical Learning* (Princeton, N.J., 1981).

84. This can be assumed from physicians' claims for payment in court, which usually covered long periods of time, often referring specifically to this kind of arrangement. For example, in 1588 the physician Giovanni Bernardi explained to the Protomedicato how, "I having treated Francesco del Medico many times in the past, we finally settled that he should give me one *castillata* of grapes per year, as my yearly salary for treating himself and his family" (A.S.B., Coll. Med., b. 197, case of Bernardi vs. Del Medico estate). A "castillata" was equivalent to 1,785.931 liters (A. Martini, *Manuale di metrologia* [Turin, 1883], 92).

This type of agreement—involving a yearly stipend for medical services—was also widespread in the seventeenth and eighteenth century: see A.S.B., Coll. Med.—b. 341, case of Gotti vs. Sgargi (1684); b. 352, case of Coltellini vs. Panzacchia (1703); b. 349, case of Del Buono vs. Bertuccini (1746). In Renaissance Florence, confraternities, convents, hospitals, and so on customarily hired a doctor as a provider of medical service for their members; see Park, *Doctors and Medicine,* 99–109, 141. For physicians kept on retainer in medieval Aragon, see McVaugh, *Medicine before the Plague,* 174–75; for similar arrangements in medieval Provence, see Shatzmiller, *Jews, Medicine, and Medieval Society,* 124–25.

85. The statutes of the Medical College of Mantua prohibited physicians from

making agreements with individual patients but allowed such agreements when made with groups and institutions: "We allow [physicians] to enter into agreements with communities such as convents or nunneries, hospitals, magistrates and their dependents, our court, heads of families, for the purpose of treating that community or family. If a member of the college makes an agreement with somebody else, he will be fined a gold scudo plus the amount he earned from the agreement" (Carra and Zanca, "Gli Statuti del Collegio dei Medici di Mantova," 31).

Zacchia (*Quaestiones medico-legales,* 467), who disapproved of cure agreements as beneath the dignity of the medical profession, argued that it was perfectly legitimate for a physician to negotiate a contract enabling him to serve as a town doctor. Several members of the College of Medicine of Bologna served as town doctors in other municipalities, even after joining the college. They include Pompeo Bolognetti, a collegiate admitted in 1651, the son of a noble family, who was town doctor in Budrio and Sarzana (G. Fantuzzi, *Notizie degli scrittori bolognesi* [Bologna, 1786–90], 2:253–54); Alessandro Recordati, admitted in 1603, who was town doctor in Rocca Bianca (A.S.B., Coll. Med., b. 196); and Giovanni Albani, who joined the college in 1622 and became the town doctor of Cento in 1632 (Fantuzzi, *Notizie* 1:91). There were many more cases, indicating that indeed even the medical elite did not spurn such hiring agreements as beneath their exalted station.

86. On the issue of the continuity (or discontinuity) between medieval town physicians and the public physicians of the ancient world, see V. Nutton, ":Continuity or Rediscovery? The City Physician in Classical Antiquity and Medieval Italy," in *The Town and State Physician in Europe from the Middle Ages to the Enlightenment,* ed. A. W. Russell (Wolfenbüttel, 1981), 9–46; on the diffusion of town doctors in Italian municipalities, see 24–34. In 1324, the city of Venice employed eleven physicians and seventeen surgeons (Monticolo, *Capitolari* 1:354). On the importance of town physicians, see also Park, *Doctors and Medicine,* 90–91.

R. Palmer ("Physicians and the State in Post-Medieval Italy," in Russell, *Town and State Physician,* 47–61) maintains that the institution of town doctors disappeared from large Italian cities in the sixteenth century. I find this thesis rather questionable: even if the city itself no longer employed town doctors, smaller groups such as parishes, confraternities, and so on still hired physicians for their members. This was certainly the case in Bologna in the sixteenth and seventeenth centuries (see chap. 4, below, pp. 106–7).

87. A photograph of this document (from the Archivio di Stato di Siena) is printed in A. Garosi, *Siena nella storia della medicina* (Florence, 1958), tav. 1. Barbers also seem to have been hired on a retainer system, usually on a yearly basis. The Modenese statutes of the fourteenth century include a petition by the city barbers who asked to be allowed to "habere aliquos homines affitatos, quos radere debeant, ad annum vel aliter pro certa quantitate pecunie vel blaudi" (*Corpus statutorum italicorum, Respublica mutinensis 1306–7,* ed. E. P. Vicini [Milan, 1952], 2:214).

The custom of retaining a private physician seems to be very ancient. It existed in the Roman world (see Nutton, "Archiatri," 209 n. 127). Evidence of this practice has been found also for medieval England, as indicated by J. B. Post, "Doctor versus Patient: Two Fourteenth-Century Lawsuits," *Medical History* 16 (1972): 296–300. Post presents cases in which patients sued their physicians for neglecting to respond to summons. For similar cases, see E. A. Hammond, "Incomes of Medieval English Doctors," *Journal of the History of Medicine and Allied Sciences* 15, no. 2 (1960): 159 ff.

88. Rawcliffe ("Profits of Practice," 62–64) indicates that English doctors in the late Middle Ages typically had two sources of income: a yearly, fixed salary from working on retainer with families, guilds, convents, or townships; and a fluctuating income from treating individual patients.

89. Sarti and Fattorini, *De claris Archigymnasii professoribus* 2:214.

90. Guerra-Coppioli, "Capitolati medici," 135. Another case: Master Giacomo da Pistoia, doctor of medicine, was hired as town doctor by the municipality of Prato. He received a fixed annual salary with the agreement that he could not request more than two *grossi* per day from his patients. See M. Socinus [M. Socini], *Consilia, seu potius responsa* (Venice, 1579), vol. 2, consilium 196, fols. 56r, 56v; the jurist's *consilium* concerned a dispute between the doctor and the municipality.

91. B.A.R., MS. 2208, "Diario del medico Giuseppe Giuli." Also, the celebrated physician Francesco Redi carefully recorded all the gifts from his patients in his "Libro di ricordi" (Del Guerra, "Gli onorari dei medici," 388).

92. The contract signed on November 21, 1590, by Gianbattista Fabi, a physician from Bologna, and the village of Argenta expressly established that the physician "cannot spend the night out of the jurisdiction without specific authorization of the *Consoli*" (A.S.B., Coll. Med., b. 199). The residency requirement was typical of the *patti di condotta*: see Naso, *Medici e strutture sanitarie,* 37, 40, for cases in which the physician could leave the place only with the patient's authorization ("licencia egrotantium" or "licentia ipsius infirmi"). For the same clause, see also the patto di condotta reported by M. Abbate, "I medici obbligati di Carmagnola, 1591–1691," in *Studi in memoria di Luigi Dal Pane* (Bologna, 1982), 393; and Guerra-Coppioli, "Capitolati medici," 135–36.

93. For example, A.S.B., Coll. Med., b. 352, case of Puppini vs. Cremonini, 1709.

94. Molière, *Monsieur de Pourceaugnac* (1669), act 1, scene 5.

95. M. Bloch, *The Royal Touch* (London, 1973), 158–59, 166–67.

96. A.S.B., Assunteria di Studio, Diversorum, b. 100, n. 10.

97. A.S.B., Coll. Med.— b. 341, the patients' testimonials; b. 320, license issued to Nannini on July 7, 1689. There were ten testimonials, of which three were signed with a cross.

The protomedici often questioned the validity of such testimonials. In the case of Francesco Nannini, the dean of the college conscientiously wrote in the "Liber secretus" (the college's diary): "Francesco Nannini, who treats scrofula, came to me, requesting to be allowed to continue to practice; and since reliable surgeons told me that the man, although ignorant, is nevertheless able to treat scrofula effectively with some kind of powder applied topically, I turned a blind eye and let him continue" (A.S.B., Coll. Med., b. 221, "Liber secretus, 1661–1693").

The issuing of licenses to charlatans on the basis of testimonials from their patients was a widespread practice throughout Europe. See G. Albi Romero, *El Protomedicato en la España ilustrada, Catálogo de Documentos del Archivio General de Simancas* (Valladolid, 1982), 93; M. Pelling, "Tradition and Diversity: Medical Practice in Norwich, 1550–1640," in *Scienze, credenze occulte e livelli di cultura* (Florence, 1982), 167, 170; Monticolo, *Capitolari* 1:322–26, 328–29, 332, 339, 368, 371.

98. A.S.B., Coll. Med., b. 340.

99. C. Saccardino, *Libro nomato la verità di diverse cose, quale minutamente tratta di molte salutifere operationi spagiriche, et chimiche* (Bologna, 1621); H. Cardanus [G. Cardano], *De vita propria* (Paris, 1643), chap. 40, pp. 188 ff.

100. E. Leclair, *Histoire de la chirurgie à Lille,* vol. 1, *Documents* (Lille, 1911), 77, 89, 92–93, 98–100; for other licenses issued in 1736, 1739, and 1751 because of patients' testimonials, see ibid., 151–52, 157, and 198–99, respectively.

101. Tension between the city authorities and the medical college over the granting of medical licenses also occurred in Bologna; see chap. 1, p. 11.

102. Leclair, *Histoire de la chirurgie* 1:98–99. The surgeons appealed to the Parliament of Tournai against the ruling. However, the parliament upheld the decision on the ground that the town's magistrates had full authority over medical licensing, which was a "matière de police" (100). One century earlier, in 1577, a similar dispute between an unlicensed healer, named Hureau, and the guild of physicians and apothecaries of Orléans ended with a decision in favor of the physicians and against the healer. The jurist representing the physicians' association, Anné Robert, left a noteworthy summary of the arguments of the lawyers of both parties (A. Robertus, *Rerum Judicatarum libri 4* [Geneva, 1604], bk. 1, chap. 5, "De empiricis qui conceptis precum et verborum formulis morbos curare profitentur," pp. 51–81). Robert's text is significant because it provides an example of how early modern jurists interpreted Roman law on the issue of the regulation of medical practice. It is clear that the defense lawyer was perfectly aware—just as historians are today—that the concept of professional licensing did not exist in Roman culture and that, according to Roman law, people could choose whomever they wished as a physician, without having to make sure that he had been licensed by a college: "Iurisconsultus medicorum constituendorum arbitrium non Praesidi provinciae, sed popularibus cuiusque civitatis concedi dixit" (see the law "De decretis ab ordine faciendis," cited in n. 61, above). "Quod si unicuique nostrum libere licet eos eligere, quorum ministerio et industria vestiri, exhiberi aut nutriri velimus: quid erit iniquius quam si cogar uti eo medico, qui mihi sit ingratus, si modo collegio et ordini sese utcumque probaverit" (55). In other words, just as the laws let us choose where to buy our clothes and food, so they let us choose our physician; and what would be more unjust than forcing somebody

to select a physician whom he doesn't like, just because that physician has been approved by the professional association?

The physicians' lawyer objected to this freedom of choice: "Indeed, the patient should not be allowed to choose indiscriminately whomever he wants to treat his illness" ("Neque vero aegrotis permittendum est quem voluerint medicum, indiscreta voluntate ad morbi curationem advocare") (69). All of this obviously relates to the issue of the two sources of legitimization for medical practice: the medical authorities and the patients themselves.

103. A.S.B., Coll. Med., b. 197. A similar case is described by Monticolo (*Capitolari* 1:369): in 1330, the Major Council of Venice allowed a physician, although he did not have the guild's license, to keep treating a patient who had expressed trust *(devocionem)* in him. Throughout the early modern age, patients pleaded with the medical authorities to allow practice by unlicensed healers. For example, in the late eighteenth century Alfonso Galli, Angiola Quinta, and Annunziata Befassi sent an appeal to the Magistratura di Sanità in Milan, requesting that a certain friar be allowed to treat their children (A.S.M., Sanità, parte antica, b. 243–44).

104. A.S.B., Coll. Med., b. 197.

105. A.S.B., Coll. Med., b. 233. This is the only printed verdict that I found in the college's records.

106. The cases heard by the college around 1570 were often deferred to the college by another court or magistracy. Ulisse Aldrovandi, a protomedico in those years, described some of these cases in a manuscript on the Protomedicato's jurisdiction: "We handed down a sentence against a weaver, who had treated a woman for breast cancer. We sentenced him to return all the money within ten days, and we admonished him not to practice medicine in the future, or he would have to pay fifty gold scudi for each violation. This case was assigned to us by the Prolegate" (B.U.B., Manoscritti di Ulisse Aldrovandi, MS. 21, vol. 3, c. 106).

107. This should be compared, for instance, with the situation in Norwich, where at the end of the sixteenth century the officers of the company of barber-surgeons were only allowed to testify as experts on disputes over payment, while the municipal courts kept the power of sentencing (Pelling and Webster, "Medical Practitioners," 214). This seems also to have been the case in northern Italian cities in the late Middle Ages. "In some cases, the statutes of the medical colleges requested the intervention of public officers to enforce statutory rules. The intervention of the municipal authority *[podestà]* was necessary, for instance, to make sure that delinquent patients paid their debts to their physicians" (Naso, *Medici e strutture sanitarie,* 220).

On the fact that an ordinary judge, rather than the medical college, would usually hear cases concerning medical fees, see also Pesenti Marangon, *"Professores chirurgie,"* 19, which reports the following episode: in 1435, Giovanni da Monteforte, a "physician-surgeon" *(medico ciroico)* from Verona, spent five days in Venice to treat Antonio "de Trecio" of Noventa; since the patient was unwilling to pay, the healer's fee was decided by a judge of the neighboring municipality of Padua.

108. "Attento maxime, sanatus est mediante eius opera et industria." A.S.B., Coll. Med., b. 197, Ulisse Parmi vs. Domenico Barilli.

109. Blaming the patient's negligent behavior for the failure of treatment seems to have been a typical reaction of healers. For instance, in 1433, in the case of Mathew Rillesford, surgeon of York, vs. Richard Ayreton, a clergyman of York, "Richard complained that Mathew in applying his cure *[in apponendo curam suam]* was so negligent that Richard's whole body became infected, and Mathew, on the other hand, alleged that Richard used to take unwholesome food which had been forbidden by him and hindered the actions of the medicines enjoined for his cure and emptied them out" (*Notes on Religious and Secular Houses of Yorkshire,* Record Series of the Yorkshire Archaeological Society, vol. 17 [York, 1895], 1:78). I thank Karen Reeds for referring me to this document.

110. A.S.B., Coll. Med., b. 197.

Chapter 3: The Medical System as Seen by the Doctors

1. *Liber pro recta administratione Protomedicatus* (Bologna, 1666), 23. For legal proceedings against charlatans accused of wearing medical garb, see A.S.B., Coll. Med.—b. 318, June 24, 1607; b. 319, May 27, 1659.

On doctors' clothing in Renaissance iconography, see A. Corsini, *Il costume del medico nelle pitture fiorentine del Rinascimento* (Florence, 1912). On doctors' clothing in Bologna, see M. L. David-Danel, *Iconographie des saints médecins Côme et Damien* (Lille, 1958), 182–85.

2. Data collected in 1606 (A.S.B., Coll. Med., b. 318).

3. A.S.B., Coll. Med., bb. 197, 350.

4. A.S.B., Coll. Med., b. 320.

5. A.S.B., Coll. Med., b. 319.

6. The numbers of doctors, apothecaries, and barber-surgeons in 1630 are taken from the lists of practitioners working in the plague hospitals; see P. Moratti, *Racconto de gli ordini e Provisioni fatte ne' lazaretti in Bologna e suo contado in tempo di contagio* (Bologna, 1631), 74–78. For the case of Norwich, see M. Pelling, "Tradition and Diversity: Medical Practice in Norwich, 1550–1640," in *Scienze, credenze occulte e livelli di cultura* (Florence, 1982), 163–65.

7. The number of healers per thousand residents was 6.74 in 1727, 7.30 in 1744, and 6.98 in 1772 (based on data in table 5).

8. The number of healers per thousand residents becomes 1.7 in 1727, 1.8 in 1744, and 1.8 in 1772, when calculated over the population of the diocese, thus including the Bolognese countryside (for the population of the diocese, see Bellettini, *La popolazione di Bologna,* table 1, pp. 25–28).

9. On the basis of the records of a 1630 survey conducted by the Ufficio di Sanità of Florence, Cipolla has calculated "a ratio of at least one university-trained

physician and more than one surgeon for every 10,000 people" in the territory of the Granducato of Tuscany; see C. M. Cipolla, *Public Health and the Medical Profession in the Renaissance* (Cambridge, 1976), 69, 81. However, a study of the countryside of Pisa in 1671 found that the number of medical practitioners was three times as high as the one indicated by Cipolla (D. Pesciatini, "Maestri, medici, cerusici, nelle comunità rurali pisane nel XVII secolo," in *Scienze, credenze occulte e livelli di cultura* [Florence, 1982], 130).

10. On the hospitals of Bologna, see *Sette secoli di storia ospedaliera a Bologna* (Bologna, 1961). The presence of "parish physicians" is often mentioned by patients testifying in the Protomedicato. For example, see A.S.B., Coll. Med., b. 338, deposition of Anna Caterina Masini, December 5, 1663, parish of San Biagio. In 1570, a decree by Cardinal Paleotti mandated that each parish should have a physician for the care of the poor (b. 233). The presence of parish physicians during the plague of 1630 is also documented (Moratti, *Racconto,* 14 ff).

As for confraternities, the physicians employed by the Ospedale della Vita, which was managed by a congregation of the same name, were requested to treat the members of the confraternity and the hospital employees, in addition to the regular inmates of the hospital (B.U.B., MS. 184, "Dell'elettione, e qualità de' medici e loro ufficio nell'Ospedale della Vita"). In Rome, the confraternity of Santissimo Sagramento regularly employed a physician to treat the sick residents of the Vatican parish; see G. Moroni, *Dizionario d'erudizione storico-ecclesiastica* (Venice, 1847), 43:117–18.

11. The epitaph is mentioned by M. Sarti and T. Fattorini (*De claris Archigymnasii Bononiensis professoribus* [Bologna, 1769–72], 1:526), who took it from G. N. Alidosi (*Instruttione delle cose notabili della città di Bologna* [Bologna, 1621]). The inscription no longer existed in the eighteenth century, when Sarti and Fattorini wrote.

12. On the "medicalization" of the Sant'Orsola Hospital in Bologna during the eighteenth century, see F. Giusberti, "Tra povertà e malattia: Il S. Orsola a Bologna dal XVII al XVIII secolo," *Annali della Fondazione Luigi Einaudi* 13 (1979). On a miracle at the Ospedale della Vita, see B.U.B., MS. 207 B, b. 8, "Ristretto informante circa il preteso miracolo della restituzione della lingua ad Antonio Prandi per intercessione della Beata Vergine della Vita" (1710); and A.C.A.B., Miscellanea vecchia, cart. 32, fasc. I 182 134h.

13. On the importance of this classical tripartition in seventeenth-century medicine, see Giulio Cesare Claudini, *De ingressu ad infirmos* (Venice, 1628). This therapeutic manual, written by a Bolognese physician, was very popular in the seventeenth century and later. In the eighteenth century, the noted Giovanni Maria Lancisi, physician to the pope, carefully summarized it for his personal use (B.L.R., MS. 88, "Compendium Claudini de ingressu ad infirmos"). On Lancisi, see P. De Angelis, *Giovanni Maria Lancisi, la Biblioteca Lancisiana, l'Accademia Lancisiana* (Rome, 1965).

14. Claudini, *De ingressu ad infirmos,* 156–65.

15. "Nihil exhibeat per os." See A.S.B., Coll. Med., bb. 195, 197, for examples of licenses carrying this prohibition.

16. On the meaning of this distinction in surgical practice, see G. Pomata, "Barbieri e comari," in *Medicina, erbe e magia* (Milan, 1981), 174–75.

17. "Conventioni Frà l'Eccellentiss. Collegio de' Medici, & l'Honorabile Compagnia delli Speciali Medicinali di Bologna" (1606), in *Liber pro recta,* 32.

18. P. Zacchia, *Quaestiones medico-legales* (Lyons, 1662), lib. 6, tit. 1, quaest. 8, p. 467.

19. R. Bozzoni, *I medici e il diritto romano* (Naples, 1904), 23–24, 162. According to Celsus, a Roman medical author of the first century A.D., the tripartition of diet, drugs, and surgery was introduced after Hippocrates (A. C. Celsus, *De medicina, Proemium,* 9; cited by O. Temkin, "Introduction," in *Soranus' Gynecology* [Baltimore, 1956], xi). According to Soranus (second century A.D.) midwives should be trained in all the three branches of therapy (Temkin, *Soranus' Gynecology,* 6). For the idea that the division of surgery and medicine was present in the ancient world (with surgery seen as manual practice and medicine as a superior, scientific liberal art), see L. Löwenfeld, "Inästimabilität und Honorierung der artes liberales nach römischem Recht," in *Festschrift für Max Planck* (Munich, 1887).

20. On the use of the terms *medicus chirurgus* and *medicus barberius* in medieval sources from Bologna, see Sarti and Fattorini, *De claris Archigymnasii professoribus* 1:520–22. For the same in Venice and Padua, see T. Pesenti Marangon, "*Professores chirurgie, medici ciroici,* and *barbitonsores* a Padova nell'età di Leonardo Buffi da Bertipaglia," *Quaderni per la storia dell'Università di Padova* (1978): 1–38.

On the use of the term *medica* for women in Bologna, see Sarti and Fattorini, *De claris Archigymnasii professoribus* 1:522; for Venice, see G. Monticolo, *I capitolari delle arti veneziane* (Rome, 1896), 1:341; and for Florence, see K. Park, *Doctors and Medicine in Early Renaissance Florence* (Princeton, N.J., 1985), 71–72.

21. A.S.B., Coll. Med., b. 219, statutes of 1507, rubr. 32.

22. On the inability of the London medical college to establish and maintain its hegemony over lower practitioners, see M. Pelling and C. Webster, "Medical Practitioners," in *Health, Medicine, and Mortality in the Sixteenth Century,* ed. C. Webster (Cambridge, 1979), 168 ff; and, more generally, H. J. Cook, *The Decline of the Old Medical Regime in Stuart London* (Ithaca, N.Y., 1986).

23. E. Benveniste, "La doctrine médicale des indo-européens," *Revue de l'histoire des religions* 130 (1945): 5–12. See also J. Filliozat, *La doctrine classique de la médecine indienne* (Paris, 1949).

24. Bruce Lincoln, *Myth, Cosmos, and Society: Indo-European Themes of Creation and Destruction* (Cambridge, England, 1986), 100. Lincoln's argument is based on Hippocrates' Aphorism VII, 87: "Those diseases that medicines do not cure are cured by the knife. Those that the knife does not cure are cured by fire. Those that fire does not cure must be considered incurable" (*Hippocrates,* trans. W.H.S. Jones, Loeb Classical Library [Cambridge, Mass., 1967], 4:217). The superior remedy here is fire,

which substitutes for magic. Lincoln offers an interesting interpretation: "The substitution of fire for charms in the top position is an innovation that results from the Hippocratic campaign to rationalize medical practice, to rid it of 'magical' elements. In locating something to take the place of unacceptable 'spells,' the text has recourse to an item with priestly associations: fire, purifying agent and sacrificial medium, central to public and domestic cults" (100).

25. Benveniste has argued that in the Indo-European languages the root *med,* from which the term *medicus* derives, generally denoted the imposition of a proper order on something or someone, by an individual endowed with knowledge and authority ("La doctrine médical," 5–7).

26. *Liber pro recta,* 12 (decree issued in 1594). In contrast, trade partnerships between physicians and apothecaries were allowed in medieval Bologna; see Sarti and Fattorini, *De Claris Archigymnasii Bononiensis Professoribus* 1:438. For such partnerships in Florence, see Raffaele Ciasca, *L'Arte dei medici e degli speziali nella storia e nel commercio fiorentino dal XII al XV secolo* (Florence, 1927), 315.

27. A.S.B., Coll. Med., b. 219, statutes of 1507, rubr. 17.

28. A.S.B., Coll. Med., b. 261, "Responsio petitionis factae ab Academia parisiensi Collegio medicorum Bononiae circa usum approbationis chirurgorum."

29. C. Malagola, *Statuti delle Università e dei Collegi dello Studio bolognese* [Bologna, 1888], 516–17, statutes of 1410, rubr. 24. See also F. Cavazza, *Le scuole dell'antico studio bolognese* (Milan, 1896), 208. On the patron saints of the three professional groups and their days of celebration, see A. di P. Masini, *Bologna perlustrata* (Bologna, 1666), 466–67, 262–63.

30. A.S.B., Coll. Med., bb. 214, 319. However, the barbers' guild kept the prerogative of allowing the opening of new shops, thus creating for prospective barbers a double licensing system, involving both the guild and the college.

31. A.S.B., Coll. Med., b. 320.

32. See A.S.B., Coll. Med., b. 350, for petitions of barbers asking to be exempted from the Protomedicato's control. For the seizure of surgical instruments from unlicensed barber-surgeons, see b. 340.

33. See A.S.B., Capitano del Popolo, Società d'Arti, b. 4, for the statutes of 1320, which contain numerous rules regarding the medical tasks of barbers (for example, how to draw blood from different parts of the body). For the statutes of 1557, see A.S.B., Codici Miniati; B.U.B., MS. 3873, "Statuti antichi dell'Arte de Barbieri di Bologna approvati dall'eccelso Senato," 1557; T. Garzoni, *La piazza universale di tutte le professioni del mondo* (Venice, 1588), 825, 856–57.

34. A.S.B., Coll. Med., b. 214.

35. A.S.B., Coll. Med., b. 350.

36. A.S.B., Coll. Med., b. 214.

37. A.S.B., Coll. Med., b. 350. It was the same in York; see M. Barnet, "The Barber-Surgeons of York," *Medical History* 12 (1968): 24.

38. M. Douglas, *Purity and Danger* (London, 1966). Jacques Le Goff, in his es-

say on the medieval classification of trades and crafts ("Mestieri leciti e mestieri il-leciti nell'Occidente medioevale," in *Tempo della chiesa, tempo del mercante* [Turin, 1977], 55), talks about a "taboo of blood," which also involved "surgeons, barbers or apothecaries who practiced bloodletting."

39. Pomata, "Barbieri," 174.

40. A.S.B., Coll. Med., b. 261, "Responsio petitionis." This document has been published by G. A. Gentili, "Cerusici e chirurgia a metà del secolo XVIII in una lettera del Collegio dei medici di Bologna all'Accademia di medicina di Parigi," *Rivista di storia delle scienze mediche e naturali* 1 (January–April 1952). Gentili is wrong in stating that the company of barbers was a religious confraternity; in fact, the company was one of the city guilds.

On the Académie Royale de Chirurgie and the edict of 1743, see T. Gelfand, "From Guild to Profession: The Surgeons of France in the Eighteenth Century," *Texas Reports on Biology and Medicine* 32, no. 1 (spring 1974). The Académie Royale de Chirurgie became a model of professional organizations for surgeons all over Europe (Gelfand, "From Guild to Profession," 128). See also idem, *Professionalizing Modern Medicine: Paris Surgeons and Medical Science and Institutions in the Eighteenth Century* (Westport, Conn., 1980).

The organizational and professional success of the Parisian surgeons was probably due also to the relative weakness of the Medical Faculty, on which see C. Gillespie, *Science and Policy in France at the End of the Old Regime* (Princeton, N.J., 1980), 212–18.

41. On the reform of surgery in Bologna, see Pomata, "Barbieri," 179–81. For France, see Gelfand, *Professionalizing Modern Medicine;* for Prussia, see C. Huerkamp, "Ärzte und Professionalisierung in Deutschland," *Geschichte und Gesellschaft* 6, no. 3 (1980); for Austria, see C. Steiner, *Die Bader und Barbiere (Wundärzte) in Wien zur Zeit Maria Theresias, 1740–1780* (Vienna, 1975); for Spain, see A. Carreras Panchón, "Las actividades de los barberos durante los siglos XVI al XVIII," *Cuadernos de Historia de la Medicina Española* 13 (1974).

42. *Liber pro recta,* 5–8. For the manuscript Tassa issued by the guild of the apothecaries in 1555, see A.S.B., Coll. Med., b. 338. The first Tassa issued by the Protomedicato was printed in 1587: *Nuova Tassa e dichiaratione del prezzo delle cose medicinali* (Bologna, 1587) (b. 235). Such Tasse were printed at regular intervals throughout the seventeenth and eighteenth centuries: for instance, *Tassa de' medicinali* (Bologna, 1667) (b. 235); *Tassa de' medicinali, semplici, composti e spagirici* (Bologna, 1693) (b. 341); and *Tariffa de' medicinali* (Bologna, 1776) (b. 260).

43. Such reports for the years 1605–1702 and 1744–76 can be found in the "Acta Prothomedicatus" (A.S.B., Coll. Med., bb. 318–27); for the reports for 1633–54, see A.S.B., Reggimento, Assunteria di Studio, b. 149.

44. For the granting of the title of "viceprotomedico" to the town doctors, see *Liber pro recta,* 9; and A.S.B., Coll. Med., b. 319, several cases. For the decision to discontinue this title "ob absurda quae incidebant," see A.S.B., Coll. Med., b. 258,

"Ristretto degli atti e decreti più notabili fatti nel Collegio e Protomedicato di Medicina dell'anno 1562 all'anno 1792," July 17, 1694.

45. A.S.B., Coll. Med., b. 319.

46. *Riforma degli Statuti dell'Onoranda Compagnia de' Speziali di Bologna* (Bologna, 1690). On the Academy of the Apothecaries, see G. Fantuzzi, *Notizie degli scrittori bolognesi* (Bologna, 1786–90), 1:23; and M. Medici, *Memorie storiche intorno le Accademie scientifiche e letterarie della città di Bologna* (Bologna, 1852), 12.

47. C. Webster, *The Great Instauration: Science, Medicine, and Reform, 1626–1660* (New York, 1976), 273–82. On the London Paracelsians and their attack on Galenism, see also P. M. Rattansi, "The Helmontian-Galenist Controversy in Restoration England," *Ambix* 12 (1964): 1–23.

48. A.S.B., Coll. Med., b. 341. Another rebellious *spagirico* was Costantino Saccardino, executed for heresy in Bologna in 1622. He was the author of *Libro nomato la verità di diverse cose, quale minutamente tratta di molte salutifere operationi spagiriche et chimiche* (Bologna, 1621), in which he attacked Galenic medicine, in line with the followers of Paracelsus. On Saccardino, see C. Ginzburg and M. Ferrari, "La colombara ha aperto gli occhi," *Quaderni storici*, no. 38 (May–August 1978): 631–39.

49. The incorporation was official only in the Antidotario of 1770, which divided medicines into two classes, Galenic and chemical. See E. Rosa, *Medicina e salute pubblica a Bologna nel Sei e Settecento* (Bologna, 1978), 28. In the early eighteenth century, however, several physicians who were members of the Accademia degli Inquieti were very interested in pharmaceutical chemistry; see M. Cavazza, "Accademie scientifiche a Bologna: Dal *Coro Anatomico* agli *Inquieti, 1650–1714*," *Quaderni storici*, no. 48 (December 1981): 906–7.

50. On the subordination of the apothecaries to the jurisdiction of the college, see *Liber pro recta*, 26, 39 (in particular, rubr. 22 of "Convenzioni fra l'Arte e il Collegio," of 1606). See also A.S.B., Reggimento, Tribuni della Plebe, Libro Azzurro, c. 283.

On the controversy regarding the apothecaries' guild's assumption of the title of "college," see B.C.A.B., MSS. B. 2463–67. The phrase quoted comes from a memorandum sent by the medical college to the cardinal legate (B.C.A.B., MS. B 2465).

51. In the seventeenth century, cases of doctors filing charges against other practitioners are few and far between. For example, in 1623, Petronio Fabiano, town doctor of Minerbio, denounced the barber Giuliano Malucillo, "who treats as a physician those who call him, draws blood, applies cupping glasses and gives medications by mouth . . . every day and freely," without license or leave from an approved doctor. In this case, however, the barber was acquitted by the protomedici, as a result of other doctors' testimony in his favor. (A.S.B., Coll. Med., b. 319). In 1698, the town physician Cesare Nanni filed charges against an unlicensed healer, Giacomo Valeriani of Bertirolo, who "wanders . . . through these mountains and draws blood for every sort of illness . . . in spite of being an ignorant man" (b. 342).

52. For example, in a petition of 1752 to the Protomedicato, Alessandro Guidetti stated that he "practiced as a surgeon in Budrio as a simple free-lancer, without a salary from the public, and with the disadvantage of having in town two doctors who routinely draw blood" (A.S.B., Coll. Med., b. 349). On such conflicts and the changes in the stratification of the medical professions, see also Pomata, "Barbieri," 179 ff.

53. A.S.B., Coll. Med., b. 342. In 1709, the community of Sant'Agostino filed charges in the Protomedicato against Angelo Sorghi, a surgeon who gave medications by mouth (b. 352). A similar case occurred in 1745, when the community of Sant'Agata denounced the surgeon Aurelio Flandoli (bb. 322, 349).

54. A.S.B., Coll. Med.—b. 349, for the charge; b. 326, for the Protomedicato's sentence. When inspecting apothecary shops in the villages, the protomedici often reminded the local authorities to lend their support to the prerogatives of the public physician. See, for instance, the reports of the inspection at Castelfranco on June 14, 1745 (b. 322) and at Castelbolognese on August 22, 1746 (b. 323).

55. A.S.B., Coll. Med., b. 349.

56. A.S.B., Coll. Med., bb. 352, 342.

57. It must be said, of course, that the Protomedicato allowed the communities to solve these conflicts on their own because the communities never questioned in any way the college's authority over medical licensing. It was different elsewhere. For instance, in Sardinia, in the eighteenth and nineteenth centuries, communities often claimed the right to choose their medical practitioners regardless of whether those practitioners had been licensed by the Protomedicato of Cagliari, the main town. Such a claim would have been unthinkable in Bologna. In 1770, the Protomedicato of Cagliari reported that

"the abuses discovered in medical practice concern mainly surgeons who, in the teeth of all laws, insist on practicing also as physicians; and yet the Protomedicato cannot prosecute them, for lack of people willing to bear witness against them. . . . In several villages, moreover, unlicensed healers have long been practicing because there are no surgeons; and when a licensed surgeon tries to set up shop there, the community opposes him, preferring to leave the practice in the hands of the unlicensed healers. Therefore, infinite complaints are issued by the certified surgeons, and in spite of some punishment already given by order of His Eminence, it has been impossible to eradicate this abuse." (A.S.C., Regia Segreteria di Stato e Guerra, 2d ser., b. 863, "Relazione del Protomedicato di Cagliari sulle incumbenze appoggiategli," 1770)

The archives of the Protomedicato of Cagliari (especially A.S.C., Regia Segreteria di Stato e Guerra, 2d ser., bb. 863–71) contain numerous reports of such conflicts between communities, claiming the right to choose their healers, and the Protomedicato, which defended the rights of licensed surgeons and town doctors. For general information on the Sardinian Protomedicato, see G. Pinna, *Sulla pubblica sanità in Sardegna dalle sue origini fino al 1850* (Sassari and Cagliari, 1898), 22 ff. In Cagliari in the seventeenth century, physicians and surgeons shared a common association — the confraternity of Saints Cosmas and Damian (see V. Atzeni, "Les ordinacions de la Confraria dels gloriosos metges Sant Cosme y Sant Damia dels Doctors en medicina y Mestres de Silurgia de la ciutat de Caller," *Humana Studia* [1953]: 192–227; this essay includes an appendix containing the statutes of the confraternity).

58. The records of this trial are filed in A.S.B., Assunteria di Governo delle Comunità, Recapiti, b. 8 (1783–95). I am grateful to Bernardino Farolfi for pointing out these records to me.

59. The Protomedicato's ruling is enclosed with the trial records cited in n. 58.

60. See above, chap. 2, n. 108. I have excluded trials of apothecaries and third-degree surgeons because, for obvious reasons, these practitioners could not be considered popular healers.

61. A.S.B., Coll. Med., b. 214, trial of Francesco Sangalli.

62. A.S.B., Coll. Med., b. 233, *Bando del Protomedico per Roma, e per tutto lo Stato ecclesiastico,* 1614: "Those who have a license to sell specific things, such as *angelica, corallina,* oils, waters, and other things, shall not distribute broadsheets or any other writings, printed or handwritten, or display tables or posters describing the virtues and qualities of such things."

On the charlatans' cultural world, see P. Burke, "Rituals of Healing in Early Modern Italy," in *The Historical Anthropology of Early Modern Italy* (Cambridge, England, 1987), 207–20; and A. Klairmont Lingo, "Empirics and Charlatans in Early Modern France: The Genesis of the Classification of the *Other* in Medical Practice," *Journal of Social History* 9, no. 4 (summer 1986).

63. On the norcini, see Garzoni, *La piazza universale,* 825. Several norcini were regularly employed in the hospitals of Bologna (see L. Samoggia, "Empirici, litotomi e oculisti negli Ospedali della Vita e della Morte in Bologna nel 1600 e 1700," in *Sette secoli di vita ospedaliera in Bologna*) and in those of Rome (see I. Pappalardo, *Litotomi e oculisti preciani e norcini* [Rome, 1963]).

64. On local "bloodletting schools," see the manual written by the barber-surgeon Pietro Paolo Magni: *Discorsi sopra il modo di sanguinare* (Rome, 1586), 9–10; for more information about this manual and bibliographic references on Magni, see Pomata, "Barbieri," 167–68, 183. On the Gascon origins of most French surgeons, see T. Gelfand, "Cultural Diversity, Professional Unity: The Surgeons of France in the Eighteenth Century" (paper read at Davis Center seminar, Princeton University, December 8, 1978).

65. A.S.B., Coll. Med., b. 350, trial of Lorenzo and Andrea Adriani, 1666.

66. A.S.B., Coll. Med., b. 214, trial of Antonio the Roman, 1657. Inspections of the apothecary shops in the countryside were usually the occasion for the protomedici to exert their control over folk healers. For example, during their visit to the apothecary shop in Castel San Pietro, in 1698, the protomedici reprimanded a

midwife for administering oral remedies and for prescribing bloodletting from the foot to pregnant women (b. 320).

67. Manuals for barber-surgeons—such as the one by Magni cited above (n. 64)—often offered instructions on how to prepare ointments and balsams to apply to wounds. Magni also explained how to find or prepare rarer ingredients so that one did not need to buy them from the apothecaries (Magni, *Discorso sopra il modo di sanguinare*).

68. A.S.B., Coll. Med., b. 340.

69. A.S.B., Coll. Med., b. 236.

70. A.S.B., Coll. Med., b. 340.

71. The only restriction placed on midwives' competence with regard to the female body, in the second half of the seventeenth century, concerned their traditional authority to "establish the loss of virginity testifying on the matter of rape and deflowering, without the advice of a licensed physician" (A.S.B., Coll. Med., b. 214). The authority to establish a woman's virginity—a quality very important to her social status—was taken away from the midwives and given to the surgeons. The medico-legal texts written for a surgeon's use in this period teach how to write official reports on cases of violation and rape of women and children. See, for instance, A. Ciucci, *Il Filo d'Arianna: Overo fedelissima scorta alli esercenti di chirurgia per uscire dal Laberinto delle Relazioni e Ricognizioni dei vari morbi e morti* (Macerata, 1689).

72. A.S.B., Coll. Med., b. 352.

73. A.S.B., Coll. Med., b. 340.

74. A.S.B., Coll. Med., b. 213.

75. "Medendi medicamentis extrinsecé applicandis varia genera morborum extrinsecé apparentium" (A.S.B., Coll. Med., b. 214).

76. A.S.B., Coll. Med., b. 349, trial of Maria la Romana, 1763.

77. On Pier Paolo Molinelli and the first chair of surgery at the University of Bologna, see E. Gualandi, "Notizie sulla scuola di chirurgia in Bologna," *Studi e memorie per la storia dell'Università di Bologna* 4 (1918).

78. The marginalization of women healers in Bologna in the eighteenth century seems to have been the rule in spite of the fact that a few women—Anna Morandi Manzolini, Laura Bassi, and Maria Dalle Donne—managed to earn the doctoral degree in medicine and even teach at the university on medical matters. Laura Bassi is perhaps the most interesting case. She not only graduated in philosophy and medicine in 1732 but was also admitted as a member by the College of Philosophy on the strength of her status as *virgo famosa*. However, her membership was merely an honorary title, which did not allow her to enjoy the full rights of a collegiate, for instance, the privilege to draw an income from the college's activities. The collegiates considered her admission extraordinary—"extraordinaria res in Statutis non comprehensa" (A.S.B., Coll. Med., b. 238)—comparable to the acceptance in the college of an eleven-year-old child, Luigi Magni, in 1663. Fantuzzi (*Notizie* 5:120–22) compares the woman prodigy to the child, praising his hometown of

Bologna for "giving birth to young people with a prodigious knowledge, and today even a woman." For information about Magni, see also Masini, *Bologna perlustrata*, pt. 3, p. 257; and A.S.B., Coll. Med., b. 353, "Civilitatis Probationes" of Luigi Magni. On Laura Bassi, see Paula Findlen, "Science as a Career in Enlightenment Italy: The Strategies of Laura Bassi," *Isis* 84 (1993): 441–69. For Maria dalle Donne, who graduated in medicine and philosophy in 1799 and became the director of the school for midwives, see O. Sanlorenzo, *L'insegnamento di ostetricia nell'Università di Bologna* (Bologna, 1988), 53–61; and idem, "Maria Dalle Donne e la Scuola di Ostetricia nel secolo XX," in *Alma Mater Studiorum: La presenza femminile dal XVIII al XX secolo* (Bologna, 1988), 147–56. On Anna Morandi Manzolini, see Fantuzzi, *Notizie* 5:113–16; and V. Ottani and G. Giuliani-Piccari, "L'opera di Anna Morandi Manzolini nella ceroplastica anatomica bolognese," in *Alma Mater Studiorum,* 81–93.

79. A.C.A.B., Miscellanea vecchia, cart. 32, contains records of inquests regarding miraculous images of the Virgin Mary, from 1585 to 1796. In particular, the late-sixteenth-century records include numerous descriptions of healing miracles performed by several images of Mary in cases of demonic possession, most of them in women. See fasc. I/182/134a, "Miracoli avanti l'immagine di Maria Vergine posta in un cancello tra Porta S.Isaia e Porta Lame" (1585); fasc. I/182/134b, "Miracoli e grazie per intercessione della Beata Vergine dell'Olmo" (1589); fasc. I/182/135c, "Miracoli e grazie per intercessione della B.V. di Piano di Medicina" (1598–99); fasc. I/182/134d, "Miracoli della B.V. in Vidilatico" (1612); fasc. I/182/134e, "Miracoli e grazie della B.V. di Boccaderio" (1637). All of these files contain reports of the miracles, as told by the people who had been cured. Other instances of miraculous healing attributed to the image of the Virgin in the Church of Saint Luca were chronicled by Sister Diodata Malvasia, *La venuta et i progressi miracolosi della S.ma Madonna dipinta da S. Luca posta sul monte della Guardia dall'anno che ci venne 1160 sin all'anno 1617* (Bologna, 1617).

80. Manuscript records of Caterina Vigri's canonization proceedings are in A.C.A.B., Atti e processi per Beatificazione e Santificazione, 1473–1725, 737, 738, 739, 740. Portions of the proceedings were printed as *Acta bononiensis canonizationis B. Catharinae a Bononia* (Bologna, 1712).

81. G. B. Melloni (*Atti, o Memorie degli uomini illustri in santità nati, o morti in Bologna* [Bologna, 1773], 5:544–65) lists a long series of Caterina's healing miracles. A recurring motif in the cures is the apparition of the saint to the sick person in a dream. This motif may derive from the pre-Christian tradition of *incubatio,* or the healing by a god during sleep. The Christian developments of incubatio raise intriguing questions, which of course cannot be dealt with here.

82. See Melloni, *Atti, o Memorie,* about the healing miracles attributed to Diana degli Andalò (6:250–52) and Paola Mezzavacca (3:214–18). On Prudenziana Zagnotti, see A.C.A.B., Atti e processi per Beatificazione e Santificazione, 1473–1725, 741, 742, 743, 744. About Anna Callegari Zucchini, see A.C.A.B., Atti e processi per Beatificazione e Santificazione, 1473–1725, 746/1, fasc. k/499/1, "Attestati di diversi,

narrazioni di fatti giurati, e pretese grazie ottenute dal Signore Iddio per intercessione di Madonna Anna Callegari Zucchini si' in vita che dopo morte della medesima" (1742–43); the document lists 186 miracles, including many cures. About Rosa Torregiani, see A.C.A.B., Atti e processi per Beatificazione e Santificazione, 1473–1725, 745, fasc. k/498/16 (1765–66).

In *Storie di un anno di peste* (Milan, 1984), which was published in English as *Histories of a Plague Year* (Berkeley, Calif., 1989), Giulia Calvi has stressed the prominence of a holy woman, Domenica da Paradiso, among the supernatural healers sought out by the people of Florence during the plague of 1630. Calvi rightly contrasts this prominence of women among the heavenly healers to the overwhelmingly male medical establishment on earth.

83. A.S.B., Coll. Med., b. 342, case of Cavazza vs. Gualandi, 1698.

84. A.S.B., Coll. Med., b. 342, case of Atti vs. Golinelli, 1701.

85. For an example of a midwife who believed that it was her duty to wash and dress the corpse of one of her patients, a peasant woman, see A.S.B., Coll. Med., b. 352, trial of Chiara Marchetti, 1711. For more details of this case, see Pomata, "Barbieri," 178.

86. A.S.B., Coll. Med., b. 213. Of the trial of Rodolfo Vacchettoni, only the sentence remains, which summarizes the charges against him. Vacchettoni was sentenced to five years of exile.

87. A.S.B., Coll. Med., b. 341, trial of Gio. Batta Terrarossa, 1689. In addition to being exiled, Terrarossa was sentenced to return the money he had received from one of his patients and to pay the cost of the trial. The surgeon (whose license had been granted in 1665) had been convicted of exceeding the limits of his profession in 1670 and had been suspended temporarily from practicing (b. 338 for the license; b. 213 for the trial of 1670).

88. The story of Sebastiano Poggi has been reconstructed here from the records filed in A.S.B., Coll. Med., bb. 213, 223, 345, 348, 351.

89. The Malvezzi family inherited this privilege from the Campeggi. The Campeggi had died out, for lack of male heirs, in 1727, and "their inheritance, honors and privileges" went to the marquises of the Malvezzi family, which took the name Malvezzi-Campeggi (G. B. Guidicini, *Cose notabili della città di Bologna* [Bologna, 1870], 3:121).

90. A hermit friar ("habitu heremitarum") who had received his medical degree from the Marquis Malvezzi was charged with practicing illegally in 1734 (A.S.B., Coll. Med., b. 346). Gio. Batta Terrarossa, the surgeon exiled by the Protomedicato in 1689 (see n. 87, above), also maintained that he had graduated *in camera*.

Doctoral degrees *in camera* were also granted in other cities. In Milan, for example, the surgeon of the Tribunale di Sanità (Health Board) admitted in 1631 that he had received his degree "by virtue of the *Privilegium palatinatus*" rather than from a public university (A.S.M., Sanità, parte antica, b. 68). Such degrees were also awarded in Padua; see Pesenti Marangon, *"Professores chirurgie,"* 23; and A. Cavalieri

Ragazzi, "I dottorati di Giacomo Zeglar, polacco (1433) e di Noè Acerbi, bergamasco (1450)," *Quaderni per la storia dell'Università di Padova* 9–10 (1976–77): 247–50.

91. In 1712, two representatives of the college complained to the legate about a license issued to a charlatan who was practicing both as a physician and as a surgeon (A.S.B., Coll. Med., b. 258, "Ristretto degli atti e decreti," June 23, 1712).

92. *Liber pro recta,* 20. The prohibition did not extend to the public lecturers hired directly by the Senate, such as lithotomists and norcini, and those who had been practicing for years and were "generally accepted as physicians." For instance, Marino Marini, a norcino charged in 1638 with illegal practice, mentioned in his defense the *in camera* doctorate he had received in Dozza one year earlier (A.S.B., Coll. Med., b. 319). Marini was acquitted and continued practicing in Bologna for twenty more years (as stated in a document written in 1668 by his nephew, Giacomo Marini, when applying for a job as lithotomist at the Ospedale della Vita). On this document, see Samoggia, "Empirici, litotomi e oculisti," 188.

93. The graduation ceremony in the college is described in the statutes of 1507 (rubr. 20). The doctrinal issues *(puncta)* to be discussed were chosen from Galen's *Liber Tegni* and Hippocrates' *Aphorisms* and were assigned to the candidate three days before the examination, during sunrise Mass in the cathedral (A.S.B., Coll. Med., b. 219).

94. A copy of the portrait is included with the trial's proceedings (A.S.B., Coll. Med., b. 351).

95. During the trial of 1719, Prince Hercolani spoke to the protomedici on Poggi's behalf (A.S.B., Coll. Med., b. 223).

96. A.S.B., Coll. Med., b. 319.

97. A.S.B., Coll. Med., b. 318.

98. A.S.B., Coll. Med., b. 321.

99. On Michele Zanardi, see A.S.B., Coll. Med., b. 319. The same happened to several other charlatans: for instance, Martino Grimaldi in 1616 (b. 318); Gioseffo Garofalo in 1617 (b. 318); Gian Filippo Robilandi in 1686 (b. 320); the distiller Matteo Ferrante in 1694 (b. 320); and the *spagirico* Gioseffo Vignudelli in 1705 (b. 321).

100. For the town physician's charge against the Baccolinis, see A.S.B., Coll. Med., b. 349. For their license, see b. 324. The same happened to Rinaldo Cavicchioli, who was interdicted from practicing in 1771 but in the following year was issued a license to practice as a first-degree surgeon (bb. 349, 327).

101. A.S.B., Coll. Med., b. 321.

102. A.S.B., Coll. Med., b. 322.

103. A.S.B., Coll. Med., b. 322. Similarly, Angiola Tarozzi, of Anzola, was tried on June 8, 1764, and licensed on October 13 of the same year (b. 326).

104. For instance, in 1682 the pills illegally prepared by the apothecary Lazzaro Trebbi were given to the Ospedale di Sant'Orsola (A.S.B., Coll. Med., b. 320). The same hospital also received the entire stock of medicines confiscated from Giuliano Nucci, whose shop did not have a licensed master apothecary or a licensed appren-

tice (b. 321). Also, the lancets taken away from the barber Rinaldo Piccinini in 1683 were given to the hospital (b. 320). The money collected from fines for illegal practice was also donated to charitable and religious institutions, such as the sisters of the convents of San Bernardino, Sant'Elena and Corpus Christi, the orphanage of San Bartolomeo, the Convertite nuns, and, in the eighteenth century, the nuns of Santa Maria Egiziaca.

105. In 1747, the Protomedicato ordered "midwives, charlatans, tooth drawers," and other lesser healers (inferiores medicinae ministros) to take an examination in order to be certified (A.S.B., Coll. Med., b. 323, "Costituzione su chirurghi, ostetriche, circolatori," 1747).

106. For licenses issued in 1818 and 1819 for infime operazioni, see A.S.B., Archivio dello Studio, Pontificia Università, bb. 450, 516–17, 629.

107. According to the statutes of the barbers' guild, women were not allowed to practice as barber-surgeons (B.U.B., MS. 3873, "Statuti antichi dell'Arte de Barbieri di Bologna approvati dall'Eccelso Senato di Bologna," 1557; a copy of this document can also be found in B.C.A.B., MS. Gozzadini 220). The rolls of licensed barber-surgeons (masters and apprentices) periodically published by the Protomedicato from the end of the sixteenth century to the end of the eighteenth do not include any female names. However, a few women barbers probably practiced unofficially. For instance, we know that in 1630 Susanna Ricci, barbiera (female barber), treated women in the plague hospital; see A. Pastore, Crimine e giustizia in tempo di peste nell'Europa moderna (Bari, 1991), 123. In 1766, in Milan, a list of barbershops included the names of "the masters' sons and daughters," suggesting that a barber's daughter could occasionally practice. However, of 265 names, only one was a woman's; see A.S.M., Sanità, parte antica, b. 243/44: "Nomi de' Signori Maestri, figli e figlie de' Maestri professori di chirurgia e barbieri, che hanno aperta bottega in Milano, e suoi borghi l'Anno 1766."

108. A.S.B., Coll. Med., b. 324. For the certification issued by her instructors regarding her internship at the Ospedale della Vita, see b. 349. Her teachers included the renowned doctor Giovanni Antonio Galli, who wrote on her behalf in very supportive terms.

109. In 1807 (one year after the French had introduced in Italy new regulations on the health professions), a similar case had a very different ending. A midwife who had requested a permit to practice as surgeon, after attending the regular courses in surgery, was denied the license and ordered to keep within the boundaries of obstetrics. On this case, see Pomata, "Barbieri," 182.

110. A.S.B., Coll. Med., b. 214. The undated broadsheet was printed for Fulvio Baroncini, Martino Grimaldi's heir, who was granted a license to continue selling the medication.

111. For the periodic renewal of licenses to the Grimaldi heirs, see A.S.B., Coll. Med., bb. 318–24; A.S.B., Assunteria di Studio, Diversorum, b. 100, no. 10, "Notizie diverse in ordine all'Elettuario che si fabbricava da Martino Grimaldi e pos-

cia da altri soggetti, 1616–1643." The Grimaldi license was also renewed periodically by the Senate.

112. A copy of the broadsheet is included among the Protomedicato records in A.S.B., Coll. Med., b. 214; the interdiction from practice, and the subsequent issuing of the license to Gioseffo Garofalo, can be found in b. 319. Other charlatans' broadsheets in b. 214 include that of Francesco Nava, also known as "the Orvietan." His broadsheet, exalting the power of an elixir "against all poisons live or dead, hot or cold," was printed in Rome, Perugia, and Bologna in 1649. Also in b. 214 is the broadsheet advertising the "Bezoardic electuary against poisons, live and dead," sold by Girolamo Siancano da Fano, also called "Aromatario Fanese" (the Apothecary from Fano). For another example of such broadsheets, see *Considerazioni del dott. Giuseppe Rosaccio sull'anno* (Bologna, 1624) (B.U.B., Aula V, Tab. I F II vol. 409/16).

113. Zacchia, *Quaestiones medico-legales,* 409: "Quam inanis est, Deus bone, haec secretorum remediorum persuasio! Et tamen non in vulgus tantum, sed in cuiuscumque generis viros, immo (inquam) in ipsos medicos surrepsit."

114. Ludovico Settala (*Animadversionum et Cautionum Medicarum libri septem* [Padua, 1628], lib. 1, chap. 14, p. 5) urged doctors not to keep medical secrets but instead to share them ("secreta remedia non habeat, sed communicet").

115. A.S.B., Coll. Med., b. 353 *quater.* The manuscripts containing medical secrets are numberless. To mention just a few examples in Bologna: B.U.B.—MS. 595, Miscell. F, 2, "Secreti di Virginio Grillenzoni," seventeenth century; Miscell. L, 11, "Secreti vari antichi," 1575; Miscell. FF, 40, "Secreti medicinali," seventeenth century. Recipes and secrets were also transcribed in diaries; see, for instance, the manuscript diary of an apothecary from Bologna, Ercole Dal Buono (B.U.B., MS. 408, I, 1600–18). In general, on the literature of secrets and its significance in early modern learning, see William Eamon, *Science and the Secrets of Nature: Books of Secrets in Medieval and Early Modern Culture* (Princeton, N.J., 1994).

116. G. Pitré, *Medici, chirurghi, barbieri e speziali antichi in Sicilia, secoli XIII–XVIII* (Florence, 1942), 329–33.

117. The report of this inspection is in A.S.B., Assunteria di Studio, b. 149.

118. A.S.B., Coll. Med., b. 338, *Alcuni Avvertimenti per la dispensa, e preparatione de gl'Ingredienti della Triaca da farsi pubblicamente dalla Honoranda Compagnia de gli Speciali di Bologna in quest'anno M.DC.LXIII d'Ordine dell'Eccellentissimo e Venerando Collegio de' Medici dell'istessa Città* (Bologna, 1663).

119. See G. Olmi, "Farmacopea antica e medicina moderna: La disputa sulla teriaca nel Cinquecento bolognese," *Physis* 19 (1977).

120. See G. Watson, *Theriac and Mithridatium: A Study in Therapeutics* (London, 1966), 102–5. On theriac, see also A. Benedicenti, *Malati, medici e farmacisti: Storia dei rimedi attraverso i secoli e delle teorie che ne spiegano l'azione sull'organismo* (Milan, 1925), 2:1017–30; and A. Corsini, *Medici ciarlatani e ciarlatani medici* (Bologna, 1922), 33–37.

121. The heads and tails of vipers were discarded because they were thought to contain the largest quantity of poison—which was supposed to be used in the compound only in diluted form. This belief lasted well into the second half of the

eighteenth century, long after Francesco Redi had shown that a viper's head and tail were innocuous and that the poison was located in a bag near the teeth. See Watson, *Theriac and Mithridatium,* 102.

122. A.S.B., Coll. Med., b. 322.

123. A.S.B., Coll. Med., bb. 345, 349.

124. Watson, *Theriac and Mithridatium,* 142–7; on the *Encyclopédie,* see Olmi, "Farmacopea antica," 215.

125. Watson, *Theriac and Mithridatium,* 17, 72–74.

126. A.S.B., Coll. Med., b. 341, *Le virtù e facoltà principali della Triaca di Andromaco Seniore* (Bologna, 1692). Some doctors, however, held an unfavorable opinion of theriac: see, for instance, Alessandro Petroni, *Del viver delli Romani et del conservar la sanità* (Rome, 1594), 297–98. According to Petroni, theriac did not prolong life and could actually be harmful: "spesso confonde l'intelletto all'huomo, e per molti semplici con le quali si compone, che sogliono empire il capo et anco per li trocisci fatti con carni di vipera. . . . Quando spesso si prende, prima fa l'huomo come embriaco, poi pien di sonno, poi gli leva affatto il sonno; all'ultimo fa impazzire" ("It often disturbs man's intellectual faculties, due to its many ingredients, which tend to go to one's head, and because of the pills made of viper's meat. . . . If taken too often, at first it makes men act as if they were drunk, then sleepy, and after that it makes them sleepless; and finally, it drives them crazy").

127. A.S.B., Coll. Med., b. 353 *bis.*

128. See, for instance, the recipe submitted by a Venetian charlatan, Angelo Cortilio in 1605, when applying for permission to sell his electuary (A.S.B., Coll. Med., b. 318). The same ingredients (herbs plus theriac) also appear in Francesco Nava's recipe for the Orvietan (b. 214), mentioned above. However, many patent medicines dispensed by popular healers were made exclusively of herbal ingredients: see, for example, the liniment prepared by one Antonio Arconanati, made of wine "medicated with roe herb *[erba capriola],* cardoon leaves *(foglie di cardo santo)* and rosemary roots" (b. 248).

129. A.S.B., Coll. Med., b. 345.

130. A.S.B., Coll. Med., b. 340.

131. The historian Pierre Goubert mentions the case of Charles Dionis, a member of the Medical Faculty of Paris in the mid–eighteenth century, who bought from a family of herbalists the royal privilege to sell the Orvietan. See P. Goubert, "L'art de guérir: Médecine savante et médecine populaire dans la France de 1790," *Annales E.S.C.* 32, no. 5 (September–October 1977). See also Paulmier, *L'orviétan* (Paris, 1892), 95–107.

132. Molière, *Amour médecin,* act 2, scene 7.

133. Public anatomy lessons were also occasions to celebrate the medical establishment. Such lessons were organized as a spectacle for the city's nobility (see G. Ferrari, "Public Anatomy Lessons and the Carnival: The Anatomy Theater of Bologna," *Past and Present,* no. 117 [November 1987]).

134. A.S.B., Coll. Med., b. 327.

135. G. Simmel, *On Individuality and Social Forms* (Chicago, 1971), 305. N. D. Jewson suggested a similar explanation for the quick turnover of therapies in eighteenth-century medicine: there were many competing theories, all based on the same assumptions (N. D. Jewson, "Medical Knowledge and the Patronage System in Eighteenth Century England," *Sociology* 8 [1974]: 380–81).

136. M. Bakhtin, "Language of the Marketplace," in *Rabelais and His World*, trans. Helene Iswolsky (Bloomington, Ind., 1984), 159. On street cries and advertising, see also P. Bojatyrev, *Semiotica della cultura popolare* (Verona, 1982), 211–26.

137. Bakhtin, *Rabelais,* 153–54, 180.

138. A.S.B., Reggimento, Tribuni della Plebe, Libro Azzurro—October 9 and 16, 1630 (meat inspection); June 12, 1630 (wheat inspection); September 7, 1633 (inspection of salami). On traditional medical views about the role of contaminated food in causing epidemics, see E. Lieber, "Galen on Contaminated Cereals as a Cause of Epidemics," *Bulletin of the History of Medicine* 44, no. 4 (1970).

139. *Direttorio del Magistrato dei Tribuni della Plebe* (Bologna, 1645); G. B. Rossi, *L'attioni memorabili fatte da . . . Confalonieri del popolo et Massari delle Arti già dominanti la città di Bologna raccolte da diversi manoscritti et autori* (Bologna, 1681).

140. In a legal sentence pronounced by the Protomedicato, we find the statement "Medicamenta sub nomine alimenti sunt consideranda" ("Medicines are included under the category of food") (see A.S.B., Coll. Med., b. 223, case of Lenzi vs. Fabbri, 1711).

141. A.S.B., Reggimento, Tribuni della Plebe, "Libro morello," fol. 185: "Collegio fatto dai Protomedici sopra le bestie malsane"; for inspection of suspicious cooked fish, see fol. 78, 90, 136; Lib. B 5, fol. 629; Lib. B 1, fol. 55 e 83, Lib. B 4, fol. 30: "cibi di farina di castagne cotti e fritturi atti a generare corrutione nel sangue sono proibiti a vendersi" ("cooked or fried foods prepared with chestnut flour and likely to generate corruption in the blood shall not be sold").

Among the Protomedicato's records I found an injunction addressed to a fisherman, forbidding him the sale of a particular fish "for eating," but allowing him to "convert it into oil" (A.S.B., Coll. Med., b. 353, 1659). The medical college was also occasionally asked about the proper way of baking bread; see O. Montalbani, *L'honore de i Collegi dell'Arti della città di Bologna* (Bologna, 1670), 51.

142. A.S.B., Coll. Med., b. 327, February 14, 1775.

143. E. P. Thompson, "The Moral Economy of the English Crowd in the Eighteenth Century," in *Customs in Common* (New York, 1991), 185–258. See also W. Reddy, "The Textile Trade and the Language of the Crowd at Rouen, 1752–1871," *Past and Present* 74 (1977).

144. A. Guenzi, *Pane e fornai a Bologna in età moderna* (Venice, 1982), 139–41. As Guenzi has insightfully noted, however, the fixed price of bread imposed by the city authorities was only occasionally a concession to popular need; most often it represented a compromise, based on secret negotiations, between the interests of the landowners (i.e., the city's nobility) and those of the bakers.

145. In 1690, Cardinal Negrone tried unsuccessfully to terminate this ritual. On that occasion, the local nobility defended it as "a very ancient custom in Bologna" (A.S.B., Assunteria dei Magistrati, Diversorum, b. 13).

146. Dorothy and Roy Porter also speak of "a moral economy of health" for eighteenth-century England (*Patient's Progress: Doctors and Doctoring in Eighteenth-Century England* [Stanford, Calif., 1989], 214).

CHAPTER 4: PATIENTS' RIGHTS AND THE DOCTORS' PRESTIGE

1. *Liber pro recta administratione Protomedicatus* (Bologna, 1666), 12.

2. Such was the case, for instance, in 1574, when the college doctors were called to decide the dispute between Paolo Vitali and the surgeon Parmi (see chap. 2, above, pp. 53–54). In 1573, the college was asked to arbitrate the lawsuit between a physician, Pietro Paci, and Count Ramazzotti, who refused to pay the practitioner. This case presumably involved a broken agreement for a cure, as did the case of Parmi vs. Vitali (A.S.B., Coll. Med., b. 217, "Liber secretus, 1504–1575"). In 1628, the vice-legate referred to the Protomedicato the case filed by one Dr. Scotti against a merchant whom he had treated for two years without receiving payment (b. 296)— yet another proof that both practitioners and patients were still bringing their disputes to the ordinary civil court and not to the protomedici, in spite of the latter's newly acquired jurisdiction over such cases.

3. Thomas Actius, *De infirmitate eiusque privilegiis et affectibus* (Venice, 1603), 46: "Judex summarie tenetur providere, ut merces medicis solvatur, ministrisque aegrorum." See also G. Fichtner, *Dissertatio de Infirmitatis commodis* (Altdorf, 1720), 23.

The delinquent party had to pay trial expenses in addition to the practitioner's fee. By the mid–eighteenth century, trial expenses ranged from one lira and seven soldi (A.S.B., Coll. Med., b. 349, Cantelli vs. Montesani, 1744) to eight lire and five soldi (b. 329, Coralli vs. Vanduzzi, 1751). The case of Coralli vs. Vanduzzi dragged on for almost two years—an exceptionally long time. This case was originally brought to an ordinary court, but the legate referred it to the protomedici.

4. Occasionally, one or both parties turned to lawyers, usually during longer trials or when courts other than the Protomedicato were involved. This happened in 13 percent of the cases (17 out of 131).

5. This happened in 34 percent of the cases. The extrajudicial settlement was sometimes recorded in the Protomedicato's books; see, for instance, A.S.B., Coll. Med., b. 223—the cases of Livizzani, 1723; and Gaudenzi and Pedretti vs. Monari, 1725. More often, such settlements went unregistered. One simply finds no trace of the case in the records other than the account of the first meeting of the parties.

6. A.S.B., Coll. Med., b. 350. The daily fee was based on the number of visits—usually two, one in the morning and one in the evening. Two daily visits were considered routine for surgical and physical treatments and were often mentioned to

prove that the practitioner had acted according to standards. For example, the barber Arcangelo de Bono, who filed a suit to obtain payment for services in 1603, claimed to have visited his patient twice a day: "bis in die accedebat et operabat" (A.S.B., Coll. Med., b. 197). Recovering patients were visited only once a day.

Hospital patients were also visited twice a day—in the morning and the evening—by physicians as well as surgeons (B.U.B., MS. 184, no. 13, "Dell'elettione, e qualità de' medici e loro ufficio nell'Ospedale della Vita").

Another item influencing fees was the distance to the patient's residence.

7. For example, see the *notula* (bill) issued by the barber-surgeon Franzosi in 1701 (A.S.B., Coll. Med., b. 342, case of Franzosi vs. Natali).

8. For example, see A.S.B., Coll. Med., b. 320, case of Aldrovandi vs. Masini, 1668.

9. A.S.B., Coll. Med., b. 342.

10. A.S.B., Coll. Med., b. 350, case of Bossi vs. Morandi, 1665. When the Protomedicato ruled that the barber-surgeon was entitled to a fee of one hundred lire for his services, Atti's heir filed an appeal with the Rota, the main civil court of Bologna.

11. A.S.B., Coll. Med., b. 350, case of Bossi vs. Morandi, 1665, deposition of Dr. Gallerati.

12. A.S.B., Coll. Med., b. 325.

13. See A.S.B., Coll. Med., b. 341, for Dr. Gotti's request for payment and for the proceedings of the case. See b. 320 for the sentence of the Protomedicato, dated September 30, 1684.

14. A.S.B., Coll. Med., bb. 351, 223.

15. A.S.B., Coll. Med., bb. 323, b. 349.

16. A.S.B., Coll. Med.—b. 342, request for payment by barber-surgeon Trebbi in the case of Trebbi vs. Sani, 1695; b. 340, request by surgeon Gioseffo Arzelli, 1687.

17. See A.S.B., Coll. Med.—b. 340, for Arzelli's request; b. 320, August 14, 1687, for the Protomedicato's sentence.

18. A.S.B., Coll. Med., b. 351. For the most difficult cases, third-degree barber-surgeons would sometimes request two or three lire per visit even in the city (for example, see b. 351, case of Redi vs. Droghi's Heirs, 1732; b. 346, case of Cantelli vs. Sarti, 1734).

19. For example, in 1725 the surgeon Cosmo Gaudenzi and the physician Gaetano Pedretti requested payment for surgical treatment from the same patient (A.S.B., Coll. Med., b. 345).

20. The physician and the surgeon in service at the Ospedale di Sant'Orsola in the 1720s received the same salary. I owe this information to Maura Palazzi, who kindly allowed me to see the as yet unpublished results of her research on the accounting books of the Bolognese Opera dei Mendicanti, which ran the Ospedale della Vita.

21. See A.S.B., Coll. Med.—b. 342, for Cattani's written request; b. 321, for the Protomedicato's sentence.

22. A.S.B., Coll. Med., b. 223.

23. A.S.B., Coll. Med., b. 325, case of Casignoli vs. Ugolini, 1756.

24. G. B. Codronchi, *De christiana ac tuta medendi ratione* (Ferrara, 1591), 89: "Stipendium medici conveniens, ac iustum metiri habeamus, considerato modo curationis, labore Medici, et industria, item facultatibus aegroti, ac consuetudine loci." Before ruling over cases involving people from villages or towns in the Bolognese territory, the protomedici did at times send for information on "the patient's condition and the local customs." (Such was the procedure adopted, for instance, before establishing the *tassa*, or fair fee, for the surgeon Arzelli of the village of Mirandola in 1687; see A.S.B., Coll. Med., bb. 340, 320.)

25. For example, in 1753, "ad instantiam infirmi" (upon the patient's request), the protomedici discussed the nature of the wound treated by one Dr. Righi (A.S.B., Coll. Med., b. 234). In 1770, they took some time to deliberate over the fee owed to one Dr. Silvani "pro difficillimi cujusdam morbi curatione" (for the cure of a very difficult disease) (b. 226).

26. A.S.B., Coll. Med., b. 321.

27. P. Zacchia, *Quaestiones medico-legales* (Lyons, 1662), lib. 6, tit. 1, quaestio 8, 20, p. 468: "Denique dubitatur, an in morbis desperatis, & incurabilibus Medicus licite mercedem recipiat: et videtur quod non, quia nemo debet recipere mercedem laboris quem incassum sciebat se insumere; sed sic est quod in desperatis, & incurabilibus morbis Medicus scit, ac manifeste cognoscit, se frustra laborem suscipere in curandis; ergo non debet ex suo labore ullam mercedem recipere." Zacchia, however, added that if the physician did not conceal from the patient the fatal nature of his illness, and the patient still requested treatment, the practitioner had the right to be paid.

28. A.S.B., Coll. Med., b. 320: "DD. decreverunt sibi dari lir. 30 pro mercede sui laboris, et hoc non obstat quod ipse Cavatia sit Barbitonsor Parochiae, quia fuit curatio maximi momenti." Before establishing the tassa, the protomedici routinely inquired whether the practitioner was a town doctor or surgeon. In such a case, he would be entitled to a lower fee, inasmuch as he was already salaried by the community. In 1675, when the barber-surgeon Gioseffo Cavalieri from the village of Medicina requested payment for treating a wound, the protomedici ruled that he was to have ten lire if he were the town surgeon, and fifteen lire if he were not (b. 342).

29. For Gotti's plea and the new tassa, see A.S.B., Coll. Med., b. 339.

30. A.S.B., Coll. Med., b. 323. Another sentence that took into account a patient's financial situation was pronounced in the case of Landuzzi vs. Frabetti, in 1747 (b. 323: "ex quo agitur de paupere rustico" ["since one is dealing with a poor peasant"]). Payment in installments was permitted in several other cases: see, for instance, Poli vs. Todeschini, 1732 (b. 346); Dotti vs. Calcina, 1745 (b. 322); and Landini vs. Gamberini, 1749 (b. 324).

31. A.S.B., Coll. Med., b. 352.

32. A.S.B., Coll. Med., b. 352.

33. A.S.B., Coll. Med., b. 342.

34. A.S.B., Coll. Med., b. 351.

35. A.S.B., Coll. Med., b. 323, case of Lodi vs. Malvasi-Masi, 1746–47. The fee initially requested by the barber-surgeon was fifty-seven lire and ten soldi.

36. Records of the proceedings in this case, that of Landi vs. Costa, are filed in A.S.B., Coll. Med., b. 351 (for other related documents, see also bb. 214, 223).

37. Landi was a lecturer in logic, philosophy, and theoretical and practical medicine from 1712 to 1738 (A.S.B., Assunteria di Studio, Requisiti dei Lettori, vol. 14, n. 9). His father was not a Bolognese citizen, and therefore he could not have been admitted to the medical college.

38. A.S.B., Coll. Med., b. 351, case of Landi vs. Costa, March 23, 1719, deposition of the apothecary Filippo Lindri.

39. Ibid., deposition of Michele Costa, May 17, 1720.

40. Copies of all these documents are filed with the lawsuit's records (A.S.B., Coll. Med., b. 351).

41. A fee of two lire and ten soldi per visit was granted by the protomedici to the surgeon Cantelli in 1734 (A.S.B., Coll. Med., b. 346). This was the highest fee ever awarded by the protomedici to a surgeon.

42. To what extent did the Protomedicato try to enforce a system of price-control for medicines? The sources I have examined do not allow me to answer this question. I have the impression, however, that the official price of medicines, or Tassa, was fixed by the protomedici in collusion with the apothecaries, often deferring to the latter's interests. Price variations usually followed fluctuations in the costs of imported drugs. For example, on November 25, 1766, the protomedici increased the prices of some medicines on the basis of business correspondence submitted by the apothecaries (A.S.B., Coll. Med., b. 326). Occasionally, price-fixing was mandated for popular remedies. During a fever epidemic in 1729, the protomedici lowered to one soldo the price for a daily dose of febrifuge (made of gentian roots and peel of pomegranate) and the cost of a laxative draught (a compound of wine tartar and sugar). The purpose of this price-fixing was "to give relief from the current epidemics — which are nevertheless to be considered nondangerous, and rather benign, and from which one can recover with the sole aid of Nature and time — to the field laborers of the Bolognese territory, so that they can recover their strength and properly return to till the soil" (b. 345, "Ordine agli speziali").

43. In 1678, in the case of Antoni vs. Bruzzi (A.S.B., Coll. Med., b. 320), the protomedici ruled that the bill for medicines presented by the apothecary Antoni should not be paid because he had not prepared the remedies according to standards.

44. In the case of Balotta vs. Del Sole (1717), a bill for 414 lire and 11 soldi was set at 410 lire and 9 soldi by the tassatore, but at 300 lire by the Protomedicato (A.S.B., Coll. Med., b. 351). In the case of Zanetti vs. Mazzoni (1742), a bill of 208 lire and 4 soldi was reduced to 198 lire and 19 soldi by the tassatore and to 149 lire by the Protomedicato (b. 351).

45. N. Elias, *The Court Society,* trans. E. Jephcott (New York, 1983), 102–3.

46. For disputes between the medical doctors and the jurists on matters of rank and precedence, see A.S.B., Coll. Med., b. 209.

47. A.S.B., Coll. Med., b. 233. The presence of a physician in each parish is documented during the plague of 1630 (see P. Moratti, *Racconto de gli ordini e Provisioni fatte ne' lazaretti in Bologna e suo contado in tempo di contagio* [Bologna, 1631], 14 ff). Many patients's depositions to the protomedici mentioned a "parish physician" (for example, see b. 338, deposition of Anna Catterina Masini, 1663).

48. A.C.A.B., Miscellanea vecchia, "Segreteria e Foro," b. 42, I/192/214, "Visite delli Infermi, et Poveri della Città di Bologna visitati dalla Congregatione eretta dal Ill. mo et R. S. Cardinale Paleotti . . . arcivescovo." This manuscript source includes a list of the patients receiving medical care from the congregation, and the sums given to them in charity every month, from 1593 to 1595.

49. A.C.A.B., Raccolta degli Statuti, cart. 12, fasc. 176, *Statuti della ven. Confraternita della Regina dei Cieli detta de' Poveri Riformati* (Bologna, 1627), 11: "And this company was specifically founded as a charitable institution for its members, that is, to help the brothers and sisters of the company who are sick; for this reason, a medical practitioner is chosen by the company and is paid a yearly salary to visit the sick, in addition to the ordinary visitors, chosen at appointed times, as prescribed by the statutes, for the purpose of visiting the sick and giving them the usual alms."

The physician's yearly salary was thirty-six lire. By the end of the sixteenth century, the company included thirteen hundred men and almost the same number of women: 4.23 percent of the population of Bologna. See Istituto per la Storia di Bologna, "Gli archivi delle istituzioni di carità e assistenza attive in Bologna nel Medioevo e nell'età moderna," *Atti del IV Colloquio dell'Istituto per la Storia di Bologna* (Bologna, 1984), 1:140. See also M. Fanti, *La chiesa e la Compagnia dei Poveri in Bologna* (Bologna, 1977).

50. A. di P. Masini, *Bologna perlustrata* (Bologna, 1666), 25; *Sacro Ragguaglio a tutto il mondo della particolare Institutione della Compagnia de gl'Agonizanti canonicamente erreta nella chiesa di S. Isaia di Bologna l'anno M DC XXVII* (Bologna, 1635); and *Regole de i fratelli e sorelle della pietosiss. Confraternità delli Agonizanti, canonicamente eretta, e fondata nell'Altare di S. Carlo, posto nella Chiesa di S. Isaia di Bologna* (Bologna, 1640).

51. *Regole e Capitoli della Pijssima Congregatione degli Agonizzanti di Bologna sopra la distributione dell'Eredità del già Sig. Valerio Brunellini, in sovvenimento de' poveri cittadini infermi* (Bologna, 1684). A copy of this document is in A.C.A.B., Statuti 1684–1771, cart. 1, fasc. 3.

52. B.C.A.B, A.V., RI, caps. 82; 61, *Distribuzione di medicinali che facevasi ogni anno dalla Congregazione degli Agonizzanti ai poveri infermi delle Parrocchie di Bologna.* (This document is a printed broadsheet, with a handwritten note dating it earlier than 1696.)

53. A.C.A.B., Miscellanea vecchia, "Congregazioni in città," cart. 185A, Congregazione degli Agonizzanti in S. Isaia (the document includes the yearly figures for the amount of money paid for medicines distributed to the poor in 1766–71 and 1783–91).

54. *Regole et ordinationi di tutta la Pijssima Confraternita de gli Agonizanti eretta primariamente in Bologna* (Bologna, 1642), 12–13.

55. A.S.B., Ospedale di S. Maria della Morte, Instrumenti e Processi, Aggiunte, Lib. 10, n. 25, "Invito a caritatevoli cittadini," 1720.

56. B.U.B., MS. 207B, b. 8, "Relatione del Trasporto degl'Infermi fatto dall'Arciconfraternita di S. Maria della Vita dallo Spedale Vecchio allo Spedale Nuovo," 1725.

The poor and indigent did respond to the ostentatious charity of the upper classes. Requests for help in cases of sickness were directed not only to the Protomedicato but also to other governmental boards, such as the Assunteria di Sanità. For example, see the plea filed by a widow, Colomba Polessi Ferraresi, to obtain "some help for a condition which cannot be relieved in any hospital," and other similar appeals by poor patients, in A.S.B., Assunteria di Sanità, Recapiti, 1782–84.

57. In the records of the Protomedicato and of the college, there are only two brief references to a charge of malpractice brought against a physician. In both cases, however, there is no mention of a trial. In 1648 the dean of the college wrote in his journal, or "Liber secretus," that a supernumerary member had been reprimanded for prescribing a dose of medicine exceeding the proper dose (A.S.B., Coll. Med., b. 219, "Liber secretus, 1626–1630"). In 1653, another entry in the books of the college briefly stated that a foreign doctor had been suspended from practicing for having prescribed too large an amount of some medications ("suspenditur a medendo ob excedentem dosim medicamentorum") (b. 299). In neither case is the name of the accused physician reported. In a broadsheet printed in 1654, perhaps related to the latter case, the medical college publicly defended an unnamed physician against the charge of having administered an excessive dosage of *spirito di vitriolo* to a patient affected by kidney stone (b. 234).

58. A.S.B., Coll. Med., b. 319, trial of the apothecary Domenico Sirani, deposition of Angelica Matuliani and Elena Mangini. *Mal mazzucco* was the term used to describe a fever accompanied by a bad cold, catarrh, and other symptoms of what today we refer to as the flu. *Petecchie* (petechia) denoted a rash characterized by tiny round spots.

59. Ibid., deposition of the priest Giovanni Masi.

60. Ibid., deposition of Dr. Valentino Montalto.

61. Ibid., deposition of the apothecary Domenico Sirani.

62. A.S.B., Coll. Med., b. 349, trial of Alessandro Guidetti.

63. Ibid., b. 349, for Guidetti's petition; and b. 326, for the response of the Protomedicato.

64. *Liber pro recta,* 15. A decree of Cardinal Alberoni in 1741 allowed the Protomedicato not only to impose fines but also to impose corporal punishment in case of "the most serious and deadly crimes, such as the one committed by persons ignorant of the medical art, causing the death of a patient by ill-advised prescriptions" (A.S.B., Coll. Med., b. 348).

65. Giacoma's words in the next several paragraphs are from A.S.B., Coll. Med., b. 197, trial of Marina Rondoni, 1588, deposition of Giacoma Gandolfi.

66. For example, see G. B. Ferminelli, *Il cauto flebotomista* (Bologna, 1817), 14.

67. Zacchia, *Quaestiones medico-legales,* lib. 6, tit. 1, quaest. 9, p. 470: "Sic & cum, subjectam arteriam venam jecorariam aperientes, incidunt, & in causa sunt, ut Aneurysma excitetur; & cum partes inurentes capita muscolorum, et nervos subjectos laedunt, aut tumorem aperientes eandem noxam aegris conciliant unde in causa sunt, ut partium motus in futurum aut diminuantur, aut depraventur, aut etiam in toto amittantur. . . . Pro his in judicium trahi possunt."

68. *Piumazzolo* was a pad used over the opening of the vein after bloodletting. On its use, see P. P. Magni, *Discorsi sopra il modo di sanguinare* (Rome, 1586), 10.

69. For the examination of Pernazza, see A.S.B., Coll. Med., b. 351; for the verdict of acquittal after warning, see b. 225, "Liber secretus, 1738–1755," dated August 31, 1738: "reprehensus inhibitusq., ex lege est dimissus."

70. A.S.B., Coll. Med., b. 339.

71. A.S.B., Coll. Med., b. 342, trial of Taddeo Azzoguidi, 1701, deposition of Orsola Alberici.

72. A.S.B., Coll. Med., b. 349, trial of Pietro Paolo Melloni, 1770, deposition of Antonio Zamboni, massaro of Sant'Agostino.

73. Ibid., deposition of Andrea Giovannini.

74. See A.S.B., Coll. Med., b. 349, for the sentence: "Quoad ad aliud vero caput, nempe extractionis violentae fetus, et violentae curatae deplicationis mercurii, dicimus et declaramus satis non constitisse nec constare de iisdem, ideoque reservamus iura quaecumque Tribunali pro prosequendo Processu et Actis contra eundem Melloni."

75. A.S.B., Coll. Med., b. 349: "Absolvimus a pena contra eum in sententia pred. demandata nempe scutorum quinquaginta auri, nec non ab ulteriori processu propter mercurium prestitum et extractionem fetus ex quo non fuit satis constitutum de praedictis."

76. See A.S.B., Coll. Med., bb. 324, 326, for the Protomedicato's previous warnings to Melloni.

77. Panormitanus [N. de Tudeschi], *In IV et V Decretalium librum interpretationes* (Lyons, 1547), chap. 19, "Tua nos," fol. 131v: "sic potius remittat infirmum manibus Dei, quam eum exponat dubiae medicinae"; A. de Clavasio, *Summa Angelica de casibus conscientiae* (Venice, 1487), s.v. "medicus," 235r: the physician's behavior is sinful whenever "quoad licet peritus non tamen sequitur traditiones artis: sed fantasiam sui capitis vel experimenta nova."

78. Countenancing such ruthless attitude toward a patient was definitely a new outlook. Behavior such as Melloni's anticipated the harsh methods that were used on hospital patients in the nineteenth century. On the new attitude toward hospital patients in the nineteenth century, see K. Figlio, "The Historiography of Scientific Medicine: An Invitation to the Human Sciences," *Comparative Studies in Society and History* (1979): 267–73, 283–85.

In the second half of the eighteenth century, the Protomedicato usually supported the claims of obstetric surgeons for payment of their attendance at childbirth. For example, in one such lawsuit filed in 1756 by a surgeon, the protomedici ruled that the surgeon had the right to request the balance of his fee for "extracting the fetus," although the woman's husband and a priest—both present during delivery—stated that the fetus had come out spontaneously, without the surgeon's intervention. In this case, the "fair fee" established by the protomedici for the obstetrician's services was unusually high: fifteen lire (A.S.B., Coll. Med., b. 325, case of Brizzi vs. Masetti, 1756).

79. The first legal treatise on the "privileges of the sick" that I have been able to trace was written by a jurist of the Papal States, *auditor* (judge) of the Rota Picena (the civil tribunal for Piceno, in the Papal State): Tommaso Azzio, *De infirmitate eiusque privilegiis et affectibus* (Venice, 1603). Like Zacchia's *Quaestiones medico-legales,* this text was repeatedly quoted in later tracts, including those written in Protestant countries. This legal literature on the *privilegia infirmorum* spread throughout Europe. M. Lipenius [M. Lipen] (*Bibliotheca realis juridica* [Leipzig, 1757], s.v. "aegritudo, aegrotus") listed the following works: I. V. Bechmann, *Dissertatio de aegritudine eiusque Juribus et privilegiis* (Jena, 1668) (Qu N 299.1, 15); J. H. Bergerus [J.-H. Berger], *Dissertatio de privilegiis aegrotorum* (Wittenberg, 1687) (Qu N 142.8, 35); H. Bodinus [H. von Bode], *Dissertatio de Juribus infirmorum & aegrotorum singularibus* (Halle, 1693) (Li 540); G. Fichtnerus [G. Fichtner], *Dissertatio de infirmitatis commodis* (Altdorf, 1720) (Re 78, 11). The call numbers following the facts of publication refer to the Herzog-August Bibliothek, Wolfenbüttel, where I consulted these rare books. I was not able to consult C. Friedlibius, *Dissertatio de aegrotorum Jure ac privilegiis in genere* (Zurich, 1676); and I. Ph. Streitius, *Dissertatio de Jure aegrotantium* (Erfurt, 1719), both cited by Lipenius. See also J. Calvinus, *Lexicon Juridicum: Juris caesarei simul, et canonici,* 3d ed. (Hanover, 1619), s.v. "aeger."

80. Fichtner, *De infirmitatis commodis,* 11 ff; Berger, *De privilegiis aegrotorum,* D2–F; Bechmann, *De aegritudine,* cap. 3.

81. Azzio, *De infirmitate,* 186 (on the loss of patria potestas); Bodinus, *De Juribus infirmorum,* 21 (on the husband's loss of rights to the dowry) and 254 (on the loss of patria potestas); J. J. Mühlpfort, *Dissertatio inauguralis juridica circa morbum et curam aegrotorum* (Strasburg, 1671) (H.A.B.W., Qu N 299. 1, 16), pp. 38–39 (on the loss of patria potestas and of rights to the dowry). These texts also discuss the duty of masters to provide medical care for sick servants and to pay servants' salaries during an illness.

82. Berger, *De privilegiis aegrotorum,* A2: *privilegium* was defined as "jus singulare in certae personae vel causae gratiam a Superiore constituto." See also Azzio, *De infirmitate,* chap. 9. For a general definition of the concept of privilegium, or "ius singulare," see Sebastianus Medicus, "De definitionibus," in *Tractatus . . . de variis verbis Juris* (Venice, 1584), t. 18, 295v.

83. In canon law, a medical practitioner's accountability for the death of a patient was discussed in connection with the problem of *irregularitas,* that is, that set of

circumstances which made a man ineligible for holy orders. If death was accidentally caused by a healer's negligence or ignorance, the healer would be considered *irregularis* and consequently disqualified from becoming a priest.

According to Agostino Trionfo, three conditions must be met to prevent a healer's incurring "irregularity" in the case of his patient's death: he must have acted "recta scientia," that is, knowing and applying the rules of the medical art; he must have avoided all forms of negligence or fraudulent intention (he must have acted "recta conscientia"); and he must have avoided illegal or morally unacceptable medicines ("rei decentia"). See A. de Ancona Triumphus [A. Trionfo], *Summa de potestate ecclesiastica* (Augsburg, 1473), quaestio 109; and also de Clavasio, *Summa*, s.v. "medicus," 235r: "Medicus tripliciter potest esse in culpa de morte infirmi. Prio ante factum, si quando intromittit se de eo quod ignorat: vel ad ipsum non spectat vel non sufficit ad agendum solus. Secundo in facto quoad licet peritus non tamen sequitur traditiones artis: sed fantasiam sui capitis vel experimenta nova. . . . Tertio post factum quando est negligens circa custodiam infirmi." On this issue, see the survey by P. Diepgen, *Die theologie und der ärztliche Stand* (Berlin, 1922), 41 ff.

F. Ripa (*De peste* [Lyons, 1564], 27r) summarizes the discussion of the earlier canonists on this issue, as does Zacchia (*Quaestiones medico-legales,* lib. 8, tit. 1, pp. 621–60), without adding anything new. The seventeenth-century legal tracts on patients' "privileges," instead, gave a new twist to the issue of the healer's responsibility in a patient's death. Of the three conditions that make a healer morally guilty, they especially stressed the first one — adopting a treatment that goes beyond the healer's professional competence. Their object was clearly to censure those lower practitioners who did not respect the limits of their profession. Thus the discussion about a medical man's liability was turned into one more argument against illegal medical practice. See Fichtner, *De infirmitatis commodis,* 22: "the condition for a medical practitioner not to be considered responsible for a patient's death is that the practitioner not overstep the limit of his profession, because in doing so he would be guilty of interfering with things that do not concern him."

84. According to the "lex Aquilia," medical practitioners were liable for the damages caused by their negligence or lack of skill: "Imperitia culpae adnumeratur, veluti si medicus ideo servuum tuum occiderit, quod eum male secuerit, aut perperam ei medicamentum dederit" (Digest, I, 4, 3, 7). However, this same law established that they could be prosecuted solely in civil court, the only remedy being a claim for damages. On the "lex Aquilia," see A. Berger, *Encyclopedic Dictionary of Roman Law,* Transactions of the American Philosophical Society, n.s., vol. 43, pt. 2 (Philadelphia, 1953), 352.

In Roman law, criminal prosecution of a medical practitioner was possible only if there was evidence of foul play, as for instance in the case of poisoning (in which case, the practitioner would be charged under the "lex Cornelia de sicariis et veneficiis"). On this issue, see R. Bozzoni, *I medici e il diritto romano* (Naples, 1904), 210–34, esp. 228–30. A more detailed survey of the same issue is offered in K. H. Below, *Der Arzt im römischen Recht* (Munich, 1953), 120–34. A brief (and not very clear) summary is given by D. W. Amundsen, "The Liability of the Physician in Roman Law," in *International Symposium on Society, Medicine and Law*, ed. H. Karplus (Amsterdam, 1973), 17–30.

Pre-Justinian legislation did admit the criminal liability of a medical practitioner in case of manslaughter, which was punishable with exile or even the death penalty; see Paulus, *Sententiae*, 5.23, 19: "Si ex eo medicamento quod ad salutem hominis vel ad remedium datum erat, homo perierit, is qui dederit, si honestior sit, in insulam relegatur, humilior autem capite punitur." This law, however, was not included in the Digest, which substituted in its place a milder rule: "Medical practitioners should not be held liable for [a patient's] death, but for everything they committed as a result of lack of skills" (Digest, I, 18, 6,7).

85. E. Speckham, *Quaestionum juris caesarei, pontifici et saxonici Centuria Prima* (Wittenberg, 1611), quaestio 24. See also Rodericus à Castro, *Medicus-politicus, sive de officiis medico-politicis Tractatus* (Hamburg, 1614), xxiii; Gailius [A. Gail], *Practicarum Observationum ad processum iudiciarium libri duo* (Cologne, 1580), lib. 2, observ. 3, num. 26.

In the Hapsburg Empire, however, a constitution promulgated by Charles V in 1532 established that a medical practitioner could be tried for manslaughter in criminal court, if the magistrate so willed (J. J. Speidel, *Speculum juridico-politico-philologico historicarum observationum* [Nuremberg, 1657], s.v. "Artzney, Doctor," p. 75; I. Fischer, *Ärztliche Standespflichten und Standesfragen: Eine historische Studie* [Vienna, 1912], 158–59).

86. Zacchia, *Quaestiones*, lib. 6, quaestio 1, p. 445.

87. Fichtner, *De infirmitatis commodis*, 20–21. After repeating, with most authors, that "in criminal cases, accidental fault or neglect should not be equated to deliberate injury," Fichtner argues that "physicians and surgeons who do not use the utmost care, or who make mistakes out of neglect or lack of skills—for example, abandoning the patient, prescribing useless remedies, etc.—are not only liable for damages under the Aquilia law but can also be tried criminally by decision of the judge." This rule, however, he adds, should be applied only to unlicensed healers, such as "Empirici, Circumforanei, Errones, Impostores, ceterique experimenta per mortem facientes Medicastri, qui non verentur in hominum vitas ac corpora grassari."

88. For the right of victims of medical error to file suit, see the "lex Aquilia" (Digest, I, 4, 3 § 7), on which see n. 84, above. Discussing the case of an unlicensed healer tried for a patient's death, the jurist Io. F. Schenardi (*Consilia, seu Responsa Juris* [Milan, 1616], consilium 8, fol. 43r) argued for the applicability of the "Aquilia" law and, therefore, the healer's liability for damages.

89. It would be interesting to compare the Protomedicato's sentences in cases of malpractice with those of other law courts. A very interesting case of malpractice in seventeenth-century London was recently examined in detail by Harold J. Cook (*Trials of an Ordinary Doctor: Joannes Groenevelt in Seventeenth-Century London* [Balti-

more, 1994]). Interestingly, in this case, the London College of Physicians adopted a very severe attitude, not only heavily fining the culprit but even committing him to imprisonment in Newgate for twelve weeks. The severity exhibited in this case, however, seems to be due to the fact that Groenevelt, a foreign physician with a largely surgical practice, had opposed the views of the conservative Fellows of the college in several ways and was held in disfavor by many of them.

For the Middle Ages, see M. P. Cosman, "Medieval Medical Malpractice: The Dicta and the Dockets," *Bulletin of the New York Academy of Medicine* 49, no. 1 (January 1973): 22–47. This study describes cases heard by the mayor and city councillors in medieval London (who also consulted with the officers of the guild of barber-surgeons). The verdicts against medical practitioners in these cases seem to be more severe than those delivered by the Bolognese Protomedicato. Those healers found guilty of malpractice were sentenced not only to return the advance deposited by the patient but also to pay damages and, sometimes, to serve prison terms (27, 40–41). See also M. P. Cosman, "Medical Malpractice and Peer Review in Medieval England," *Transactions of the American Academy of Ophthalmology and Otolaryngology* 80, no. 3, pt. 1 (1975): 293–97; and idem, "The Medieval Medical Third Party: Compulsory Consultation and Malpractice Insurance," *Annals of Plastic Surgery* 8, no. 1 (1982): 152–62. On malpractice trials in the United States in the nineteenth century, see K. A. De Ville, *Medical Malpractice in Nineteenth Century America* (New York, 1990).

90. Molière, *L'amour médecin,* act 2, scene 4: "A dead man is but a dead man, and not of much consequence, but a neglected formality is harmful to the entire medical profession."

Chapter 5: The Medical System as Seen by the Sick

1. In reconstructing the patients' view of the medical system, I have found most helpful the ethnographic questionnaire by E. Ackerknecht ("On the Collecting of Data," in *Medicine and Ethnography* [Stuttgart-Wein, 1971], 117–19). For an anthropological approach to this issue, see also A. Kleinmann, *Patients and Healers in the Context of Culture* (Berkeley, Calif., 1980). A model ethnographic description of the relationship between healer and patient was offered by V. Turner, "A Ndembu Doctor in Practice," in *Magic, Faith, and Healing,* ed. A. Kiev (London, 1974), 230–63. For a fascinating account of the relationship between a sixteenth-century healer and his patients, see M. MacDonald, *Mystical Bedlam: Madness, Anxiety, and Healing in Seventeenth-Century England* (Cambridge, England, 1981). Also centered on the physician-patient relationship is a brilliant study by B. Duden, *Geschichte unter der Haut* (Stuttgart, 1987), which offers a detailed reconstruction of women patients' perception of body and illness in eighteenth-century Germany. It was published in English as *The Woman under the Skin: A Doctor's Patients in Eighteenth-Century Germany* (Cambridge, Mass., 1991).

2. A.S.B., Coll. Med., b. 340, trial of Fabrizio Ingegneri, 1678, deposition of Giovanni Bongianini.

3. For examples of charges brought simultaneously against a healer by several patients, see A.S.B., Coll. Med.—b. 342, *contra Antonium Mondini,* 1689; b. 351, trial of the barber Domenico Toni, 1742.

4. A.S.B., Coll. Med., b. 350, trial of the distiller Vincenzo Allegri, 1663.

5. A.S.B., Coll. Med., b. 341, trial of the surgeon G. B. Terrarossa, 1670.

6. A.S.B., Coll. Med., b. 350, trial of the distiller Aurelio Righettini, 1669, deposition of Antonio Monti.

7. A.S.B., Coll. Med., b. 341, trial of Antonio Mazzetti, 1691.

8. A.S.B., Coll. Med., b. 341, trial of the surgeon G. B. Terrarossa, 1689.

9. P. Zacchia, *Quaestiones medico-legales* (Lyons, 1662), 409.

10. A.S.B., Coll. Med., b. 339, trial of Fabrizio Ingegneri, 1672, deposition of Ippolita Riccioli.

11. A.S.B., Coll. Med., b. 213, deposition of the physician Bartolini, 1601.

12. F. Giusberti, "Tra povertà e malattia: Il S. Orsola a Bologna dal XVII al XVIII secolo," *Annali della Fondazione Luigi Einaudi* 13 (1979): 135, 147. The stock of words used by the people of Bologna to indicate illness seems rather limited and standardized. For a very different case, see C. O. Freke, "The Diagnosis of Disease among the Subanum of Mindanao," *American Anthropologist* 63 (1961); in a culture where the official role of healer barely existed and the sick routinely resorted to self-therapy, the anthropologist found an extremely varied and diversified terminology of disease.

13. A.S.B., Coll. Med., b. 319, license issued to Caterina Panzacchia, 1647; cf. b. 321, license issued to Anna Beloi, 1697.

14. Dorothy and Roy Porter (*Patient's Progress: Doctors and Doctoring in Eighteenth-Century England* [Stanford, Calif., 1989]) found the same in eighteenth-century England. Their study indicates that medical self-help was common among the English upper classes; on self-treatment, see 35, 38, 110, 209; on self-diagnosis, see 78.

15. A.S.B., Coll. Med., b. 342, *contra Annam,* 1698, deposition of Cattarina Rambotti.

16. A.S.B., Coll. Med., b. 350, deposition of Benedetto Rubbi, 1663.

17. A.S.B., Coll. Med., b. 339, trial of Fabrizio Ingegneri, 1672.

18. Ibid.

19. Ibid.

20. In the case of women, sexual honor was an ulterior motive for the presence of kin or friends during a medical visit. Ippolita Riccioli insisted on being visited by Fabricio in her daughter's presence. "Many times the women in my household have opened the door to this Fabricio, but they never saw what he did, because when he treated me there was no one around but one of my daughters, whose name is Caterina" (ibid.).

21. Ibid. Ingegneri had already been tried in 1666 by the Protomedicato and had been forbidden to practice (A.S.B., Coll. Med., b. 350).

22. A.S.B., Coll. Med., b. 320, sentence of Fabrizio Ingegneri, November 4, 1672. Ingegneri was tried again by the Protomedicato in 1678, after a patient filed charges against him (b. 350). I was not able to locate the verdict in this later trial.

23. A.S.B., Coll. Med., b. 339, trial of Fabrizio Ingegneri, 1672.

24. A.S.B., Coll. Med., b. 342, trial of Fanti, 1695, deposition of Angelo Ratti.

25. Ibid.

26. A.S.B., Coll. Med., b. 236, *Catalogo de Signori Dottori tanto bolognesi che forestieri che di presente ponno praticare la professione di Medicina in Bologna,* 1698.

27. According to Ivan Waddington, at the end of the eighteenth century in England the truly important distinction of medical roles was not the conventional distinction between physician, surgeon, and apothecary, but that between general practitioner and consultant. General practitioners formed the lower level of the medical hierarchy, while consultants, to whom patients turned for medical advice, were at the top. This seems somewhat similar to what I find in early modern Bologna. See I. Waddington, "General Practitioners and Consultants in Early Nineteenth-Century England: The Sociology of an Intra-Professional Conflict," in *Health Care and Popular Medicine in Nineteenth Century England,* ed. J. Woodward and D. Richards (London, 1977), 164–88.

28. A lucid and immensely suggestive description of two such "models of healing" has been drawn by Peter Brown in relation to early Christianity. I believe that Brown's outline of two "therapeutic systems"—a "vertical" one, based on "a high-pitched idiom of relationships of dependence"; and a "horizontal" one, based on self-help — are applicable well beyond the context he analyzed and are in fact a persistent aspect of the history of healing in European history. See P. Brown, *The Cult of the Saints: Its Rise and Function in Early Christianity* (Chicago, 1981), 113–20.

29. Barbers who applied for a license in the middle of the seventeenth century had to take an official examination that asked, among other things, "whether they draw blood only on the order of a physician, or also by request of the sick and their relatives" (A.S.B., Coll. Med., b. 213). For many cases of patients who had themselves bled without first consulting a physician see G. Pomata, "Barbieri e comari," in *Medicina, erbe e magia* (Milan, 1981), 166, 179.

There is ample evidence that bloodletting was also a popular form of self-therapy in early modern England; see Porter and Porter, *Patient's Progress,* 45, 50, 66, 170.

30. A.S.B., Coll. Med., b. 340, case of Negrini vs. Marocchi.

31. The statutes of the Medical College of Mantua (1559), rubr. 25, ruled: "Physicians should not treat themselves. Since we believe that it is very dangerous for somebody affected by a serious illness to treat oneself, we order that no physician, in any kind of illness, medicate himself or prescribe his own medicines; but that he turn to another physician for treatment" (G. Carra and A. Zanca, "Gli Statuti del Collegio dei medici di Mantova," in *Atti e memorie dell'Accademia Virgiliana di Mantova* [Mantua, 1977], 33). On this prohibition, see also Rodericus à Castro, *Medicus-politicus, sive de officiis medico-politicis Tractatus* (Hamburg, 1614), chap. 15. Zacchia (*Quaes-*

tiones medico-legales, lib. 6, quaestio 7, 31, p. 464) acknowledges that this is the common opinion but specifies that self-therapy for a physician is not a true "sin" but a simple "imprudence" ("Videndum, an Medicus curando se ipsum . . . aliquo modo erret; et in hoc quidem vulgi opinio est, hoc Medico non licere. . . . At ego quidem, ut ex mea sententia loquar, magis imprudentiae, quam peccati cuiuspiam insimulandum censeo, qui sibi ipsi in gravioribus praecipue morbis medetur").

On the attitude of eighteenth-century English physicians toward their patients's self-help, see Porter and Porter, *Patient's Progress,* 134–37: although critical of self-therapy, physicians had to put up with it in everyday life.

32. Harold J. Cook has similarly argued that the physician's role in early modern England was often a "pastoral" one, limited to giving advice about an appropriate regimen; see his "Good Advice and Little Medicine: The Professional Authority of Early Modern English Physicians," *Journal of British Studies* 33 (1994): 1–31.

33. A.S.B., Coll. Med., b. 349, trial of the charlatan Boschetti. Boschetti was licensed to sell ointments for external use; see b. 325 for his license.

34. On G. A. Galli, see S. Mazzetti, *Repertorio de' Professori antichi e moderni dell'Università e dell'Istituto di Bologna* (Bologna, 1847), 136–37.

35. The quotations are taken, respectively, from A.S.B., Coll. Med.—b. 350, deposition of Agata Aspertini, 1633; b. 349, trial of the surgeon Simone Gordini, 1759, deposition of Pietro Manfrara, tailor; b. 342, trial of the healer Francesco Rasponi, 1702, deposition of Carlo Pedrazzi; and b. 340, deposition of Caterina Casoli, midwife, tried for administering oral remedies, 1677.

The traditional notions of disease moving inside the body and of the use of bloodletting to control its movement emerge also in the testimony of another midwife, in 1781: "The hemorrhage stopped, and the delivery also stopped, and the belly of the woman swelled a great deal, so that she died of major inflammation after a few days, although surgeon Bazzano tried in every possible way to draw labor back *[richiamare il parto],* with fomentations and sweet almond oil, and finally, by opening the foot vein" (A.S.B., Assunteria di Governo delle Comunità, Recapiti, b. 8, trial of the surgeon Domenico Bazzani, deposition of Anastasia Bergonzini).

36. A patient specified, for instance, that his disease was "the French disease, that is to say bad blood" (A.S.B., Coll. Med., b. 342, *contra Antonium Mondini,* deposition of Antonio Golino, 1696).

37. A.S.B., Tribunale criminale del Torrone, "Fasciculum diversorum processuum criminalium fabricator. contra diversos tempore epithemico pro conservanda sanitate, annor. 1630, 1631, 1632," cc. 576–84.

38. Ibid.

39. A.S.B., Coll. Med., b. 340, trial of the barber Carlo Marocchi, 1687, deposition of Domenico Negrini, plaintiff. In 1670, Bonaventura Gamma filed charges against the surgeon Terrarossa, arguing that the electuary prescribed by the surgeon had brought about results opposite to those of any good medicine—that is, it had hindered evacuation (b. 341, trial of G. B. Terrarossa, 1670).

The belief that "the clap" *(scolatione)* could be trapped inside the body, with very dangerous consequences to health, was still widespread in the nineteenth century among peasants from the Umbria region. See Z. Zanetti, *La medicina delle nostre donne* (Foligno, 1892; reprint, 1978), 241.

40. A.S.B., Coll. Med., b. 350, trial of the distiller Gioseffo Braccesi, 1662, deposition of Marco Antonio Trebbi.

41. A.S.B., Coll. Med., b. 341, trial of Andrea Volta, 1691, deposition of the defendant.

42. A.S.B., Coll. Med., b. 341, trial of G. B. Terrarossa, surgeon, 1670, deposition of the defendant.

43. Ibid.

44. A.S.B., Coll. Med., b. 350, trial of Carlo Marocchi, barber, 1662, deposition of the defendant.

45. A.S.B., Coll. Med., b. 341, trial of G. B. Terrarossa, 1670, deposition of the defendant.

46. On these ancient and long-lived healing techniques, see A. Benedicenti, *Malati, medici e farmacisti: Storia dei rimedi attraverso i secoli e delle teorie che ne spiegano l'azione sull'organismo* (Milan, 1925), 2:984–92. The use of cauteries is described in a barber-surgeon's handbook: P. P. Magni, *Discorso sopra il modo di fare i cauterij o rottorij a corpi humani* (Rome, 1588).

47. On the dichotomy of hot and cold in humoral theory, see M. H. Logan, "Selected References on the Hot-Cold Theory of Disease," *Medical Anthropology Newsletter* 6, no. 8 (1975). For a general overview of these symbolic opposites in Greek medicine, see G.E.R. Lloyd, "The Hot and the Cold, the Dry and the Wet in Greek Philosophy," *Journal of Hellenistic Studies* 84 (1964).

On the survival of the hot-cold dichotomy in present-day popular medicine, see R. L. Currier, "The Hot-Cold Syndrome and Symbolic Balance in Mexican and Spanish-American Folk Medicine," *Ethnology* (1970); and W. Madsen, "Value Conflicts and Folk Psychotherapy in South Texas," in Kiev, *Magic, Faith, and Healing,* 423. See also E. Messer, "Hot-Cold Classification: Theoretical and Practical Implications of a Mexican Study," *Social Science and Medicine* 15B (1981): 133–54.

48. M. Vegetti, "Metafora politica e immagine del corpo nella medicina greca," in *Tra Edipo e Euclide: Forme del sapere antico* (Milan, 1983), 46.

49. M. Bakhtin, *Rabelais and His World,* trans. Helene Iswolsky (Bloomington, Ind., 1984), 355–61.

50. Ibid., 357, translation slightly modified.

51. Ibid., 317, 339.

52. A.S.B., Coll. Med., b. 339, trial of Fabrizio Ingegneri, 1672, deposition of Ippolita Riccioli. *Ascites* was the learned word for dropsy. *Mal d'oppilatione* (oppilation disease) was a term commonly used in early modern Bologna; for instance, in a chronicle of the healing miracles performed by an image of the Virgin in early-seventeenth-century Bologna, we find the case of a woman, Lucia de Passarini, suffer-

ing from "male d'opilatione" (described as "a contraction of nerves so that, crouching and swollen, she looked like a balloon"); see Sister Diodata Malvasia, *La venuta et i progressi miracolosi della S.ma Madonna dipinta da S. Luca posta sul monte della Guardia dall'anno che ci venne 1160 sin all'anno 1617* (Bologna, 1617), 178.

53. In classical Latin, *oppilare* means to close a door or to obstruct a flow. In early modern Italian, the term kept its primary semantic association with the obstruction of flowing waters, but it was often employed with a medical meaning. The Italian lexicologist Niccolò Tommaseo (*Dizionario della lingua italiana* [Turin, 1861–79], vol. 8, s.v. "oppilare") lists several examples of such medical uses of the word: "Per li tristi cibi, e bever acque crude, e dormir al sereno, vennero la maggior parte a cadere in alcune febbri continue; per le quali la maggior parte di loro vennero ad oppilare, e dalle oppilazioni a gonfiare" ("Because of bad food, and unboiled water, and sleeping outside, most of them fell ill with continuous fevers; in consequence of which many suffered from oppilation, and the oppilation made them swell"); "Io medicai un giovinetto, che per alcune terzane bastarde si aveva oppilato; e per le oppilazioni si aveva enfiato tutto di modo che era quasi idropico" ("I medicated a young lad, who got oppilated following some tertian, bastard fevers; and in consequence of the oppilation he was so swollen that he was almost hydropic").

For examples of the medical use of the term see also *Oxford English Dictionary*, under "oppilation." At the entry "oppilare," Du Cange's dictionary of medieval Latin lists an interesting variant of the term's meaning, from Gregory of Tours (*Historiae Francorum*, bk. 10, chap. 8): "Concubinae ejus, instigante, ut quidam asserunt, invidia, maleficiis sensum ejus oppilaverunt." In this case, the word meant to hinder ejaculation, or cause impotence. In early modern Italy, the term *oppilation* was used to refer to illnesses affecting both men and women, but it often indicated the female condition of amenorrhea; see, for one example of this use of the term, R. Merzario, "La donna e il suo corpo: Un tentativo di analisi (Diocesi di Como, 1550–1650)," in *L'erba delle donne* (Rome, 1978), 72.

54. An apt reminder of this view of disease comes from the printed advertisement for Acqua di Nocera—a mineral water imported and sold in mid-seventeenth-century Bologna for its curative properties—which stated that the water's "primary activity and energy" consisted in "making the humors of the body more fluid, and opening up the body's channels" (A.S.B., Coll. Med., b. 351).

55. The medieval idea of "humidum radicale," ("radical moisture") implied a perception of the flowing of life as a gradual process of desiccation; see M. McVaugh, "The Humidum Radicale in Thirteenth Century Medicine," *Traditio* 30 (1974); T. S. Hall, "Life, Death, and Radical Moisture," *Clio Medica* 6 (1971); P. H. Niebyl, "Old Age, Fever, and the Lamp Metaphor," *Journal of the History of Medicine and Allied Sciences* 26 (1972).

56. G. Bollème, "L'enjeu du corps et la Bibliothèque bleue," *Ethnologie française* 6 (1976): 288. The *Bibliothèque bleue* was a series of printed booklets for popular readership in early modern France.

57. *Sancti Antonini Summa theologica,* pt. 3, p. 281: "Et haec (poenitentia) est confectio quasi reubarbarum, quod facit vomere"; "Purgativa humorum malorum, id est expulsiva vitiorum, hoc est paenitentia."

58. *Preparamento del Pastarino, per medicarsi in questi sospettosi tempi di peste* (Bologna, 1577), 16. This text is mentioned in P. Camporesi, *Il pane selvaggio* (Bologna, 1980), 67–68.

59. L. A. Muratori, *Del governo della peste* (Modena, 1714), 32.

60. On the connection between evacuation therapies and self-help, see also Porter and Porter, *Patient's Progress,* 39, 160 ff.

61. There is, however, one exception to this pattern — exorcism. The ritual of exorcism had strong analogies to evacuative therapy, and yet the exorcist, being a priest, obviously held a role of authority over the patient. The similarities between exorcism and medical evacuation are pointed out by Aline Rousselle in a fascinating study of Saint Martin's healing miracles ("Du sanctuaire au thaumaturge: La guérison en Gaule au IVe siècle," *Annales E.S.C.* 31 [1976]: 1098; see also her *Croire et guérir: La foi en Gaule dans l'Antiquité tardive* [Paris, 1990]). In order to exorcise a possessed man, for instance, Martin put his fingers in the man's mouth, and the demon, incapable of exiting from that opening, was evacuated from below with a belly discharge. The saint, Rousselle observes pointedly, adopted the most traditional of medical treatments — evacuation (1104).

On the practice of exorcism between the sixteenth and the seventeenth centuries, as reconstructed through the trials of the Inquisition Tribunal of Modena, see M. O'Neil, "Sacerdote ovvero strione: Ecclesiastical and Superstitious Remedies in Sixteenth Century Italy," in *Understanding Popular Culture,* ed. S. Kaplan (Paris, 1984); for a general overview, see also O. Franceschini, "L'esorcista," in *Cultura popolare in Emilia Romagna. Medicina, erbe e magia* (Milan, 1981), 100–115.

62. On the function of evacuation as the shedding of corporeal surplus, see Zacchia, *Quaestiones medico-legales,* 405: "Omnium quae superfluunt salubris suo tempore est evacuatio, quia Naturam velut a sarcina sublevat, quae aliquando ex se, ipsum superfluentem sanguinem, et ipsissimum semen nonmodo absque noxa, se maximo cum commodo sponte excernit."

63. On the slow decline of Galenism, especially in the field of therapeutics, see O. Temkin, *Galenism: Rise and Decline of a Medical Philosophy* (Ithaca, N.Y., 1973), 165 ff. In early-eighteenth-century Bologna, Morgagni still used Galen's texts to teach medical students (168).

64. Vegetti, "Metafora politica," 55–56; see also idem, "Modelli di medicina in Galeno," in *Tra Edipo e Euclide* (on the Galenic doctrine as a synthesis of Hippocratic and Aristotelian themes). For a general survey of the political metaphors of the body, see O. Temkin, "Metaphors of Human Biology," in *The Double Face of Janus* (Baltimore, 1977), 271–83. On the symbolic link between the image of the body and urban space in an early modern context, see N. Z. Davis, "The Sacred and the Body Social in Sixteenth-Century Lyon," *Past and Present,* no. 90 (February 1981).

65. "Hippocratic clinical practice was not concerned with the 'good management' of physiology and its organicist, politic models. In fact, the Hippocratic Corpus lacks one of the basic requisites for such a theory, namely a view of nature as an active, purposeful entity" (Vegetti, "Metafora politica," 54). In contrast, a providential view of nature was present in the Aristotelian-Stoic tradition, in which the Galenic doctrine was rooted (Vegetti, "Modelli di medicina," 122 ff). For a general study of the doctrine of the healing power of nature, see M. Neuburger, *The Doctrine of the Healing Power of Nature throughout the Course of Time* (New York, 1926).

66. A.S.B., Coll. Med., b. 352, case of Zamboni vs. Bonfiglioli, 1705, deposition of Dr. Lodovico Bartoli.

67. Let it be recalled, incidentally, that seventeenth-century medicine was deeply interested in the study of metabolism, as shown, among other things, by the influential work of Santorio Santorio (*De statica medicina* [Venice, 1614]).

68. A.S.B., Coll. Med., b. 352, case of Zamboni vs. Bonfiglioli.

69. As a patient said: "I observed the rule of life that he gave me" (A.S.B., Coll. Med., b. 340, cure testimonial of Gio. Solieri on behalf of Dr. Ottavio Pellini, 1675). The prescription of a "rule of life" was acknowledged as a specific therapeutic performance that deserved remuneration (b. 195, charge filed by Iulio Dondini against the false physician Alfonso Riccoboni, 1599: "I paid him three *piastre* several times, as his fee for prescribing me a rule of life").

70. On social rules about food as a "relational idiom," see H. Medick and D. Sabean, "Interest and Emotion in Family and Kinship Studies: A Critique of Social History and Anthropology," in *Interest and Emotion: Essays on the Study of Family and Kinship,* ed. H. Medick and D. Sabean (Cambridge, England, 1984), 13–15; and D. Sabean, "The Bonds of Social Unity: 'Community' through the Eyes of a Thirteen-Year-Old Witch," in *Power in the Blood: Popular Culture and Village Discourse in Early Modern Germany* (Cambridge, England, 1984), 94–112. For a classic anthropological analysis of dietary rules, see M. Douglas, "Deciphering a Meal," in *Implicit Meanings: Essays in Anthropology* (London, 1975).

71. B.C.A.B., Fondo Inquisizione, MS. b. 1882, cc. 134–38 (italics added).

72. B.C.A.B., MS. B 1883, "Contra Rosam Paleottam, exturcam baptizatam ob esum carnis diebus ab ecclesia vetitis," 1699.

73. The verdict in her case also specified that, in addition to the above, she had to recite the rosary three times (ibid., c. 599).

74. Just like medical prescriptions, these certificates of exemption from fasting were supposed to be signed only by a physician, and not by a lower practitioner. Several specimens of such certificates are located among the Protomedicato's papers (A.S.B., Coll. Med., b. 353 *bis*). The Catholic physician's proper conduct vis-à-vis Lenten rules is discussed by Zacchia (*Quaestiones medico-legales,* lib. 5, tit. 1, quaest. 1, "De ieiunio et Quadragesima"). See also the entry under "jeunes" in *Dictionnaire d'archéologie chrétienne et de la liturgie* (Paris, 1927), 7:2481–502.

75. *Relazioni degli Ambasciatori veneti al Senato,* ed. M. Alberi, ser. 2, vol. 3 (Flo-

rence, 1846), quoted in C. King, "The Liturgical and Commemorative Allusions in Raphael's 'Transfiguration and Failure to Heal,'" *Journal of the Warburg and Courtauld Institute* 45 (1982): 152 ff.

76. See P. Zacchia, *Il vitto quaresimale* (Rome, 1636); and A. Petroni, *De Victu Romanorum, et sanitate tuenda* (Rome, 1581); and idem, *Del viver delli Romani et del conservar la sanità* (Rome, 1592). Both Petroni and Zacchia argue that fasting during Lent is beneficial not only from a religious but also from a medical viewpoint, because it purifies the body and prevents illnesses. "This rule [Lenten fasting] has been established for the season of spring, when the body, overfilled in the wintertime, needs to be depleted. . . . Thanks to Lenten fasting, human bodies expurge slowly, without the damage that can derive from medically induced evacuation, which is sudden and can endanger the body even to the point of death" (Petroni, *Del viver delli Romani,* 266). Once again, we see that penance (Lent) is associated with evacuation. On Petroni and Ignatius Loyola, see G. Bardi, *Medicus politico-catholicus* (Genoa, 1644), 226–32; and G. Moroni, *Dizionario d'erudizione storico-ecclesiastica* (Venice, 1847), 42:134.

77. *Sancti Antonini Summa theologica,* 281: "medicina conservativa, ut electuarium, hoc est heucharistia."

78. Innocentius Quartus Pont. Maximus, *Super Libros Quinque Decretalium* (Frankfurt-am-Main, 1570), tit. 12, cap. 19, "Tua nos," fol. 512v: "De infirmo autem videtur, quod non peccat, si non obediat medico, quia nec praelatus est eius, nec aliter tenetur sibi obedire."

This opinion is shared by Panormitanus, *In IV et V Decretalium Librum Interpretationes* (Lyons, 1547), 131r: "Infirmi non oboedientes medicis non incurrunt crimen inoboedientiae"; I. Andrea, *In Quintum Decretalium Librum Novella Commentaria* (Venice, 1581), 63r; and Felinus, *Super Decretal. Lib. j,* tit. 32, cap. 19, "Tua nos," 206v: "Infirmus non oboediens medico non peccat."

79. G. B. Codronchi, *De christiana ac tuta medendi ratione* (Ferrara, 1591), 139–43: "Infirmus non obediens Medico . . . peccat." Thus Codronchi gave a religious sanction to the patient's duty to obey the doctor. By contrast, sixteenth-century medical deontology had justified the patient's duty to obey the physician on purely practical and professional grounds, with no religious overtones. See for instance L. Botallo, "Tractatus de medici et aegri munere," in *Opera Omnia* (1512; Lyons, 1660), 41–45; published in Italian as L. Botallo, *I doveri del medico e del malato,* ed. L. Careri and A. Boggetti Fassone (Turin, 1981).

80. The behavior of the archpriest Petroni is described in A.S.B., Coll. Med., b. 341, trial of G. B. Terrarossa, 1689, deposition of Michele Pellegrini.

When the charlatan Ulivieri brought his remedies to the Protomedicato for inspection, he described them as "all composed of herbal juices, without any corrosive ingredients." To prove it, he offered to "freely eat and swallow them" (A.S.B., Coll. Med., b. 236). This charlatan offered to do spontaneously what was sometimes officially required by the medical authorities. For example, the statutes of the Medical College of Mantua established that "the peddler, after disclosing the ingredients of the electuary to the Head Officer of the Apothecaries with a solemn oath, will then proceed to taste a little of that electuary in the presence of the same Officer" (Carra and Zanca, "Gli Statuti del Collegio dei Medici di Mantova," 36).

81. A.S.B., Coll. Med., b. 349, trial of Alessio Porta, apothecary, March 10, 1746, deposition of Pietro Volta.

82. By definition, the idea of a weak boundary between the body and the world is ambivalent. For an anthropological analysis of this issue, see B. J. Colby, "Psychological Orientations," in *Handbook of Middle American Indians* (Austin, Tex., 1967), 427; and L. Paul, "Work and Sex in a Guatemalan Village," in *Woman, Culture, and Society,* ed. M. Rosaldo and L. Lamphere (Stanford, Calif., 1974), 299.

CHAPTER 6: THE DISAPPEARANCE OF THE AGREEMENT FOR A CURE

1. A.S.B., Coll. Med., b. 219, "Liber secretus, 1626–30," January 4, 1633. The protomedici occasionally met at the dean's house (usually when the dean was ill). This specific case was concluded with an extrajudicial settlement mediated by the protomedici.

2. A.S.B., Coll. Med., b. 233, *Bando del Protomedico per Roma, e per tutto lo Stato Ecclesiastico, mediate, & immediate, sottoposto alla Santa Sede Apostolica* (Rome, 1614).

3. This text was a fragment by Ulpian inserted in the Digest under the heading "De variis et extraordinariis cognitionibus." The right to appeal to a magistrate in order to obtain payment for medical services was granted to "those who promise a cure for a given part of the body or for a given disease," but was denied to those who "employ magic or exorcism," because "these practices do not belong to medicine" (Digest, 50, 13; see above, chap. 2, n. 55, for a citation of the entire passage). The significance of this law in the origins of medical licensing is yet to be studied; as far as I know, no study of the professionalization of medicine takes it into account. Of course, I do not mean to suggest that the intent of Ulpian's text was to introduce a form of professional licensing. I simply want to point out that this text was re-interpreted and used in early modern jurisprudence against all unlicensed practitioners.

Ulpian's original intent might have been very different and should be reconstructed contextually (which cannot be done here). One might ask, for instance, which healers the Roman lawmakers of the third century were trying to disqualify by ruling that they had no right to payment. An interesting answer was suggested in 1577, in a suit over illegal practice filed by the guild of the apothecaries and physicians of Orléans against an unlicensed healer named Hureau (see chap. 2, n. 102, above). The lawyer for the guild, Anné Robert, wrote a summary of the arguments used by both parties. See A. Robertus, *Rerum Judicatarum,* libri 4 (Geneva, 1604), lib. 1, cap. 5, "De empiricis qui conceptis precum et verborum formulis morbos curare profitentur," pp. 51–81. Hureau, defined by the physicians as a charlatan, treated his patients with medicines but also with prayers and words. The doctors therefore accused him of practicing magic, which was not to be considered part of medicine according to the law "De variis et extraordinariis cognitionibus." Hureau's lawyer retorted that with this law, Ulpian had excluded prayers and exorcisms from medicine because, as a pagan, he wished to oppose Christian healers. "Exorcisationes in morbis reiicit Ulpianus sed cum paganus esset, christianos criminari et impostorum nota calumniari voluit" (59). I find this hypothesis interesting.

4. J. Verdier, *Essai sur la jurisprudence de la médecine en France* (Alençon, 1762), 93. The same rule also applied in the Kingdom of Sardinia. For example, in 1768 the surgeon Antiogo Serra asked the protomedico of Cagliari to set the "fair price" for his surgical services, so that he could demand payment from his patients. The protomedico decided that "since he did not have a license as a surgeon, as he himself confessed, he had no right to be paid" (A.S.C., Regia Segreteria di Stato, 2 serie, b. 863).

5. In France, too, apparently, the sums requested by charlatans for their services were often reduced by the medical authorities (Verdier, *Jurisprudence,* 96).

6. A.S.B., Coll. Med., b. 219.

7. A.S.B., Coll. Med.—b. 341, for the interrogation of Guarnieri; b. 320, for the protomedici's sentence.

8. A.S.B., Coll. Med., b. 233. The same rule can also be found in other European countries. In 1717 a barber of Dresden filed claims for nonpayment against a patient whom he had treated with oral medications. The barber lost his case and was sentenced to a fine for exceeding the limits of his profession. See G. C. Bastineller, *De medico ex voluntate aegroti perperam curante* (Wittenberg, 1719) (H.A.B.W., Qu N 142.8 36), pp. 7–9. Similar cases are reported in J. C. Hasenest, *Des medicinischen Richters oder Actorum physicomedico-forensium Collegii medici Onoldini* (Onolzbach-Ansbach, 1756), vol. 1, casus 14, pp. 100–117; vol. 2, casus 22, pp. 108–34; vol. 2, casus 26, pp. 166–72.

9. In 1678, the apothecary Antoni asked the protomedici to revise a bill for medicines which a patient had refused to pay. The protomedici ruled that it was not possible to establish the "fair price" that was due to the apothecary because one of the medicines had not been prepared according to the rules of the Antidotario, and the apothecary therefore had no right to payment (A.S.B., Coll. Med., b. 320).

The same thing happened in the case of a patient who filed a suit against the apothecary Nucci in 1696. The patient had found a bill questionable and asked the Protomedicato to establish the "fair price." The court ruled that no payment was required because the apothecary had neglected to ask for a physician's written prescription before preparing the medicines (A.S.B., Coll. Med., bb. 342, 321, case of Barbieri vs. Nucci, 1696).

10. As stated in the Roman Protomedicato's decree of 1614: "No one, practicing any part of medicine, shall turn for payment to any court other than ours" (A.S.B., Coll. Med., b. 233).

11. "Ex quo ipse Marochius absque licentia medicandi est contra formam

decreti Collegii" (A.S.B., Coll. Med., bb. 340, 320, case of Marocchi vs. Mazzetti, 1678).

12. A.S.B., Coll. Med., b. 340.

13. "Licentiam et facultatem medendi non habebat nec habet" (A.S.B., Coll. Med., b. 319, case of Bugognoli vs. Quirini, 1618). One scudo was equal to five lire (A. Martini, *Manuale di metrologia* [Turin, 1883], 92).

14. A.S.B., Coll. Med., b. 319, case of Bugognoli vs. Quirini. The sentence stated that the barber should receive only 6 lire of the remaining balance of 112 lire.

15. A.S.B., Coll. Med.—b. 338, case of Terrarossa vs. Capponi, 1668, deposition of Cristoforo Capponi; b. 320, sentence in the case of Terrarossa vs. Capponi, 1668.

16. B.C.A.B., Fondo Inquisizione, MS. B 1882, c. 336.

17. A.S.B., Coll. Med.—b. 213, deposition of Dorotea Beltrami, cited in the sentence against Rodolfo Vacchettoni, norcino, 1614; b. 213, charges filed by Cesare Zanolini against the barber Andrea Comellini, 1599 (italics added).

18. S. Loriga, "Un secreto per far morire la persona del Re. Magia e protezione nel Piemonte del '700," *Quaderni storici* 18, 2, n. 53 (1983): 543. On the social meaning of accusations against individuals and groups, M. Douglas, ed., *Witchcraft, Confessions and Accusations* (London, 1970).

19. A.S.B., Coll. Med.—b. 321, case of Gualandi vs. Cavazza, 1697, minutes of the case; b. 342, deposition of the witness.

20. The Foro dei Mercanti was a court formed by five merchants, drawn by casting lots, plus a doctor of law. This court adjudicated all cases related to trading. The procedure was summary. About this court, see B.U.B., MS. 686, no. 46, "Nota de Magistrati e tribunali della città di Bologna"; S. Verardi Ventura, ed., "L'ordinamento bolognese dei secc. XVI–XVII: Introduzione all'edizione del ms. B 1114 della Biblioteca dell'Archiginnasio: *Lo stato, il governo et i magistrati di Bologna,* del Cavaliere Ciro Spontone," *L'Archiginnasio* 74 (1979): 360–61; G. Giordani, *Notizie intorno al Foro dei Mercanti, volgarmente detto la Mercanzia* (Bologna, 1837); L. Dal Pane, *Economia e società a Bologna nell'età del Risorgimento* (Bologna, 1969), 371–72; and F. Boris, "Lo Studio e la Mercanzia: I 'Signori Dottori cittadini' giudici del Foro dei Mercanti nel Cinquecento," in *Sapere e/è potere: Discipline, dispute e professioni nell'Università medievale e moderna* (Bologna, 1990). See also idem, "L'archivio del Foro dei Mercanti di Bologna: Problemi di riordinamento e prospettive di ricerca" (paper presented to the conference "'Pro Tribunali Sedentes': Le Magistrature giudiziarie dello Stato Pontificio e i loro Archivi," Spoleto, November 8–10, 1990).

21. There were seven cases in all: A.S.B., Coll. Med.—b. 340, Santini vs. Allegri, 1678; b. 340, Gotti vs. Mancutino, 1683; b. 340, Negri vs. Marocchi, 1687; b. 321, Nucci vs. Barbieri, 1696; b. 321, Gualandi vs. Cavazza, 1697; b. 352, Guerzoni vs. Rovini, 1709; and b. 223, Bella vs. Taruffi, 1716.

22. Such a study would be very time-consuming, since the cases heard in the Foro dei Mercanti were far more numerous than those heard in the Protomedicato. I

have examined the records of the Foro dei Mercanti only for those years in which I knew, from the Protomedicato records, that a suit for medical payment had been initiated in the Foro dei Mercanti. However, I found no traces of these cases in the archives of the Foro dei Mercanti. Most likely, all of the papers related to these lawsuits had been transmitted to the Protomedicato once the latter had been identified as the competent judge. This, at least, seems to be what happened for the seven lawsuits cited in n. 21, above.

23. These cases (cited in n. 21, above) were Negri vs. Marocchi, Nucci vs. Barbieri, Gualandi vs. Cavazza, and Guerzoni vs. Rovini.

24. A.S.B., Coll. Med., b. 349, trial of Carlo Gavassei, 1772. Fifteen paoli were equivalent to seven lire and ten soldi.

25. Such was the case, for instance, in the trials of the distiller Guarnieri (see n. 7, above) and Maria la Romana (A.S.B., Coll. Med., b. 349); the latter trial was described in chap. 3, pp. 78–79.

26. P. Zacchia, *Quaestiones medico-legales* (Lyons, 1662), lib. 6, tit. 1, quaest. 8, p. 466. Zacchia specified: "It should be kept in mind, however, that it is not improper for a physician to agree upon a yearly salary with princes, municipalities, communities and public institutions." In fact, in chap. 2 we saw the importance of such contracts in early modern medical practice.

A similar statement can be found in Verdier, *Jurisprudence*, 95. "According to the law, the definition of honorarium implies that it cannot be stipulated by agreement or contract. Some authorities, however, aware of men's ingratitude, did allow physicians to make agreements with patients, although most authors rejected a practice considered fitting only for charlatans." Like Zacchia, Verdier also distinguished between cure agreements with individuals and contracts with a municipality, acknowledging that the latter not only did not affect a physician's dignity but were "very useful and universally widespread" (96).

27. On the prohibition of agreements for a cure in the statutes of the colleges in the sixteenth century, see above, chap. 2, n. 82, above. Earlier statutes, in contrast, acknowledged the validity of such agreements. For example, the statutes of the College of Physicians of Milan from 1386, in the section listing fees for medical visits, specified that such fees were due "unless there be a specific agreement between the parties, in which case, both parties are required to keep to the terms of the agreement" (A. Bottero, "I più antichi statuti del Collegio dei Medici di Milano," *Archivio storico lombardo*, n.s., 7, nos. 1–4 [1942]: 42–43). In 1421, the Sicilian protomedico Antonio D'Alessandro, in establishing medical fees, authorized cure agreements in case of serious illnesses, and for specific surgical procedures such as extracting a cataract and stopping a hemorrhage (F. Orlando-Salinas, "Le tariffe per i medici nelle 'Constitutiones protomedicales' di Gian Filippo Ingrassia [1563]," *La cultura medica moderna* 9, no. 5 [1930], 9–10).

28. *Statuta Collegii Mag. DD. Medicorum Civitatis Mutinae*, rubr. 16, "Quod nullus medicus possit aliquem in ius vocare pro sua mercede nec vocari nisi coram D.

Priore"; the entire document is printed in V. Casoli, "Gli Statuti del Collegio dei Medici della Città di Modena, riformati da Giovanni Grillenzoni medico modenese," *Rivista di storia critica delle scienze mediche e naturali* 1 (1910–12): 102–3.

29. "Ut ceteri, inter medendum, non expectata sanitate" (Casoli, "Statuti," 102).

30. A.S.B., Coll. Med., b. 342, case of Cavazza vs. Lambertini, 1697.

31. A.S.B., Coll. Med.—b. 321, Acta Prothomedicatus, 1695–1702; bb. 322–27, Acta Prothomedicatus, 1744–76. For an overview of cases concerning medical payment, see chap. 4, pp. 96–104, above.

32. A.S.B., Coll. Med., b. 323, case of Lodi vs. Modona, 1747.

33. A.S.B., Coll. Med., b. 342, trial of Taddeo Azzoguidi, 1701, deposition of Antonio Campeggi.

34. A.S.B., Coll. Med., b. 225, "Liber secretus, 1738–55," trial of Nicolò Callegari.

35. Ibid.

36. A.S.B., Coll. Med., b. 349, trial of Alessio Porta, 1746, deposition of Domenico Santi.

37. A.S.B., Coll. Med., b. 349, trial of Simone Gordini, surgeon, 1759, deposition of Pietro Manfrara.

38. A.S.B., Coll. Med., b. 349, trial of Francesco Cossarini, surgeon, 1769, deposition of Pietro Schiavina.

39. A.S.B., Coll. Med., b. 351, charges filed by Felice Rossi, peasant, against the barber Domenico Toni, 1742.

40. On the changes of medical opinion on bloodletting in this period, see J. Bauer, *Geschichte der Aderlässe* (Munich, 1870), 197 ff; and for an earlier period see, for instance, D. La Scala, *Phlebotomia damnata* (Padua, 1696). In the nineteenth century, this critical attitude would become strong condemnation; see L. Angeli, *L'abuso del salasso condannato dall'autorità dei sommi pratici, della ragione, e della sperienza* (Imola, 1824); and L. Bucellati, *Cenno sui perniciosi effetti del salasso* (Milan, 1817), to mention only two of the many works written on this issue. It should be noted, however, that medical opinion on the use and abuse of bloodletting shifted constantly throughout European history. In practice, though, bloodletting seems to have enjoyed a steady popularity among patients regardless of medical theories or trends.

41. A.S.B., Coll. Med., b. 349, trial of Giuseppe Maria Pietri, also known as "Il Corso," 1764. One zecchino equaled 11.8 lire (Martini, *Manuale di metrologia,* 618–19). On lithotomy in Bologna, see G. M. Bacchettoni, *Ragguagli dell'operazione di pietra fatta in Bologna* (Bologna, 1727); about Bacchettoni, see L. Samoggia, "Litotomi, empirici e oculisti negli Ospedali della Vita e della Morte in Bologna nel 1600 e 1700," in *Sette secoli di storia ospedaliera* (Bologna, 1961), 198 ff.

The requirement that recovery be confirmed by a professional was also included in an agreement signed in Poitiers in 1620 for the treatment of a hernia (see document 7 in the Appendix, below).

42. A.S.B., Coll. Med., b. 349, trial of "Il Corso," 1764, deposition of Antonio Fossi.

43. A.S.B., Coll. Med., b. 349, trial of Il Corso, 1764: "conventiones initas in scriptura de qua in Processu tamquam minus equas et captiosas, nequaquam esse admittendas, ipsisq. etiam Approbatis non permittendas."

44. Cited in Orlando-Salinas, "Le tariffe per i medici," 22.

45. The *decisiones* were legal "reports" and not "records"; in other words, they were not official records of the courts but only reports of what was discussed by the judges. They did, however, have some value as jurisprudence. In the early modern age, sentences issued by courts usually did not include legal motivations and therefore could not be used as judicial precedents in analogous cases. Hence the increasing popularity among jurists of the collections of *decisiones;* written by a member of the court who had issued the verdicts, the *decisiones* explained the motivations behind sentences, thus providing jurists with materials for establishing juridical precedents.

For the distinction between "reports" and "records," see J. H. Baker, "Case-Law: Reports and Records," in *Englische und kontinentale Rechtsgeschichte: ein Forschungsprojekt,* ed. H. Coing and K. W. Nörr (Berlin, 1985), 49–55. About the collections of *decisiones* as a legal genre, see M. Ascheri, "Rechtsprechungssammlungen—Italien," in *Handbuch der Quellen und Literatur der neueren europäischen Privatsrechtgeschichte,* ed. H. Coing (Munich, 1976), 2:2.

46. M. de Afflictis [M. D'Afflitto], *Decisiones Sacri Regii Consilii Neapolitani, . . . Th. Grammatici, et C. Ursilli I.C. Neapolitani aureis adnotationibus, Casuumque novis quibusdam Decisionibus separatim olim editis illustratae* (Venice, 1604), decisio 123, fol. 111r.

D'Afflitto does not give the year of the sentence, but since he says that he participated in the ruling, the case must have been heard either in 1495–1501 or in 1503–6, when he was a member of the Regio Consiglio (see G. Vallone, *Le "Decisiones" di Matteo D'Afflitto* [Lecce, 1988], 115–16; on the *editio princeps* of 1509, see 127, 134).

47. H. Magonius, *Decisiones causarum tam Rotae florentinae quam Rotae Lucensis* (Venice, 1612), decisio 11, "De salario medicorum," fols. 45r–47r. In the discussion of this lawsuit, the magistrates referred to another case in which the appointment of the physician Giacomo da Pistoia had been tacitly renewed by the community of Prato. The latter case was reported by M. Socinus, *Consilia, seu potius Responsa* (Venice, 1579), vol. 2, consilium 196, fols. 56r, 56v.

48. Magonius, *Decisiones,* 47r.

49. See above, chap. 2, n. 52.

50. See above, chap. 2, n. 53.

51. All transactions and contracts vitiated by fear *(metus)* were legally invalid according to medieval jurists. Analyzing such cases, Baldus de Ubaldis [Baldo degli Ubaldi] brought the example of the "Si medicus" law: "If the physician intentionally worsens the condition of a patient, thus endangering his life in order to extort from

him illicit promises, the transaction shall be voided *ex officio judicis*" (*In tres priores libros Codicis Commentaria* [Venice, 1615], 120r).

52. Ibid.: unless the physician acts in bad faith, aggravating the disease with the wrong therapy to obtain higher fees, the agreement is legal, because the "Si medicus" law does not apply. See also J. Maynus, *De actionibus* (Venice, 1574), 218: the law "Si medicus" acknowledges the validity of agreements between patient and physician, because it concerns only those dishonest doctors who deliberately aggravate the disease. This opinion is also shared by H. Cagnolus, *In Justiniani Codicem Enarrationes* (Venice, 1586), 119; and Robertus, *Rerum Judicatarum*, lib. 1, chap. 2, sec. 17.

53. The sentence reported by d'Afflitto was used as a legal precedent in the case discussed by Magonius; it was also cited as the exemplary ruling on the issue by G. A. Marta, *Digestorum Novissimorum totius juris controversi scientiae ex omnibus decisionibus universi orbi, quae hucusque extant impressae* (Frankfurt-am-Main, 1621), 3:234: "Obligatio aegroti facta medico est valida. Quicquid aegrotus medico curanti promiserit, ab ejus haeredi deberi placuit, quoniam obligatio valida est, quando medicus salarium de publico haberet, aliter dicendum est. Ex decisione Consilii Neapolitani, n. 123, Matthaei de Afflictis."

54. A. Pinellus [A. Pinhel], *Ad rubricam et legem II Codicis de Rescindenda Venditione elaboratissimi Commentarii* (Venice, 1570), chap. 32: "Explicatur articulus a Dominis non bene tractatus de venditione aliave conventione inter medicum et aegrum," 116v–117r: "Ita intelligi debet l. Archiatri, quae male ab Afflict. et aliis restringitur ad medicum habentem salarium publicum: cum verba eius legis generalem sensum magis expriment ibi, *quos etiam patimur accipere quae sani offerunt pro obsequis, non quae periclitantes pro salute promittunt,* et sic ea lex manifeste ex verbis et ratione omnem medicum comprehendit" (117r).

55. Digest, 50, 13, "Si cui": "Si cui cautum est honorarium, vel si quis de lite pactus est: videamus an petere possit. Et quidem de pactis ita est rescriptum ab imperatore nostro, et divo patre ejus: 'Litis causae malo more pecuniam tibi promissam ipse quoque profiteris. Sed hoc ita jus est, si suspensa lite societatem futuri emolumenti cautio pollicetur. Si vero post causam actam cauta est honoraria summa, peti poterit usque ad probabilem quantitatem, etsi nomine palmarii cautum sit: sic tamen, ut computetur id quod datum est, cum eo quod debetur, neutrumque compositum licitam quantitatem excedat.'"

The law is included under the same section, "De variis et extraordinariis cognitionibus," as the law "Si medicus." The section deals with fees for liberal arts teachers, lawyers, and physicians (as well as midwives and wet-nurses). The fragment is from Ulpian's *"liber octavus de omnibus tribunalibus."*

The prohibition against lawyers entering into agreements with a client while the legal case was pending is also stated in a law of the Code of Justinian (2, 6, "De postulando," 2: "Praeterea nullum cum eo litigatore contractum, quem in propriam recepit fidem, ineat advocatus: nullam conferat pactionem").

56. Pinellus, *Ad rubricam et legem II Codicis de Rescindenda Venditione elaboratis-*

simi Commentarii, 117r: "Imo major prohibendi ratio videtur in medico cum aegro quam in advocato cum clientulo, ut constat ad sensum."

57. V. Carocius [V. Carocci], *Tractatus Locati et Conducti,* 1st ed. (Pavia, 1586); quoted from 5th ed. (Venice, 1649), pars 2, "De medico," quaestio 4, "An medicus, chirurgicus, et similes pacisci possint cum infirmo pendente infirmitate," fols. 122r–122v: "Dici poterit fortasse semper invitus aegrotus contrahens, quasi violentatus a spe recuperandae sanitatis, ut clientulus evictione litis" (122v).

58. In addition to Carocci, others who shared Pinhel's opinion were F. Bursatius [F. Borsati], *Consiliorum sive Responsorum Liber* (Venice, 1573), consilium 72, n. 11; P. Granutius, *Communes conclusiones utriusque juris* (Venice, 1582), theorema 12, fol. 62v (the agreement is considered "inefficax"); A. Fachineus [A. Fachinei], *Controversiarum juris Libri novem* (Ingolstadt, 1598), lib. 2, chap. 25, pp. 263–64; the Jesuit canonist J. Azorius [Juan Azor], *Institutiones morales,* 2d ed. (Lyons, 1613), vol. 3, pars 3, lib. 6, caput 14, col. 419: "Prohibetur advocatus lite durante contrahere cum his qui litigant, lex 'quisquis' Codicis 'De postulando'; Medicus cum infirmo, quem curat, durante infirmitate contrahere nequit, lex 'si medicus', ff. 'De var. et extraord. crimin.' *[sic!]*."

E. Soarez (*Thesaurus receptarum sententiarum, quas vulgus interpretum communes opiniones vocat* [Venice, 1569], 164v), quotes approvingly Pinhel's opinion: "Medicus cum aegroto nullam pactionem, nullamque conventionem interim dum ille cum morbo conflictatur, facere potest, ut verius et receptius accurate profitetur Arius Pinellus." But he adds somewhat contradictorily: "Nec ante praemium ullum exigeat, quam sanitas infirmo restituatur." In this obviously sloppy compilation, the author has assembled as *communes opiniones* two ideas that are clearly at odds with each other: the old principle of paying a physician only upon successful treatment, and the new idea that the cure agreement is an invalid transaction.

By the middle of the eighteenth century, the Spanish jurist M. E. Muñoz, in a collection of all laws concerning the Protomedicato and medical practice, argued that the cure agreement was legally invalid according to jurists' *communis opinio* (*Recopilación de las leyes, pragmáticas, reales decretos, y acuerdos del Real Proto-Medicato* [Valencia, 1751], cited in J. Tate Lanning, *The Royal Protomedicato: The Regulation of the Medical Profession in the Spanish Empire* [Durham, 1985], 202, 93).

59. H. Lampe, *Dissertatio historico-juridica de honore, privilegiis et juribus singularibus medicorum* (Gröningen, 1736), chaps. 24–29, pp. 180–90.

60. According to Lampe (*Dissertatio,* 188–89), this is proved by the fact that under the "Si medicus" law, physicians could be sentenced to return the goods extorted from the patient; whereas the "Cincia" law (which established that lawyers could not extort gifts or other offers from clients) did not enforce the restitution of such gifts, nor did it establish penalties for this behavior. Also the "Si cui" law, which denied validity to agreements between lawyers and clients during legal cases, did not mention specific penalties for lawyers who made such agreements.

61. We find it, for example, in Cassiodorus's *Formula comitis archiatrorum* (5th–6th century A.D.): "Causarum periti palmares habentur, cum negotia defend-

erint singulorum; sed quanto gloriosius expellere quod mortem videbatur inferre et salutem periclitanti reddere, de qua coactus fuerat desperare!" (*Magnii Aurelii Cassiodori: Variarum libri XII,* ed. A. J. Fridh, Corpus Christianorum, Series Latina, no. 96 [Turnhout, Belgium, 1973], 249).

62. Odofredus, *Lectura super Codice I* (Lyons, 1562; reprint, Forni, 1968, Opera Iuridica Rariora, no. 6), 1:80v–81r:

"Signori, hec lex valde honesta est . . . Signori, custodiatis vos hic, ex quo advocatus recipit clientulum suum ad iuvandum in fide sua, non potest advocatus aliquid emere cum eo: nec alium contractum cum eo inire pendente lite. Nam vos debetis scire quod est eadem natura hominum litigantium et egrotantium: quod egrotantes et litigantes paribus passibus ambulant nam clientulus non vadit nisi ad caudam advocati diebus festivis deserit castrum suum ut sciat quod debeat facere: et vadit ad advocatum suum: hoc casu si facit aliquem contractum cum eo, non valebit: quod propter timorem litis omnia daret. . . . Et idem est in egro: nam eger non habet dominum nisi medicum: si dominus medicus emit ab egro, non valet, quod presumit lex quod eger non celebrat contractum cum medico, nisi ut liberet eum unde non valet: quod propter timorem mortis omnia daret."

63. Baldus, *In tres priores,* fol. 120r, tit. *De transact.,* l. XIII. *Interpositas:* "Transactionem vitiant metus, et dominium, seu servitus, ubi inter dominum et servum intervenit transactio . . . Transactio facta iusto metu, rata non habetur, et inter dominum, et servum non valet transactio, hoc dicit Bartolus."

All of this raises the issue of the juridical definition of contract and its changes over time—an issue too vast to be discussed here. For both Baldo and Bartolo, the concept of contract was based on equity; an agreement could not be equitable if one of the contracting parties acted in fear. Their view was very different from the early modern view, expressed by Hobbes, that "Fear and Liberty are consistent." On the waning of considerations of equity and *metus* (duress) in the theory of contract in nineteenth-century England, see F. Alaya, *The Rise and Fall of Freedom of Contract* (Oxford, 1979), 435–36. My thanks to Natalie Davis who pointed out this major issue to me.

64. Thomas Actius, *De infirmitate eiusque privilegiis et affectibus* (Venice, 1603), rubr. 49, "De salario medicorum," pp. 121–25. Azzio shared the opinion of Pinhel, Borsati, and other authors who believed that agreements between physician and patient were invalid: "Contracts made by physician and patient during an illness, just like the ones between lawyer and client during a lawsuit, are null and void *ipso iure.*"

65. H. Bodinus, *Dissertatio de iuribus infirmorum & aegrotorum singularibus* (Halle, 1693), thesis 19, p. 23.

66. Significantly, the promise for a cure was mentioned in this vast juridical literature only once, by an author who, against the dominant view, argued for the validity of good-faith agreements between healers and patients: "What has been promised to a healer on condition that the patient recovers, should be kept if health has been regained; and the person who made the promise can be sued in a court of

law either under the *'actio certa'* or the *'ex stipulatu'* procedure. However, the healer who signed the agreement cannot file a suit for payment unless the patient has been clearly returned to health"; see J. Mühlpfort, *Dissertatio inauguralis juridica circa morbum et cura aegrotorum* (Strasburg, 1671), (H.A.B.W.: Qu N 299.1 16), p. 45. This text is a dissertation for a doctorate in civil and canon law at the University of Strasburg. The author argued that "the 'Si medicus' law does not take away from private citizens the right to sign an agreement for a cure with a physician" (48). His is the only opinion favorable to the cure agreement which I found in two centuries of debate among European jurists on the issue.

67. Gloss to the "Marcius" law (Digest, 19, 2, 59). Cf. Bartolo, *In secundam Digesti veteris partem* (Venice, 1570), 136v: "Ultimo hic lex inducitur in argomentum ad questionem de medico qui promisit aliquem curare de podagra, et ipse liberatus est aliquis diebus et postea reversa est infirmitas, an debeat habere totum salarium?" Bartolo answered that it is necessary to distinguish: if the patient's relapse is brought about by the same causes that originated the first bout of illness, the physician should not be paid because he has not thoroughly cured the disease; otherwise, the physician should receive the agreed-upon salary. See also above, chap. 2, n. 22.

68. See the literature mentioned above in chap. 2, nn. 22, 23.

69. For example, Pinhel (*De rescindenda venditione,* 117r) acknowledged that the gloss supported the validity of the cure agreement and that the medieval canonist Durandus had so maintained in his *Speculum judiciale.* He admitted that the gloss, together with the authority of Durandus, would suffice to explain the decision by the Regio Consiglio of Naples (reported by D'Afflitto) to uphold the validity of the agreement. But in spite of all these authoritative precedents, Pinhel believed that agreements between physician and patient were unlawful.

Pinhel's opinion was followed by Carocci (*Tractatus locati et conducti,* 123v), who noted that "Pinellus . . . dicens ex ventre huius quaestionis colligi, et extrahi posse valere conventionem de salario inter medicum et infirmum, et sic defendi posse Afflict. in allegata decisione 123"; but he concluded that the opposite opinion, namely that such agreements were invalid, was the correct one.

70. Digest, 19, 2, 59: "Marcius domum faciendam a Flacco conduxerat: deinde operis parte effecta terrae motu concussum erat aedificium. Massurius Sabinus, si vi naturali veluti terrae motu hoc acciderit, Flacci esse periculum."

71. This had already been the opinion of medieval commentators—for instance, Bartolo, who had argued that physicians could claim their salaries not by means of an *actio locati* but by means of an *actio in factum* (*In secundam Digesti novi partem* [Venice, 1570], 239r). See also Carocci, *Tractatus locati et conducti* (Pavia, 1586), 7v: "Inter medicum et infirmum, advocatum et clientulum non esse proprie locationem, sed agi praescriptis verbis, et certe honorarium dicitur."

Legal historians have hotly debated the question of whether in Roman antiquity any physician's work could be hired by contract or whether a physician's work could only be so hired if he was a slave or a freedman. R. Bozzoni (*I medici e il diritto romano* [Naples, 1904], 208–9) summarizes the prevailing view: physicians who were slaves or freedmen could be hired under *locatio-conductio* contracts, but this was not possible with doctors who were freeborn citizens. In the latter case, the transaction between healer and patient was considered an unenforceable contract on the basis of the principle "do ut facias et facio ut des." The honorarium of the freeborn physician was given in token of gratitude and not as wages (although it was called *merces*), because the value of medical services was considered inestimable. K. H. Below (*Der Arzt im römischen Recht* [Munich, 1953]) corrects Bozzoni's conclusions on a few minor points and provides a more extensive bibliography. Among more recent studies, see F. Kudlien, "Die Unschätzbarkeit ärztlicher Leistung und das Honorarproblem," *Medizinhistorisches Journal* 14, nos. 1–2 (1979): 4–6; and M. Just, "Der Honoraranspruch des 'medicus ingenuus,'" in *"Sodalitas": Scritti in onore di Antonio Guarino* (Naples, 1984), 6:3057–75 (on the honorarium of freeborn physicians).

72. Carocius, *Tractatus locati et conducti,* 123v: "Ad materiam legis 'Martius,' Digest. 'Locat.,' an medicus, qui certa mercede conventa curavit semel infirmum, si iterum incidat in morbum, teneatur iterum curare? Quaestio haec appellatur a Doctoribus Sabbatina, et occurrere potest in medico, *multo magis in Chirurgico, et Marescalco, qui curavit animal de formidrella*" (italics added).

73. Lipenius (*Bibliotheca realis juridica* [Leipzig, 1757], s.v. "medici contractus") mentions several doctoral dissertations defended in European universities, including those of Wittenberg, Strasburg, and Danzig): Bastineller, *De medico ex voluntate aegroti perperam curante;* Io. G. Schertzius, *Dissertatio de pacto medici cum aegroto pro salute* (Strasburg, 1718); J. Schultz, *De contractu medici cum aegroto* (Danzig, 1689) (H.A.B.W.: Li 4801). Lipenius also mentions G. L. De Kornatowski, *Epistola de valida emptione venditione inter medicum et aegrotum celebrata* (Leipzig, 1739), but I was not able to locate this text.

74. "Palmarium: certa pecunia summa honorarii, seu stipendi nomine promissa, in eo casu, quo lis vincatur a cliente" (*Universa civilis et criminalis jurisprudentia* [Turin, 1827], t. 9, lib. 3, tit. 4, cap. 3, p. 184).

"Palmarium: est merces, quae datur causidico post causam actam et litem obtentam" (Ae. Forcellini, *Totius latinitatis lexicon* [Prato, Italy, 1868], vol. 4, s.v. "palmarium"). See also A. Berger, *Encyclopaedic Dictionary of Roman Law,* Transactions of the American Philosophical Society, n.s., vol. 43, pt. 2 (Philadelphia, 1953), s.v. "palmarium."

For a seventeenth-century juridical discussion on the issue, see W. A. Lauterbach, *Disputatio de palmario advocatorum* (Tübingen, 1671). Describing the history of lawyers' fees, F. Brummerus [F. Brummer] (*Commentarius ad Legem Cinciam* [Paris, 1668], 135–36) states that in order to foresee the outcome of a case and, therefore, their chance of getting a palmarium, ancient lawyers turned to divinatory practices (using snake eggs, the hair of newborn babies, and haruspex responses).

75. Numerous agreements with a promise of payment for legal services are recorded in the notarial archives of Bologna ("Libri dei memoriali") for the thir-

teenth and fourteenth centuries (*Chartularium Studii Bononiensis: Documenti per la storia dell'università di Bologna dalle origini fino al secolo XV* [Bologna, 1909–16], 7:118, 178).

76. Bartolus de Saxo Ferrato, *In tres codicis libros* (Venice, 1570), 242v; Jason Maynus, *In primam Digesti veteris partem commentarii* (Lyons, 1569), 56v: "Advocati non debent habere salarium lite durante . . . quod non debent habere salarium nisi finita causa," and "medici non debent habere salarium nisi quando est sanatus infirmus"; H. Praevidellius, *De peste eiusque privilegiis,* in *Tractatus . . . de variis verbis iuris* (Venice, 1584), 18:171v: "Sciendum est tamen, quod medici de iure non debent recipere salarium ab infirmis, sed cum sani fuerint . . . eodem modo advocati lite pendente a clientis non debent aliquid recipere." Soarez (*Thesaurus,* 8r) presents this as concurring opinion: "Advocatus non antea recte salarium exigeat, quam lis ad finem pervenerit."

Baldus de Ubaldis (*In quartum et quintum Codicis librum Commentaria* [Venice, 1615], 11r) argued instead that lawyers should receive payment when they begin working on a case: "Quando debeatur salarium advocato? Respondeo cum incipit advocare, licet non peregit: nam interim clientulus consequitur patrocinium, ergo praestat salarium. . . . Si spectaremus finem litis, magis faveremus clientulo quam advocato, & daretur manus clientulo subtrahendi salarium, quod esset inconveniens."

77. Odofredus, *Lectura super codicem,* 88r, held that the lawyer should work on a case until its final conclusion, including appeal. Baldus (*In quartum et quintum Codicis librum Commentaria,* 11r) disagreed, unless the lawyer's fee had been promised as a "palmarium."

78. See *Instructiones Curiae Hollandicae,* art. 71; *Instructiones Curiae Brabantinae,* art. 288; and *Instructiones Curiae Flandricae,* art. 154 (cited in I. Voet, *Commentariorum ad pandectas libri 50,* which I quote from the Italian translation: *Commento alle pandette* [Venice, 1846], 2:376).

79. Baldus, *In quartum et quintum Codicis librum Commentaria,* 11r: the lawyer should not be paid "ratione victoriae sed ratione simplicis patrocinii: quia de futuris incerti sumus." About the prohibition against lawyers' promising victory in legal cases, see J. Menochius [G. Menochio], *De arbitrariis judicum quaestionibus et causis* (Lyons, 1606), casus 344, p. 496; E. Speckham, *Quaestionum juris caesarei, pontifici, et saxonici, Centuria prima* (Wittemberg, 1611), quaestio 21, fols. 64r–64v.

80. Actius, *De infirmitate,* 121. The jurists' *communis opinio* on this issue shifted toward Azzio's view. For example, see A. Gabrieli, *Communes conclusiones* (Venice, 1593), 562: "Si medicus promisit aegrotum curare, non tenetur illum nisi semel curare: et propterea etiamsi aegrotus in medem. morbum reincidat ipse medicus dicitur liberatus." (Strangely enough, Gabrieli supports this thesis by citing sources such as Durante, who had in fact argued exactly the opposite: see above, chap. 2, n. 23.) The new opinion was shared by J. J. Speidel, *Speculum juridico-politico-philologico historicarum observationum* (Nuremberg, 1657), 76: "regulare et extra dubium est, quod medici se in infinitum obligare non soleant, cum vix ullus morbus sit, qui non recur-

rere valeat." See also Gregorius Tholosanus [Pierre Grégoire], *Commentaria in prolegomena syntaxeon mirabilis artis* (Lyons, 1578), lib. 18, cap. 25, no. 7; and C. Boot, *Dissertatio de privilegiis medicorum* (Duisburg, 1697), 15 (both cited in Lampe, *Dissertatio,* 203).

81. *Manuale de' confessori e penitenti . . . composto dal dottor Martino Azpliqueta Navarro* (Venice, 1659), 631; see also G. B. Codronchi, *De christiana ac tuta medendi ratione* (Ferrara, 1591), 89.

82. Zacchia, *Quaestiones medico-legales,* 400. Zacchia further stated that a physician should not be paid in exchange for recovery: "quale enim esse praemium par sanitati? Sed tantum pro labore, quem Medicus in curando impendet" (416); cf. Actius, *De infirmitate,* rubr. 49, "Medico deberi salarium pro labore, non pro sanitate."

83. E. Freidson, *Professional Dominance* (New York, 1970); idem, *Doctoring Together: A Study of Professional Social Control* (New York, 1975); I. Illich, *Limits to Medicine* (Harmondsworth, England, 1977); P. Starr, *The Social Transformation of American Medicine* (New York, 1982).

84. In the seventeenth century, a few European jurists kept to the traditional view, according to which the agreement between patient and physician was valid if there was no *metus* (fear) nor extortion. See G. B. De Luca, *Theatrum veritatis et justitiae* (Lyons, 1697), tom. 9, discursus 51, pp. 103–4; and Voet, *Commentariorum ad pandectas libri 50,* lib. 2, tit. 14, p. 376. This opinion was also adopted in a doctoral dissertation defended in 1689 at the Law Faculty of the University of Danzig: see Schultz, *De contractu medici cum aegroto,* 7–8.

85. *Universa civilis et criminalis jurisprudentia* (Turin, 1827), vol. 9, lib. 3, tit. 4, cap. 3, p. 187: "quod potissimum hodie medicorum favore credendum est, cum honestioris longe conditionis esse soleant, quam forent olim apud Romanos, apud quos medicae disciplinae operam dabant servi, aliique inferioris status, prout testantur Romanorum rerum periti, itaut non omni prorsus suspicionis labe plerique carerent."

86. The medical college of Bologna was suppressed in 1797, after the arrival of the French troops. It was replaced by the Società Medico-chirurgica. See L. Sighinolfi, *Il pensiero e l'opera della Società medico-chirurgica di Bologna nel Risorgimento italiano* (Bologna, 1924), 12. The Società Medico-chirurgica of Bologna was founded in 1802; see M. Medici, *Memorie storiche intorno alle Accademie scientifiche e letterarie della città di Bologna* (Bologna, 1852), 25. Unlike the college, which was by definition an elitist institution, the società was a professional association in the modern sense, open to everyone who practiced medicine and surgery.

The Protomedicato seems to have survived for a few years during the French occupation, but only with a purely consulting role; see B.C.A.B., Fondo Malvezzi, cart. 313, fasc. 25, "Parere del Protomedicato ai Cittadini Amministratori dipartimentali del Reno," August 20, 1800.

87. Twentieth-century Italian jurists define the relationship between physician and patient as a contractual transaction; see P. Calamandrei, "Note sul contratto tra il chirurgo e il paziente," in *Studi in onore di Riccardo Dalla Volta* (Florence, 1936),

350–66; and F. Carresi, "Il contratto concluso in stato di pericolo con particolare riguardo al contratto concluso fra il medico e il paziente," *Rivista bimestrale di diritto sanitario,* no. 6 (November–December 1969): 849–70.

88. A.S.B., Coll. Med., b. 349, trial of Boschetti, 1758, deposition of Lucia Zaffi.

89. P. Brown, *The Cult of the Saints: Its Rise and Function in Early Christianity* (Chicago, 1981), chap. 5.

90. See, for example, *Monumenti appartenenti alla guarigione di D. Maria Maddalena Mittarelli ad intercessione di Gio. Francesco Regis* (Bologna, 1738). Physicians sometimes recommended a specific saint to their patients. For example, in a healing miracle attributed to Sister Rosa Torregiani (1765), the physician himself procured for the patient a fragment of the veil belonging to the holy woman and told him to swallow it as a remedy (A.C.A.B., Processi per Beatificazione e Santificazione, 745, fasc. k/498/16).

91. Mühlpfort, *Dissertatio inauguralis juridica circa morbum et curam aegrotorum,* 45. According to this jurist, the ecclesiastic authorities responsible for the sanctuary to which the vow was made had the right to file a legal suit to claim payment of what had been promised in the vow: "Nam rector ejus loci, cui facta est pollicitatio, potest agere, ut impleta conditione praestet id, quod promisit" (45).

There are obvious analogies between the cure agreement with a healer and the vow to a saint. Here is a testimonial (1687) from the "Mirakelbuch," or book of miracles, from the Marian sanctuary of Föching, in Oberbayern: "I had a wound on my knee, and the barber said that six weeks would not be enough [for a cure]; feeling worse, I rushed to Föching to ask the Virgin Mary for help . . . ; and the knee healed in less than three weeks" (H. Ohse, *Die Wallfahrt Föching im Spiegel der Mirakelbücher* [Munich, 1969], 144–45, cited in H. Müller, "Erhaltung und Wiederherstellung körperlichen Gesundheit in der traditionellen Gesellschaft, an Hand der Votivtafelsammlung des Museums für Deutsche Volkskunde Berlin," in *Der Mensch und sein Körper von den Antike bis heute,* ed. A. E. Imhof [Munich, 1983]).

A fascinating, in-depth study of vows made by early modern communities to local saints is W. A. Christian, *Local Religion in Sixteenth-Century Spain* (Princeton, N.J., 1981). As described by Christian, the relationship between community and saint seems very similar to that between community and town doctor.

92. The inscription says, "Goya agradecido, a su amigo Arrieta: por el acierto y esmero con el que le salvó la vida en su aguda y peligrosa enfermedad, padecida a fines del año 1819, a los setenta y tres de su edad. Lo pintó en 1820." On this painting, see J. F. Moffitt, "Observations on the Origins and Meanings of Goya with the Devils in the 1820 Self-Portrait with Dr. Arrieta," *Minneapolis Institute of Arts Bulletin* 45 (1981–82): 37. My thanks to Louise Lincoln, who kindly brought this article to my attention.

Published Primary Sources

Actius, Th. (Tommaso Azzio). *De infirmitate eiusque privilegiis et affectibus.* Venetiis, 1603.

Alexander de Imola (Alessandro Tartagni: 1424–1477). *In secundam digesti novi secunda pars commentariorum.* Venetiis, 1541.

Alidosi, G. N. (1570–1627). *Instruttione delle cose notabili della città di Bologna.* Bologna, 1621.

———. *Li dottori bolognesi di Teologia, Filosofia, Medicina e d'Arti liberali dall'anno 1000 per tutto marzo del 1623.* Bologna, 1623 (ristampa Forni, Bologna, 1980).

———. *I Signori Antiani, Consoli e Gonfalonieri di Giustitia della città di Bologna dall'anno 1456 accresciuti sino al 1670.* Bologna, 1670.

Allacci, L. *Apes Urbanae, sive de viribus illustribus qui ab anno MDCXXX per totum MDCXXXII Romae adfuerunt.* Romae, 1663.

Andreae, Joannes (d. 1348). *In tertium Decretalium librum novella Commentaria.* Venetiis, 1581.

———. *In quartum Decretalium librum novella Commentaria.* Venetiis, 1581.

Angeli, L. *L'abuso del salasso condannato dall'autorità dei sommi pratici, della ragione, e della sperienza.* Imola, 1824.

Angelus de Clavasio (1411–95?). *Summa Angelica de casibus conscientiae.* Venetiis, 1487.

Antoninus, sanctus (1389–1459). *Summa theologica.* Veronae, 1740.

Archimathaeus. *De instructione Medici.* In *Collectio salernitana,* a cura di S. De Renzi. Napoli, 1852, t. V.

Arderne, John. *Treatises of fistula in ano, haemorrhoids and clysters,* ed. D'Arcy Power, London, 1910.

Ariosto, L. *Erbolato.* In *Opere minori,* a cura di A. Vallone. Milano, 1964.

Astesanus. *Summa de casibus conscientiae.* Venetiis, 1478.

Azorius, J. (Juan Azor: 1533–1603). *Institutiones morales.* Lugduni, 1613, II ed.

Bacchettoni, G. M. *Ragguagli dell'operazione di pietra fatta in Bologna.* Bologna, 1727.

Baldus, de Ubaldis (Baldo degli Ubaldi: 1327?–1400). *In tres priores libros Codicis Commentaria.* Venetiis, 1615.

———. *In quartum et quintum Codicis librum Commentaria.* Venetiis, 1615.

Bandi lucchesi del secolo XIV, tratti dai registri del R. Archivio di Stato di Lucca, per cura di S. Bongi. Bologna, 1863.

Bardi, G. (1600–1667). *Medicus politico-catholicus.* Genuae, 1644.

Bartolus de Saxo Ferrato (Bartolo di Sassoferrato: 1314–57). *In tres codicis libros.* Venetiis, 1570.

————. *In secundam Digesti veteris partem*. Venetiis, 1570.

Bastineller, G. *De medico ex voluntate aegroti perperam curante*. Vittembergae, 1719.

Bechmann, I. V. *Dissertatio de aegritudine eiusque iuribus et privilegiis*. Ienae, 1668.

Benedetti, A. (ca. 1450–1512). *De medici atque aegri officio*. In *De re medica*. Basileae, 1549.

Benincasa, C. (d. 1603). *De paupertate ac eius privilegiis*. In *Tractatus . . . de variis verbis Juris*. Venetiis, 1584, t. XVIII.

Bergerus, J.-H. (J.-H. Berger: 1657–1732). *Dissertatio de privilegiis aegrotorum*. Vittembergae, 1687.

Bertachini, Do. Ioan. *Repertorium juris utriusque Doctoris Praestantissimi*. Venetiis, 1570.

Bodinus, H. (Heinrich von Bode: 1652–1720). *Dissertatio de iuribus infirmorum & aegrotorum singularibus*. Halle, 1693.

Boot, C. *Dissertatio de privilegiis medicorum*. Duisburgi ad Rhenum, 1697.

Botallo, Ludovico. *Tractatus de medici et aegri munere*. In *Opera Omnia*. Lugduni, 1660 (1512).

Brummerus, F. (F. Brummer: 1642–68). *Commentarius ad Legem Cinciam*. Lutetiae Parisiorum, 1668.

Bucellati, L. *Cenno sui perniciosi effetti del salasso*. Milano, 1817.

Bursatius, Franciscus (Francesco Borsati). *Consiliorum sive Responsorum Liber*. Venetiis, 1573.

Cagnolus, Hieronymus (Girolamo Cagnolo: 1490?–1551). *In Constitutiones et Leges Primi, Secundi, Quinti ac Duodecimi Pandectarum . . . aurearum enarrationum Liber primus*. Venetiis, 1586.

————. *In primam et secundam Digesti veteris ac Codicis partem*. Venetiis, 1590, t. III.

————. *In Justiniani Codicem enarrationes*. Venetiis, 1586.

Calvinus, J. (fl. 1595–1614). *Lexicon Juridicum: Juris caesarei simul, et canonici*. Hanoviae, 1619, III ed.

Cardanus, H. (Girolamo Cardano: 1501–76). *De vita propria*. Parisiis, 1643.

Carocius, Vincentius (Vincenzo Carocci: fl. 1580). *Tractatus locati et conducti*. Venetiis, 1649, V ed.

Carrarius, V. (Vincenzo Carrari). *De medico et illius erga aegros officio*. Ravennae, 1581.

Cassiodorus. *Formula comitis archiatrorum*. In *Variarum libri XII*, ed. A. J. Fridh. Turnholti, 1973 (Corpus Christianorum, Serie Latina, vol. XCVI).

Catalogus omnium doctorum collegiatorum in artibus liberalibus et in facultate medica incip. ab A.D. 1156. Bononiae, 1664.

Chartularium Studii Bononiensis: Documenti per la storia dell'università di Bologna dalle origini fino al secolo XV. Bologna, 1909–16.

Ciucci, A. (fl. 1679–81). *Il Filo d'Arianna: overo fedelissima scorta alli esercenti di chirurgia per uscire dal Laberinto delle Relazioni e Ricognizioni dei vari morbi e morti*. Macerata, 1689.

Claudini, G.C. (d. 1618). *De ingressu ad infirmos*. Venetiis, 1628.

Codex Theodosianus. Lugduni,1566 (eds. T. Mommsen and P. M. Meyer. *Theodosiani libri XVI cum constitutionibus Sirmondianis et leges novellae ad Theodosianum perti-nentes.* Berlin, 1954, II ed.).

Codronchi, G. B. (1547–1628). *De christiana ac tuta medendi ratione.* Ferrariae, 1591.

Constitutiones et Capitula, necnon Regii Protomedicatus officii, ed. Paulo Pizzuto. Panormi, 1657.

Corpus juris civilis, rec. P. Krueger. Lipsiae, 1877.

Corpus statutorum italicorum, Respublica Mutinensis, 1306–7, a cura di E. P. Vicini. Milano, 1932.

Cujas, J. (1522–90). *Ad tres postremos Codicis Iustiniani libros commentarii.* In *Opera omnia.* Lutetiae Parisiorum, 1658, t. II.

De Afflictis, M. (Matteo D'Afflitto: d. 1532), *Decisiones Sacri Regii Consilii Neapolitani, . . . Th. Grammatici, et C. Ursilli I. C. Neapolitani aureis adnotationibus, Casuumque novis quibusdam Decisionibus separatim olim editis illustratae.* Venetiis, 1604.

De Burgos, Antonius. *Super utili et quotidiano titulo De emptione et venditione.* Parmae, 1574.

De Luca, Jo. Bapt. (1614–83). *Theatrum Veritatis et Justitiae.* Lugduni, 1697.

Direttorio del Magistrato dei Tribuni della Plebe. Bologna, 1645.

Dolfi, P. S. *Cronologia delle famiglie nobili di Bologna.* Bologna, 1670 (ristampa Forni, Bologna, 1973).

Durandus, Gulielmus (Gulielmus Durantis: ca. 1237–96). *Speculum Judiciale.* Bononiae, 1477.

Fachineus, A. (A. Fachinei: d. ca. 1607). *Controversiarum juris Libri novem.* Ingolstadii, 1598.

Fantuzzi, G. *Notizie degli scrittori bolognesi.* Bologna, 1786–1790.

Felinus, Sandaeus (Felino Maria Sandeo: 1444–1503). *Commentaria ad quinque Decretalium libros.* Lugduni, 1555.

Ferminelli, G. B. *Il cauto flebotomista.* Bologna, 1817.

Ferraris, L. *Prompta Bibliotheca canonica juridico-moralis theologica.* Romae, 1766.

Fichtnerus, G. *Dissertatio de infirmitatis commodis.* Altdorfi, 1720.

Frank, J. P. *Sistema compiuto di Polizia medica.* Milano, 1786.

Friedlibius, C. *Dissertatio de aegrotorum iure ac privilegiis in genere.* Gryphaei, 1676.

Fuero Juzgo, o Libro de los Jueces. Madrid, 1815.

Gabrieli, Antonio (d. 1555). *Communes conclusiones.* Venetiis, 1593.

Gailius (A. Gail: 1526–87). *Practicarum Observationum ad processum indiciarium libri duo.* Coloniae Agrippinae, 1580.

Galeno. *De praenotione ad Posthumum.* In *Opera,* ed. C.G. Kühn. Leipzig, 1823, vol. XIV.

Gandolfi, G. *Elogio di Tarsizio Riviera.* Bologna, 1807.

Garzoni, Tommaso (1549?–89). *La piazza universale di tutte le professioni del mondo.* Venetia, 1588.

Gatta, D. *Regali dispacci, nelli quali si contengono le sovrane determinazioni . . . nel Regno di Napoli.* Napoli, 1773–77, voll. 7.

Gloria, A. *Monumenti della Università di Padova, 1318–1405.* Padova, 1888, voll. 2.

Gonfalonieri del Popolo o Tribuni della Plebe dall'anno 1500 a tutto il 1769. Sassi, Bologna, 1769.

Granutius, Paulus. *Communium conclusionum utriusque juris liber primus.* Venetiis, 1582.

Gregorius Tholosanus (Pierre Grégoire: 1540–97?). *Commentaria in prolegomena syntaxeon mirabilis artis.* Lugduni, 1578.

Guidicini, G. B. *Cose notabili della città di Bologna.* Bologna, 1870, voll. 5.

Hasenest, J. C. *Des medicinischen Richters oder Actorum physicomedicoforensium Collegii medici Onoldini.* Onolzbach (Ansbach), 1756.

Hippocrates. *Aphorisms,* ed. Loeb. Cambridge, 1979, vol. IV.

Hostiensis (Henricus de Segusia: d. 1271). *Summa aurea.* Venetiis, 1586.

Innocentius Quartus Pont. Maximus (d. 1254). *Super libros quinque Decretalium.* Francofurti ad Moenum, 1570.

Lampe, H. *Dissertatio historico-juridica de honore, privilegiis et juribus singularibus medicorum.* Groningae, 1736.

La Scala, D. (1632–97). *Phlebotomia damnata.* Patavii, 1696.

Lauterbach, W. A. (1618–78). *Disputatio de palmario advocatorum.* Tübingen, 1671.

Leges ac Statuta Ampliss. Senatus Norimbergensis ad Medicos, Pharmacopoeos & alios pertinentia. Norimbergae, 1612.

Leges Visigothorum Antiquiores, ed. K Zeumer, Hannoverae et Lipsiae 1894 (also in *Monumenta Germaniae Historica, Legum Sectio I: Leges Nationum Germanicarum,* Hannoverae et Lipsiae 1902, t. I).

Liber pro recta administratione Protomedicatus. Bononiae, 1666.

Lipenius, M. (Martin Lipen: 1630–92). *Bibliotheca realis juridica post virorum clarissimorum F.G. Stravii et G.A. Ienichenii curas emendata.* Lipsiae, 1757 (1679).

Magni, P. P. (b. 1525). *Discorsi sopra il modo di sanguinare.* Roma, 1586.

———. *Discorso sopra il modo di fare i cauterij o rottorij a corpi humani.* Roma, 1588.

Magonius, Hieronymus. *Decisiones causarum tam Rotae Florentinae quam Rotae Lucensis.* Venetiis, 1612.

Malvasia, Diodata. *La venuta et i progressi miracolosi della S.ma Madonna dipinta da S. Luca posta sul monte della Guardia dall'anno che ci venne 1160 sin all'anno 1617.* Bologna, 1617.

Maranta, Robertus (d. 1540?). *Consilia sive Responsa.* Venetiis, 1591.

Marcus, Franciscus (François Marc). *Aureae decisiones in sacro Delphinatus senatu.* Francofurti ad Moenum, 1624 (1587).

Marta, G. A. (1559–1628). *Digestorum novissimorum totius iuris controversi scientiae.* . . . Francofurti ad Moenum, 1621.

Masini, A. di P. (1599–1691). *Bologna perlustrata.* Bologna, 1666.

Mazzetti, S. *Repertorio di tutti i professori antichi e moderni, della famosa Università e del celebre Istituto delle Scienze di Bologna.* Bologna, 1848.

Maynus, Jason (Giasone Dal Maino: 1435–1519). *In primam Digesti Veteris Partem Commentarii.* Lugduni, 1569.

Melloni, G. B. *Atti, o Memorie degli uomini illustri in santità nati, o morti in Bologna.* Bologna, 1773.

Menochius, Jacobus (Giacomo Menochio: 1532–1607). *De arbitrariis iudicum quaestionibus et causis.* Lugduni, 1606.

Mondeville, H. de. *Chirurgie,* trad. it. di M. Tabanelli, *Un secolo d'oro della Chirurgia francese,* vol. I: *Henry de Mondeville.* Forlì, 1969.

Montalbani, O. (1601–71). *L'honore de i Collegi dell'Arti della città di Bologna.* Bologna, 1670.

Monumenti appartenenti alla guarigione di D. Maria Maddalena Mittarelli ad intercessione di S. Gio. Francesco Regis. Bologna, 1738.

Moratti, P. *Racconto de gli ordini e Provisioni fatte ne' lazaretti in Bologna e suo contado in tempo di contagio.* Bologna, 1631.

Mühlpfort, J. J. *Dissertatio inauguralis juridica circa morbum et curam aegrotorum.* Argentorati, 1671.

Muñoz, M. E. (a cura di). *Recopilación de las leyes, pragmáticas, reales decretos, y acuerdos del Real Proto-Medicato.* Valencia, 1751.

Muratori, L. A. *Del Governo della peste.* Modena, 1714.

Navarro, M. (Martín de Azpilcueta: d. 1586). *Manuale de' confessori e penitenti . . . composto dal dottor Martino Azpliqueta Navarro.* Venezia, 1659.

Notes on Religious and Secular Houses of Yorkshire, vol. I. Record Series of the Yorkshire Archaeological Society, vol. XVII. York, 1895.

Odofredus (d. 1265). *Summa de formandis libellis,* ristampa anastatica. Torino, 1968.

———. *Lectura super Codice I.* Lugduni, 1562 (ristampa anastatica, Forni, Bologna, 1968–69, Opera iuridica rariora VI).

Orlandi, P. A. *Notizie degli scrittori bolognesi e dell'opere loro stampate e manoscritte.* Bologna, 1714.

Panormitanus (Niccolò de Tudeschi: 1386–1445). *In tertium Decretalium librum interpretationes.* Lugduni, 1547.

———. *Secunda interpretationum in primum Decretalium librum Pars.* Lugduni, 1547.

———. *In IV et V Decretalium libros interpretationes.* Lugduni, 1547.

Papa, Guido (Guy de la Pape: 1402–87). *Singularia.* Lugduni, 1533.

Preparamento del Pastarino, per medicarsi in questi sospettosi tempi di peste. Bologna, 1577.

Petroni Alessandro (d. 1585). *De Victu Romanorum, et sanitate tuenda.* Romae, 1581 *(Del viver delli Romani et del conservar la sanità.* Roma, 1594).

Pilius medicinensis (fl. 1200). *Questiones sabbatinae,* ristampa anastatica. Augustae Taurinorum, 1967 (C.G.J.C. IV).

Pinellus, Arius (Aires Pinhel). *Ad Rub. et l. ij C. de rescin. vend. elaboratissimi commentarij.* Venetiis, 1570.

Praevidellius, H. *De peste eiusque privilegiis.* In *Tractatus . . . de variis verbis iuris.* Venetiis, 1584, t. XVIII.

Regia imperatoriaque protomedicatus officii diplomata seu privilegia. Panormi, 1564.

Regole de i fratelli e sorelle della pietosiss. Confraternità delli Agonizanti, canonicamente eretta, e fondata nell'Altare di S.Carlo, posto nella Chiesa di S. Isaia di Bologna. Bologna, 1640.

Regole e Capitoli della Pijssima Congregatione degli Agonizzanti di Bologna sopra la distributione dell'Eredità del già Sig. Valerio Brunellini, in sovenimento de' poveri cittadini infermi. Bologna, 1684.

Regole et ordinationi di tutta la Pijssima Confraternita de gli Agonizanti eretta primariamente in Bologna. Bologna, 1642.

Riforma degli Statuti dell'Onoranda Compagnia de' Speziali di Bologna. Bologna, 1690.

Ripa, Franciscus Joannes de Sancto Nazario (d. 1535). *De peste.* Lugduni, 1564.

Robertus, Annaeus (Anné Robert: fl. 1596). *Rerum Judicatarum libri 4.* Genevae, 1604.

Rodericus à Castro (Estevão Rodrigues de Castro: 1559–1638). *Medicus-Politicus, sive de officiis medico-politicis Tractatus.* Hamburgi, 1614.

Roffredus, Beneventanus (ca. 1170–1243). *Libelli juris civilis,* ristampa anastatica. Augustae Taurinorum, 1968 (C.G.J.C. VI).

Rossi, G. B. *L'attioni memorabili fatte da . . . Confalonieri del popolo et Massari delle Arti già dominanti la città di Bologna raccolte da diversi manoscritti et autori.* Bologna, 1681.

Saccardino, C. *Libro nomato la verità di diverse cose, quale minutamente tratta di molte salutifere opetationi spagiriche, et chimiche.* Bologna, 1621.

Sacro Ragguaglio a tutto il mondo della particolare Institutione della Compagnia de gl'Agonizanti canonicamente erreta nella chiesa di S. Isaia di Bologna l'anno M DC XXVII. Bologna, 1635.

Santorio, S. (1561–1636), *De statica medicina et de responsione ad Staticomasticem.* Hagae Comitis, 1657.

Sarti, M.-Fattorini, T. *De Claris Archigymnasii Bononiensis Professoribus.* Bologna, 1769–72.

Schenardus, Io. Franciscus. *Consiliorum, seu Responsorum Iuris Libri duo.* Mediolani, 1616.

Schultz, J. *Disputatio Juridica de contractu medici cum aegroto.* Gedani, 1679.

Sebastianus Medicus. *De definitionibus.* In *Tractatus . . . de variis verbis Juris.* Venetiis, 1584, t. XVIII.

Settala, L. (1552–1633). *Animadversionum et Cautionum Medicarum libri septem.* Patavii, 1628.

Soarez, Emanuel. *Thesaurus receptarum sententiarum, quas vulgus interpretum communes opiniones vocat.* Venetiis, 1569.

Socinus, Marianus (Mariano Socini: 1401–67). *Consilia seu potius responsa.* Venetiis, 1579, voll. 2.

Speckham, Eberhard (d. 1627). *Quaestionum juris caesarei, pontifici et saxonici Centuria Prima.* Wittembergae, 1611.

Speidel, J. J. (d. ca. 1666). *Speculum juridico-politico-philologico historicarum observationum.* Noribergae, 1657.

Statuta civilia et criminalia civitatis Bononiae . . . illustrata a P. C. Sacco. Bononiae,
    1735–37.

Statuti delle Università e dei Collegi dello Studio bolognese, a cura di C. Malagola. Bo-
    logna, 1888.

Streitius, I. Ph. *Dissertatio de iure aegrotantium.* Erfurti, 1719.

Tiraquellus, A. (André Tiraqueau: 1488–1558). *Commentariorum in l. Si unquam. C. de
    revoc. don.* Francofurti, 1574 (1535).

Tractatus . . . de variis verbis Juris. Venetiis, 1584.

Triumphus, Augustinus de Ancona (Agostino Trionfo: 1243–1328). *Summa de Potes-
    tate Ecclesiastica.* Augustae, 1473.

*Universa civilis et criminalis jurisprudentia, juxta seriem institutionum ex naturali et romano
    jure deprompta et ad usum fori perpetuo accomodata.* Taurini, 1824.

Verdier, J. *Essai sur la jurisprudence de la médecine en France.* Alençon, 1763.

Vivius, Franciscus (Francesco Vivio: b. ca. 1532). *Communium Opinionum Doctorum
    utriusque censurae Liber primus.* Venetiis, 1566.

Voet, J. (1647–1713). *Commentariorum ad pandectas libri quinquaginta.* Bassani, 1804
    (trad. it., *Commento alle pandette.* Venezia, 1846).

Zacchias, Paulus (Paolo Zacchia: 1584–1659). *Quaestiones medico-legales.* Lugduni,
    1662 (1612–30).

———. *Il vitto quaresimale.* Roma, 1636.

INDEX OF NAMES

SUBJECT INDEX

Abortion, 22, 195n. 99
Académie Royale de Chirurgie, 67, 223n. 40
Accademia degli Inquieti, 224n. 49
Agreements for a cure: decline of, 46, 54,
148; diffusion of, 29, 198-99nn. 8, 9, 10,
210-11n. 64; disappearance of, 96, 141,
148, 151-52, 168-69, 171; endorsed by
protomedici, 54, 141-42; examples of,
27-29, 32-33, 42, 150, 154, 173-79, 198n.
7, 201n. 21; and horizontal model of healing, 140-41; jurists' view of, 156-66, 168;
legal foundation of, 37, 40; legal invalidity
of, 155, 158-59, 161, 166; legal validity of,
39, 141-42; as notarized documents, 26,
28-29, 46, 148; as obstacle to medical professionalism, 49-50, 165-66; as oral contracts, 26; patients' view of, 127, 162; and
patti di condotta, 48; physicians' view of, 34,
149; protomedici's view of, 54, 141-42,
149, 155; relapse clause, 32; time in, 42,
44, 151; in Visigothic law, 37-38; and vows
to saints, 170-71
Anatomy, as public ceremony, 233n. 133
Antidotario. *See* Pharmacopoeia
Apothecaries, 2, 7, 22, 57-60; control by
protomedici, 67-68, 88-89, 104; guild of,
63, 67, 68, 104; lawsuits for bill payment,
95-96; licensing of, 9, 68; malpractice
charges against, 108-9, 112-13; Noble
College of, 69; relationship with physicians, 61, 63; shops of, 56, 67; social and
professional mobility, 16-17, 68-69
Archiatri, 39 (*see also* Town doctors)
Arcidiacono, 1
Assunteria di Sanità, 12-13; and control of
epidemics, 12, 93
Assunteria di Studio, 4, 12-13

Barber-surgeons, 2, 22, 56, 60, 64-66; attitude to cure agreements, 127, 148, 150;
culture of, 75-76; dilemmas in practice,
152-53, 247n. 29; fees, 99, 102; fines for
being unlicensed, 64, 143; illicit practice
of, 75, 143-44, 147, 152-53; lawsuits for
payment, 96-97; licensing of, 9, 63, 68,
84; malpractice charges against, 109,
111-12, 114-15; manuals for, 75; in
Norwich, 218n. 107; number of, 57-59;
remedies used by, 75, 131-32; social
mobility of, 16-17; statutes of guild, 64,
231n. 107
Blood, as seat of disease, 30, 248n. 36
Bloodletting, 63, 64, 66, 71, 75, 97, 248n. 35,
258n. 40; as cause of aneurysm, 112;
changes in patients' perception of, 153-54;
patients' self-prescription of, 65, 127, 152;
rules about, 65, 146
Body: grotesque, 92, 133-34, 139; images of,
60, 92, 129, 132, 139-40, 251n. 64; obstructed, 133-34, 139

Canon law: on medical practitioners' ineligi-
bility for holy orders, 242-43n. 83; on
physicians' authority over patients, 253nn.
78, 79; on physicians' fees, 202n. 23, 211n.
70; on physicians' liability, 242-43n. 83;
prohibiting experimentation on patients,
138, 241n. 77
Cardinal legate, 10, 81
Charity to the sick, 106-7
Charlatans: competition with medical establishment, 91-92; control of, 72-73, 147;
culture of, 73-74; and cure agreements,
148; denied right to a fee if unlicensed,
147; and medical secrets, 86-88

Library of Congress Cataloging-in-Publication Data

Pomata, Gianna.
    [Promessa di guarigione. English]
    Contracting a cure : patients, healers, and the law in early modern Bologna / Gianna
Pomata ; translated by the author, with the assistance of Rosemarie Foy and Anna
Taraboletti-Segre.
       p.   cm.
    Includes bibliographical references and index.
    ISBN 0-8018-5858-5 (alk. paper)
    1. Medical care—Europe—History—16th century.   2. Medical care—Italy—
Bologna—History—16th century.   3. Medical care—Europe—History—17th century.
4. Medical care—Italy—Bologna—History—17th century.   I. Title.
RA483.P6613   1998
362.1'0945'4109031—dc21
                                                          98-5982
                                                           CIP